Manual on Image-Guided Brachytherapy of Inner Organs

Konrad Mohnike · Jens Ricke
Stefanie Corradini
Editors

Manual on Image-Guided Brachytherapy of Inner Organs

Technique, Indications and Evidence

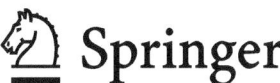

Springer

Editors
Konrad Mohnike
Department of Diagnostics
Department of Interventional Oncology
& Radionuclide Therapy
Diagnostic Therapeutic Center Berlin
Berlin, Germany

Jens Ricke
Department of Radiology
Ludwig Maximilian University (LMU)
Hospital Munich
Munich, Germany

Stefanie Corradini
Department of Radiation Oncology
Ludwig Maximilian University (LMU)
Hospital Munich
Munich, Germany

ISBN 978-3-030-78078-4   ISBN 978-3-030-78079-1   (eBook)
https://doi.org/10.1007/978-3-030-78079-1

This Springer imprint is published by the registered company Springer Nature Switzerland AG
The registered company address is: Gewerbestrasse 11, 6330 Cham, Switzerland

This is the first manual of a very unconventional method for cancer treatment, a method that has emerged from close collaboration between radiotherapy and interventional radiology. The method is currently not widely used, but it has demonstrated high effectiveness in the treatment of primary and secondary neoplasms of inner organs, and it holds promise for the near future once it has become more widely disseminated.

Image-guided interstitial high-dose-rate brachytherapy (iBT) is a local ablative therapy with a highly interdisciplinary character. Even ascertaining the indication for treatment is a cross-disciplinary procedure, involving the medical oncologist, the oncological surgeon, the radiation oncologist, the radiologist and specialists from other disciplines. Likewise, the conduct of iBT requires a highly specialised team including a radiation oncologist, an interventional radiologist, a medical physicist, radiation therapy technologists, interventional radiological technologists and specialised staff to conduct monitoring and imaging of the patient. The experienced reader will be well aware that such intensive teamwork requires a high degree of co-operation and exchange of information between all the team members involved. However, it is also important to note that none of these disciplines could perform this complex treatment on their own. Each specialist makes his or her own contribution and all do what they can do best. Yet the goal is the same for everyone involved: to perform a successful *local* treatment of primary or secondary malignancies that provides *systemic* benefit to the patient and improves the disease prognosis. This is truly a team effort.

The editors of this book are delighted that international experts from the relevant specialised disciplines have been willing to contribute as authors—experts in the field from India, Italy, Malaysia and the USA, as well as from Germany, where the editors are based. The reader who takes the time to read the entire book will immediately notice that each chapter has its own flow and perspective, depending on whether the principal authors are radiation oncologists, interventional radiologists, medical oncologists or medical physicists, and whether the contribution comes from Europe, America or Asia. This is intentional, but also unavoidable, and it adds to the complexity and richness of the content. For the same reason, we take the liberty of advising readers who only intend to pick out one or two chapters: please read the whole book anyway! That will give you a comprehensive view of the clinical possibilities of iBT as practised in Germany, Europe, America, Asia and thus worldwide.

The editors wish to thank Sabine Thürk of *alesco concepts* for her central and indispensable contribution in collating and editing the contributions to this book and for her central role in the communication between the editors, the authors and the staff of the Springer Verlag. We also thank Dr. Paul Woolley for his expert linguistic and critical review of the text of each chapter. For both of these persons, the old adage applies: If they had not existed, we would have had to invent them. Moreover, Thomas Wendland of *alesco concepts* edited many of the illustrations in this book, for which we are also grateful.

Finally, we would like to thank Springer London for the opportunity to publish this very special topic.

Berlin, Germany   Konrad Mohnike
Munich, Germany   Jens Ricke
Munich, Germany   Stefanie Corradini
March 2021

Contents

About the Editors

Jens Ricke Prof. Jens Ricke and his team invented and developed the method of interstitial brachytherapy of the lung and liver in 2002 and introduced it into clinical practice. Prof. Ricke is well-known in Germany and Europe as an expert in the field of interventional radiology. Apart from interventional radiology, his areas of expertise include in particular minimally invasive oncological surgery, interdisciplinary interventional radiology, nuclear medicine (therapeutic hybrid procedures) and image-guided radiotherapy. After 12 years at the Charité Universitätsmedizin Berlin ("Campus Virchow" Klinikum), Prof. Ricke was appointed in 2006 to the chair of Radiology and Nuclear Medicine at the Otto von Guericke University of Magdeburg. In 2011, he founded the German Academy of Microtherapy, of which he is still president. He has been a member of the Scientific Advisory Board of the German Medical Association since 2014. Since 2017, Prof. Ricke has also held the chair of Radiology and been director of the Department of Radiology at the Ludwig Maximillian University hospital in Munich.

Konrad Mohnike Since the start of his career, Dr. Konrad Mohnike has worked scientifically in the field of interstitial brachytherapy. As an interventional radiologist, he is an expert in this field, performing therapeutic procedures since 2011. Initially, he worked with Prof. Jens Ricke, including during his time as an assistant physician after qualifying in 2006, and from 2013 he was a senior physician at the Department of Radiology and Nuclear Medicine in Magdeburg. Dr. Mohnike is an accredited specialist in radiology and interventional radiology (both since 2012) and in nuclear medicine (since 2017). In 2016, he moved to the Diagnostic Therapeutic Center in Berlin, where he established the Department of Interventional Oncology and Radionuclide Therapy. In co-operation with partner hospitals, he performs brachytherapy of the liver in a private practice. In 2020, he became Medical Director of the Diagnostic Therapeutic Center. Since 2019, Dr. Mohnike has also been on the advisory board of the Berliner Krebsgesellschaft e.V. (Berlin Cancer Society).

Stefanie Corradini Dr. Stefanie Corradini is a recognised radiation oncology expert in the field of brachytherapy with a wide range of experience. Initially, she worked at the University of Tübingen and joined the Department of Radiation

Oncology at the Ludwig Maximillian University (LMU) in Munich in 2009. Dr. Corradini has been an accredited specialist in radiation oncology since 2014, and from 2015 she has been an attending physician at the LMU. She has worked in the field of radiation oncology for over 12 years, with a clinical focus on brachytherapy, surface-guided radiotherapy, MR-guided radiotherapy, gastrointestinal tumours, gynaecological tumours and breast cancer. Dr. Corradini has been head of the Brachytherapy unit at the LMU hospital since 2017, and of the MR-guided radiotherapy programme since 2019. Dr. Corradini is a senior lecturer at the LMU, where she holds a teaching license (*venia legendi*).

Introduction: Why and When Radiotherapy with iBT? When SBRT?

Konrad Mohnike, Jens Ricke, and Stefanie Corradini

Radiotherapy of the liver, lung, and other inner organs can be performed percutane-ously and noninvasively using modern *stereotactic body radiotherapy* (SBRT) strat-egies [1, 2]. SBRT offers an elegant approach for the treatment of oligometastatic disease, especially because of its unique advantage of noninvasiveness. Experience with this modality continues to grow, as there is an increasing number of publica-tions on the SBRT of liver and lung malignomas [3–8]. On the one hand, SBRT offers an opportunity for a noninvasive and effective treatment of metastases, and it carries no risk of intervention-related or peri-interventional complications such as hemorrhage [9]. On the other hand, the hypofractionated administration of large radiation doses results in a significant exposure of the surrounding tissue. Therefore, SBRT is usually restricted to lesions sized up to about 4–5 cm, and the number of lesions that can be treated simultaneously is also limited [10, 11]. Moreover, respi-ratory organ motion and the proximity to vulnerable organs at risk (OARs) may limit the dose that can be administered. As a result, the optimum balance between effective dose and safety considerations is sometimes difficult to achieve in a

K. Mohnike (✉)
Department of Diagnostics, Department of Interventional Oncology & Radionuclide Therapy, Diagnostic Therapeutic Center Berlin, Berlin, Germany

Department of Radiology and Nuclear Medicine, University Hospital Magdeburg, Magdeburg, Germany
e-mail: konrad.mohnike@berlin-dtz.de

J. Ricke
Department of Radiology, Ludwig Maximilian University (LMU) Hospital Munich, Munich, Germany
e-mail: Jens.Ricke@med.uni-muenchen.de

S. Corradini
Department of Radiation Oncology, Ludwig Maximilian University (LMU) Hospital Munich, Munich, Germany
e-mail: Stefanie.corradini@med.uni-muenchen.de

© The Author(s), under exclusive license to Springer Nature Switzerland AG 2021
K. Mohnike et al. (eds.), *Manual on Image-Guided Brachytherapy of Inner Organs*, https://doi.org/10.1007/978-3-030-78079-1_1

clinical routine. Results from various studies show a gastro-intestinal complication rate (CTCAE Grades ≥3) that ranges from 0 to 35% for Grade 3 and 0 to 25% for Grade 4, with wide variations. These complications include gastroduodenal ulceration, hepatotoxicity, nausea/vomiting, oesophagitis, and bile-duct stenosis in liver SBRT [12]. According to the current literature, radiation-induced liver disorder (RILD) occurs less frequently than with conventionally fractionated irradiation methods, but RILD remains a clinical problem, for example, in SBRT of hepatocellular carcinomas, and it has an effect on the outcome for patients [13]. However, modern MR-guided SBRT approaches allow direct visualization of the target volume and surrounding OARs and, through an online adaptive treatment approach, intrafractional anatomic variations can be taken into account [14]. This new technology offers a new opportunity to achieve durable local control rates while reducing toxicity to OARs.

Another option for the safe application of high single doses is *interstitial brachytherapy* (iBT). Here, a radioactive source, for example, iridium-192, is inserted directly into the tumor through a catheter. For liver and lung lesions, iBT was introduced into clinical practice in the early 2000s, following developments in advanced imaging (multilevel CT, CT-fluoroscopy) and 3D treatment planning methods in the 1990s, which for the first time allowed accurate placement of an applicator in parenchymal organs [15–18].

The principle of image-guided brachytherapy is the precise, CT- or MRI-guided implantation of the brachytherapy catheter in the target lesion for the subsequent introduction of the radioactive source. Since the source is positioned directly within the tumor, intrafractional respiratory motion is negligible, as the organ moves together with the catheter. This is a particular advantage when one is treating targets in the upper abdomen and lung. Usually, placement of the brachytherapy catheter is performed under CT- or MR-fluoroscopy guidance and analgosedation (fentanyl and midazolam, both i.v.) of the patient. After puncture of the target lesion, an angiography sheath is inserted by using a guidewire followed by the brachytherapy catheter (Seldinger technique). After successful positioning of the brachytherapy catheter, a contrast-enhanced planning CT or MRT is performed and the image data set is transferred to the treatment planning system. For HDR brachytherapy an iridium-192 source is frequently used. The duration of the treatment depends on the number and volume of lesions, as well as the prescription dose, and usually lasts between approximately 10 and 60 min.

With iBT, very high radiation doses can be delivered in a single fraction with a high degree of accuracy. Owing to the brachytherapy-specific dose inhomogeneity, with a very high dose close to the brachytherapy catheters, the central doses can reach more than 100 Gy in the tumor, while being as low as 25 Gy at its periphery and resulting in high mean gross tumor volume (GTV) doses. In brachytherapy, the dose gradient is very steep, which allows the administration of effective tumoricidal doses while sparing the surrounding OARs, even in very large and centrally located tumors [19, 20]. Although in plan-comparison studies the superiority of iBT in sparing the surrounding tissue appears to diminish with increasing lesion size compared with SBRT, a much more effective sparing of the surrounding liver parenchyma is usually seen in clinical routine with iBT. However, for irradiation of smaller volumes, the exposure of other OARs might theoretically be lower than with iBT—e.g., the gastric wall in lesions close to the stomach (see Fig. 1.1). Moreover, such high single doses can also induce additional therapeutic effects, such as induction of apoptosis in the endothelia of tumor-feeding blood vessels, which is associated with a subsequent antiangiogenic effect [21, 22]. In some cases, hypofractionated regimens with single doses of 10–12 Gy may be of value, for example, in the treatment of very large tumors located in the left liver close to the gastric mucosa (Fig. 1.2) [23].

The effectiveness of iBT has been confirmed for various cancer entities and locations [18–20, 24–29]. In hepatocellular carcinomas measuring up to 12 cm or more in diameter and treated with a prescription dose of 1×15 Gy, local tumor control rates of >90% have been reported at 12 months. In a randomized dose-escalation study of iBT in colorectal liver metastases, prescription doses of 1×25 Gy were associated with a very high local control rate [26, 28]. Such excellent tumor control rates have also been demonstrated in extrahepatic neoplasms, for example, pulmonary neoplasms of various origins [30].

A comparative planning study evaluated dosimetric endpoints of SBRT versus iBT in 85 patients with liver malignancies of different primaries [31]. All patients were clinically treated with iBT, and plan parameters were compared with those of virtually planned ("mock") SBRT treatments using the same prescription dose of 1×15 or 1×20 Gy. SBRT plans were generated using the original brachytherapy planning CTs with the brachytherapy catheters in place. Since no 4D datasets were available to account for respiratory organ motion, additional margins of 5 mm in a lateral direction and 10 mm along the cranio-caudal axis were added to the

Fig. 1.1 SBRT irradiation plan (**a**) according to ICRU-91 of a left-situated colorectal carcinoma metastasis and mock iBT plan, (**b**) of the same lesion with a reasonably anticipated catheter position, SBRT volume 8.1 mL, iBT volume 3.1 mL. D99.9: SBRT 25.0 Gy, iBT 25.0 Gy; D95 SBRT 25.6 Gy, iBT 34.9 Gy; D90 SBRT 26.11 Gy, iBT 40.67 Gy. V5Gy Liver (mL and percentages): SBRT 281 mL and 14%, iBT 92.39 mL and 4.96%. D1cc gastric wall: SBRT 10.3 Gy, iBT 14.0 Gy

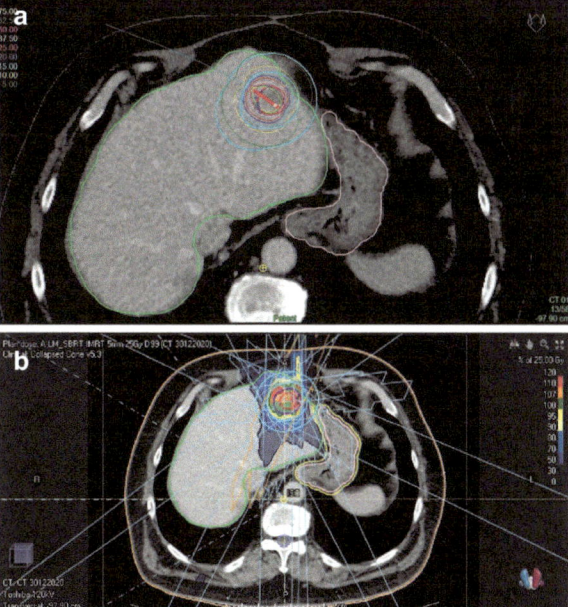

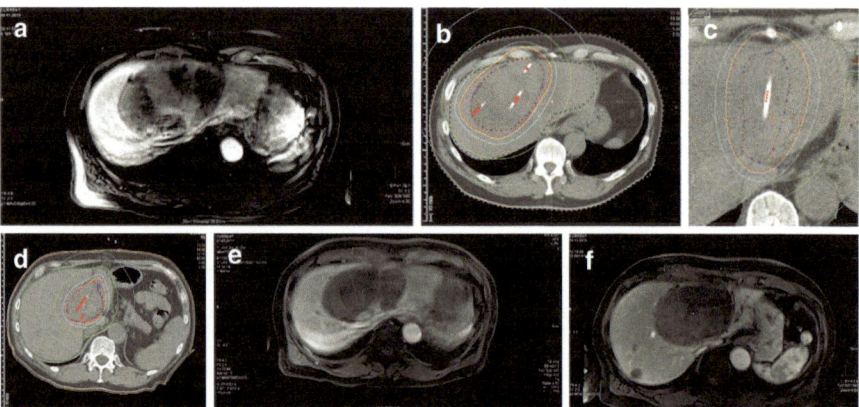

Fig. 1.2 Large hepatocellular carcinoma of both liver lobes, 14 × 8 × 8 cm. Relapse after transarterial chemoembolization. (**a**) MRI scan before iBT. (**b**) Planning CT with isodose lines, first session, Dec 2016. (**c**) Planning CT with isodose lines, second session, Jan 2017. (**d**) Planning CT with isodose lines, third session, Jan 2017. (**e**) MRI 2 months after the last session. (**f**) MRI 2 years after the first session

brachytherapy GTVs to generate planning target volumes (PTV) for SBRT treatment planning. For both techniques, the dose to the PTV was optimized to meet the aimed-for prescription dose, but it was reduced if dose constraints of OARs were violated. The median volume of the PTVs for iBT was 34.7 cm^3, with a range of 0.5–410 cm^2, and in SBRT plans it was 73.2 cm^3, with a range of 6.1–593.4 cm^2. In this comparison, the PTV target coverage with the planned prescription dose was significantly better with iBT than with SBRT. For the D99.9 (dose coverage of 99.9% of the PTV volume with the prescription dose) the values were 19.9 ± 0.4 Gy for iBT and 17.5 ± 0.5 Gy for SBRT, at a planned dose of 20 Gy ($p < 0.001$). This was also significant for the 1 × 15 Gy dose prescription group ($p = 0.003$). The difference between the two modalities was even more pronounced regarding the D90 dose coverage. Owing to the heterogeneous iBT dose distribution, the D90 at a planned dose of 1 × 15 Gy was 24.3 ± 0.8 Gy for iBT, compared with 16.5 ± 0.3 Gy for SBRT ($p < 0.001$). For a planned dose of 20 Gy, corresponding values were 29.2 ± 0.4 Gy (iBT) and 20.6 ± 0.3 (SBRT; $p < 0.001$). In the group of patients with the higher prescription dose (20 Gy), the exposure of the healthy liver was significantly higher in the SBRT than in the iBT plans. The liver volume receiving 5 Gy or more was 611 ± 43 cm^3 for iBT and 694 ± 37 cm^3 for SBRT ($p = 0.001$); these corresponded to 41.8 ± 2.5% for iBT and 45.9 ± 2.0% for SBRT ($p = 0.007$) of total liver volume [31].

In an earlier comparative study by Pennington et al., the inverse strategy was used: virtual brachytherapy plans were compared with real SBRT plans for clinical treatment of ten liver metastases. The authors found no difference between the modalities regarding target coverage of the mean PTV volume, which was reached by 100% of the prescription dose (V100%: 94.1% for iBT vs. 93.9% for SBRT, $p = 0.8$); while the mean PTV volume that received 150% of the planned dose (V150%) was 63.6%

for iBT and 0% for SBRT. The minimum dose to the PTV (D100) was 65.8% for iBT and 87.4% for SBRT ($p = 0.0002$). However, while the liver V15Gy and the mean dose to the stomach were comparable between the two techniques, the mean dose to the small intestine was higher for iBT than for SBRT (respectively 10.8% and 7.1%, $p = 0.006$). The authors of the study concluded that iBT plans resulted in a higher dose to the tumor but a decreased target volume coverage [32].

The two studies show partly contradictory results. However, the study by Pennington et al. has some limitations. First, the creation of virtual iBT plans is only partially feasible if detailed practical expertise in catheter insertion trajectories is lacking. Secondly, because of the inhomogeneity of iBT dose distribution, trained teams performing iBT in clinical routine optimize treatment plans to the minimum dose (D100 or D99.9, less often also D90). Owing to the inherently inhomogeneous dose distributions in brachytherapy, very high mean tumor doses are delivered to the target lesions. This concept has only recently been adapted for SBRT [33]. Recent reports have pointed out the importance of the mean dose in the gross tumor volume and the need to consider this in plan optimization for the best possible tumor control and outcome [34–37]. Furthermore, regarding dose constraints for organs at risk, only dose maximum values to 1 or 0.1 cm^3 are clinically considered, because of the rapid dose fall-off. Mean values are usually not considered relevant. Another uncertainty factor in SBRT is the organ motion of the liver due to respiration. Both modeling studies added PTV margins to the lesions to account for intrafractional organ motion. Obviously, the PTVs are therefore larger in SBRT and the normal tissue exposure is usually greater.

Wust et al. compared the dose distributions in iBT with those in two different SBRT techniques using a Cyberknife platform and a volumetric-modulated arch therapy (VMAT) approach with Tomotherapy. They found that iBT had the highest therapeutic ratios in terms of both high-dose and low-dose liver exposure, even in larger lesions. In this planning study, iBT was the most effective technique for treating intrahepatic lesions in a single fraction. iBT achieved mean tumor doses of nearly 60 Gy, whereas the other techniques reached only 22–34 Gy, and the conformality of iBT was still good for lesions ≥ 3 cm in diameter. However, with iBT, sparing of the surrounding tissue declined with increasing lesion size and approached the levels associated with SBRT (see also Chap. 3) [38].

When evaluating a local ablative treatment modality, the local recurrence rate (LRR) is the main criterion for measuring its efficacy. However, oncological outcome is complex, is determined by many factors, and is often only weakly associated with LRR alone. To date, available evidence suggests that iBT can achieve very good local control rates in most tumor entities, even when local recurrence or puncture-tract metastases occur [39]. Since iBT is subject to considerably fewer restrictions than other local procedures with respect to tumor location, size, and number of lesions, iBT can also be repeated [26].

The key to success is adequate patient selection with evaluation of all oncological factors. These include whether the disease is oligometastatic or whether a rapid polymetastatic progression can be expected without the potential to achieve local control. A second factor is the presence of a predisposition to severe complications.

This aspect is critical in determining whether the treatment will be beneficial to the patient. While surgical resection, thermoablation, and even SBRT involve a certain degree of inherent patient selection, the relative freedom of iBT from modality-related limitations makes an adequate patient stratification particularly significant and, in some cases, even more challenging. On the basis of the available evidence, it can be concluded that the minimally invasive technique of iBT has its advantages, especially for larger tumors and in cases where repeated treatments may be indicated. Unfortunately, prospective, multicentric, or randomized studies will not be available in the near future because the use of iBT and the necessary interventional radiology expertise are not yet widely available. However, there is a need for clinical studies that incorporate different treatment modalities and local ablative techniques to address the issue of proper patient selection.

Key Points
- The efficacy of modern, noninvasive stereotactic concepts for irradiation has been demonstrated in numerous tumor locations.
- A further possible way of treating tumors radiologically is *interstitial brachytherapy* (iBT).
- iBT allows the introduction of very high radiation doses in a single fraction.
- Evidence adduced so far indicates that this minimally invasive brachytherapy is especially advantageous in the treatment of larger tumors and because of its repeatability.

References

1. Scorsetti M, Clerici E, Comito T. Stereotactic body radiation therapy for liver metastases. J Gastrointest Oncol. 2014;5:190–7.
2. Scorsetti M, Comito T, Tozzi A, et al. Final results of a phase II trial for stereotactic body radiation therapy for patients with inoperable liver metastases from colorectal cancer. J Cancer Res Clin Oncol. 2015;141(3):543–53.
3. Andratschke N, Alheid H, Allgauer M, et al. The SBRT database initiative of the German Society for Radiation Oncology (DEGRO): patterns of care and outcome analysis of stereotactic body radiotherapy (SBRT) for liver oligometastases in 474 patients with 623 metastases. BMC Cancer. 2018;18:283.
4. Boda-Heggemann J, Jahnke A, Chan MKH, et al. In-vivo treatment accuracy analysis of active motion-compensated liver SBRT through registration of plan dose to post-therapeutic MRI-morphologic alterations. Radiother Oncol. 2019;134:158–65.
5. Gkika E, Strouthos I, Kirste S, et al. Repeated SBRT for in- and out-of-field recurrences in the liver. Strahlenther Onkol. 2019;195:246–53.
6. Han S, Yin FF, Cai J. Evaluation of dosimetric uncertainty caused by MR geometric distortion in MRI-based liver SBRT treatment planning. J Appl Clin Med Phys. 2019;20:43–50.
7. Ibragimov B, Toesca DAS, Yuan Y, Koong AC, Chang DT, Xing L. Neural networks for deep radiotherapy dose analysis and prediction of liver SBRT outcomes. IEEE J Biomed Health Inform. 2019;23:1821–33.

8. Scorsetti M, Comito T, Clerici E, et al. Phase II trial on SBRT for unresectable liver metastases: long-term outcome and prognostic factors of survival after 5 years of follow-up. Radiat Oncol. 2018;13:234.
9. Rieber J, Streblow J, Uhlmann L, et al. Stereotactic body radiotherapy (SBRT) for medically inoperable lung metastases—a pooled analysis of the German working group "stereotactic radiotherapy". Lung Cancer. 2016;97:51–8.
10. Dawson LA. Overview: where does radiation therapy fit in the spectrum of liver cancer local-regional therapies? Semin Radiat Oncol. 2011;21:241–6.
11. Scorsetti M, Arcangeli S, Tozzi A, et al. Is stereotactic body radiation therapy an attractive option for unresectable liver metastases? A preliminary report from a phase 2 trial. Int J Radiat Oncol Biol Phys. 2013;86:336–42.
12. Thomas TO, Hasan S, Small W Jr, et al. The tolerance of gastrointestinal organs to stereotactic body radiation therapy: what do we know so far? J Gastrointest Oncol. 2014;5:236–46.
13. Sanuki N, Takeda A, Oku Y, et al. Influence of liver toxicities on prognosis after stereotactic body radiation therapy for hepatocellular carcinoma. Hepatol Res. 2015;45:540–7.
14. Witt JS, Rosenberg SA, Bassetti MF. MRI-guided adaptive radiotherapy for liver tumours: visualising the future. Lancet Oncol. 2020;21:e74–82.
15. Ricke J, Wust P, Hengst S, et al. [CT-guided interstitial brachytherapy of lung malignancies. Technique and first results]. Radiologe. 2004;44:684–6.
16. Ricke J, Wust P, Stohlmann A, et al. CT-guided interstitial brachytherapy of liver malignancies alone or in combination with thermal ablation: phase I-II results of a novel technique. Int J Radiat Oncol Biol Phys. 2004;58:1496–505.
17. Ricke J, Wust P, Stohlmann A, et al. [CT-Guided brachytherapy. A novel percutaneous technique for interstitial ablation of liver metastases]. Strahlenther Onkol. 2004;180:274–80.
18. Ricke J, Wust P, Wieners G, et al. Liver malignancies: CT-guided interstitial brachytherapy in patients with unfavorable lesions for thermal ablation. J Vasc Interv Radiol. 2004;15:1279–86.
19. Collettini F, Schnapauff D, Poellinger A, et al. Hepatocellular carcinoma: computed-tomography-guided high-dose-rate brachytherapy (CT-HDRBT) ablation of large (5-7 cm) and very large (>7 cm) tumours. Eur Radiol. 2012;22:1101–9.
20. Tselis N, Chatzikonstantinou G, Kolotas C, Milickovic N, Baltas D, Zamboglou N. Computed tomography-guided interstitial high dose rate brachytherapy for centrally located liver tumours: a single institution study. Eur Radiol. 2013;23:2264–70.
21. Brown JM, Koong AC. High-dose single-fraction radiotherapy: exploiting a new biology? Int J Radiat Oncol Biol Phys. 2008;71:324–5.
22. Garcia-Barros M, Paris F, Cordon-Cardo C, et al. Tumor response to radiotherapy regulated by endothelial cell apoptosis. Science. 2003;300:1155–9.
23. Streitparth F, Pech M, Bohmig M, et al. In vivo assessment of the gastric mucosal tolerance dose after single fraction, small volume irradiation of liver malignancies by computed tomography-guided, high-dose-rate brachytherapy. Int J Radiat Oncol Biol Phys. 2006;65:1479–86.
24. Collettini F, Singh A, Schnapauff D, et al. Computed-tomography-guided high-dose-rate brachytherapy (CT-HDRBT) ablation of metastases adjacent to the liver hilum. Eur J Radiol. 2013;82:e509–14.
25. Mohnike K, Wieners G, Pech M, et al. Image-guided interstitial high-dose-rate brachytherapy in hepatocellular carcinoma. Dig Dis. 2009;27:170–4.
26. Mohnike K, Wieners G, Schwartz F, et al. Computed tomography-guided high-dose-rate brachytherapy in hepatocellular carcinoma: safety, efficacy, and effect on survival. Int J Radiat Oncol Biol Phys. 2010;78:172–9.
27. Pech M, Wieners G, Kryza R, et al. CT-guided brachytherapy (CTGB) versus interstitial laser ablation (ILT) of colorectal liver metastases: an intraindividual matched-pair analysis. Strahlenther Onkol. 2008;184:302–6.
28. Ricke J, Mohnike K, Pech M, et al. Local response and impact on survival after local ablation of liver metastases from colorectal carcinoma by computed tomography-guided high-dose-rate brachytherapy. Int J Radiat Oncol Biol Phys. 2010;78:479–85.

29. Ricke J, Wust P, Wieners G, et al. CT-guided interstitial single-fraction brachytherapy of lung tumors: phase I results of a novel technique. Chest. 2005;127:2237–42.
30. Peters N, Wieners G, Pech M, et al. CT-guided interstitial brachytherapy of primary and secondary lung malignancies: results of a prospective phase II trial. Strahlenther Onkol. 2008;184:296–301.
31. Hass P, Mohnike K, Kropf S, et al. Comparative analysis between interstitial brachytherapy and stereotactic body irradiation for local ablation in liver malignancies. Brachytherapy. 2019;18:823–8.
32. Pennington JD, Park SJ, Abgaryan N, et al. Dosimetric comparison of brachyablation and stereotactic ablative body radiotherapy in the treatment of liver metastasis. Brachytherapy. 2015;14:537–42.
33. Wilke L, Andratschke N, Blanck O, et al. ICRU report 91 on prescribing, recording, and reporting of stereotactic treatments with small photon beams: statement from the DEGRO/DGMP working group stereotactic radiotherapy and radiosurgery. Strahlenther Onkol. 2019;195:193–8.
34. Andratschke N, Parys A, Stadtfeld S, et al. Clinical results of mean GTV dose optimized robotic guided SBRT for liver metastases. Radiat Oncol. 2016;11:74.
35. Baumann R, Chan MKH, Pyschny F, et al. Clinical results of mean GTV dose optimized robotic-guided stereotactic body radiation therapy for lung tumors. Front Oncol. 2018;8:171.
36. Stera S, Balermpas P, Chan MKH, et al. Breathing-motion-compensated robotic guided stereotactic body radiation therapy: patterns of failure analysis. Strahlenther Onkol. 2018;194:143–55.
37. Zhao L, Zhou S, Balter P, et al. Planning target volume D95 and mean dose should be considered for optimal local control for stereotactic ablative radiation therapy. Int J Radiat Oncol Biol Phys. 2016;95:1226–35.
38. Wust P, Beck M, Dabrowski R, et al. Radiotherapeutic treatment options for oligotopic malignant liver lesions. Radiat Oncol. 2021;16:51.
39. Buttner L, Ludemann WM, Jonczyk M, et al. Tumor seeding along the puncture tract in CT-guided interstitial high-dose-rate brachytherapy. J Vasc Interv Radiol. 2020;31:720–7.

Stefanie Corradini, Sebastian Marschner, and Daniel Reitz

Historical Background

The history of brachytherapy began with the discovery of radium over 120 years ago in 1898, when Marie Curie's groundbreaking research culminated in the discovery of new radioactive substances. Following the discovery of the new elements, the heroic and legendary research period began [1]. After thousands of crystallisations, Marie Curie and her husband Pierre Curie succeeded in isolating almost pure radium chloride and determining the atomic weight of radium. In 1903, Marie presented the results of her work in her doctoral thesis; the examination committee expressed the opinion that her findings represented the greatest scientific contribution ever made in a doctoral thesis [2]. Later in 1903, Marie and Pierre Curie shared half of the Nobel Prize in Physics "in recognition of the extraordinary merits they have rendered by their joint researches on the radiation phenomena discovered by Professor Henri Becquerel," who was awarded the other half of the Nobel Prize for his discovery of spontaneous radioactivity. Radium as a compact source of constant, highly penetrating radiation was suitable for external and internal use, and Marie and Pierre Curie discovered early on that radium could also be used in cancer treatment [3].

In fact, the first successful clinical applications of radioisotopes had already been reported at that time. In 1901, Danlos and Bloch irradiated a case of lupus erythematosus and other dermatological conditions at the St. Louis Hospital in Paris (France) with a small borrowed radium tube containing 0.398 g of radium sulfate [4]. In 1903, two cases of basal cell carcinoma of the face were the first oncological treatments using brachytherapy known to have been performed in St.

S. Corradini (✉) · S. Marschner · D. Reitz
Department of Radiation Oncology, Ludwig Maximilian University (LMU)
Hospital Munich, Munich, Germany
e-mail: Stefanie.corradini@med.uni-muenchen.de; Sebastian.marschner@med.uni-muenchen.de;
Daniel.reitz@med.uni-muenchen.de

© The Author(s), under exclusive license to Springer Nature
Switzerland AG 2021
K. Mohnike et al. (eds.), *Manual on Image-Guided Brachytherapy of Inner Organs*, https://doi.org/10.1007/978-3-030-78079-1_2

9

Petersburg, Russia [5]. At the same time, the first gynecological brachytherapy was described by Margareth Cleaves in New York, where an inoperable cervical cancer case was treated with a glass cylinder filled with radium [6]. An early treatment result of such a historic brachytherapy performed in Switzerland in 1924 is shown in Fig. 2.1.

In the following years Marie Curie, together with André Debierne, was able to isolate radium in metallic form. In 1911, she was awarded the Nobel Prize in Chemistry for this "in recognition of her merits to the advancement of chemistry by the discovery of the elements radium and polonium, by the isolation of radium and the study of the nature and compounds of this remarkable element."

Thereafter, progress was rapid and several schools of brachytherapy were established, such as the Radium Hemmet in Stockholm (Sweden), the Memorial Hospital in New York (USA), and the Radium Institute in Paris (France). The beginning of dosimetry began in 1904 when different units for quantifying the strength, intensity, and activity of radioactivity with the "gamma-ray unit" were first described. Other units were the "milligram-hour" first described in 1909, the "curie" in 1910, and the "millicurie-destroyed per square centimetre" in 1914. Milligram-hour remained the most popular unit for radium until the ICRU recommendation of 1937 proposed to use "roentgen" as a unit for both radioactivity and X-rays [5].

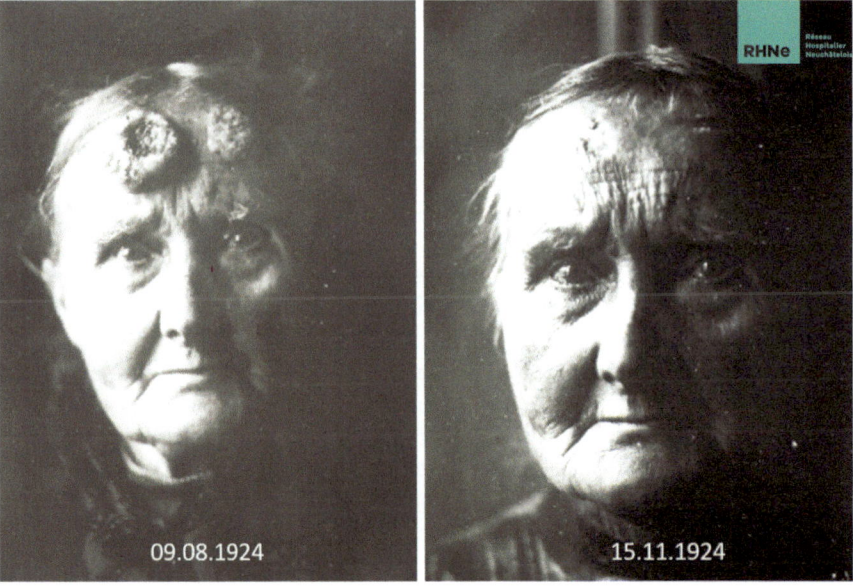

Fig. 2.1 Historical skin cancer treatment. The image on the left was taken in August 1924 and shows a female patient with exophytic skin cancer on her forehead before treatment at the Service of Radio-Oncologie at Chaux-de-Fonds in Switzerland. The treatment was performed by Dr. André Grosjean. The right-hand image shows the 3-month follow-up image, with complete remission. Published with permission of Dr. Berardino De Bari (Medecin Chef de Service, Service Radio-Oncologie, Réseau hospitalier neuchâtelois, La Chaux-de-Fonds, Switzerland)

The most important contribution regarding dosimetry was the Manchester system, established by Paterson and Parker in 1938, which first described the "radium dosage system" for brachytherapy. This was designed to deliver a uniform dose throughout the target volume by using a nonuniform distribution of the sources and following certain rules. Dosage tables and distribution rules helped to preplan and calculate the required number and placement of sources (see Fig. 2.2) [7].

Gösta Forssell coined the term "brachytherapy" from the Greek word "βραχύς – brachys," which means "short" and refers to the distance between the therapeutic agent radium and the target lesion. In a French article in the Journal of Radiology entitled "La lutte social contre le cancer" in 1931, he proposed to use the term "brachyradium" for short-distance radium treatments [3]. In fact, many early radium techniques were for surface applications, where radium tubes or needles were mounted with the help of molds made of wax, leather, or other suitable material (see Fig. 2.3).

At that time, radium was rare and expensive. Therefore, early practitioners sometimes used rather small, ineffective quantities; because of the resulting very low doses, clinical response rates could not always meet the high expectations with which the new radium therapy was regarded. This changed however when mass mining of American (later also African and Canadian) radium ore sources resulted in the availability of sufficient quantities of radium for clinical applications. Radium sources remained in widespread clinical use until the 1960s, even if their use declined over the years owing to the problem of exposure of medical staff to radiation through the manual application of radioactive sources, and also to technical advances in external-beam treatments and surgical techniques [8]. The first interstitial treatments were performed in Munich by H. Strebel in 1903 by inserting radium needles with a trocar through a skin incision directly into the tumor.

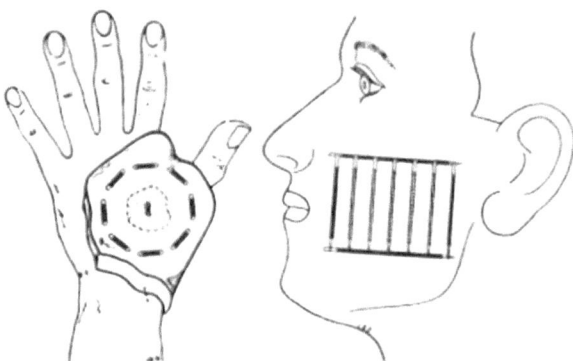

Fig. 2.2 Arrangements of radium sources following the Manchester system devised by Paterson and Parker in 1938. The arrangements were applicable for surface molds, as well as to interstitial brachytherapy treatments with needles implanted in a single plane (from "A Century of X-Rays and Radioactivity in Medicine: With Emphasis on Photographic Records of the Early Years" R.F. Mould, with permission)

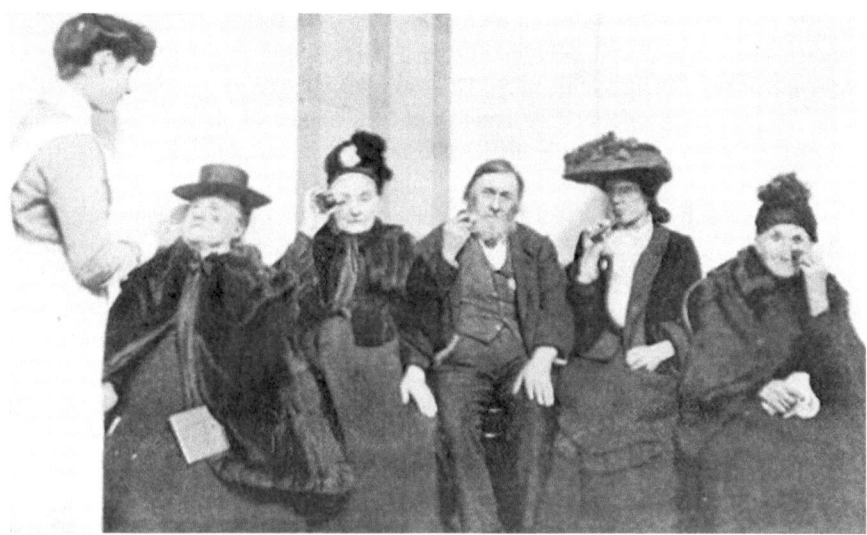

Fig. 2.3 Treatment with radium plaques in 1905 in the Dermatology Department, St. Vincent Hospital, Melbourne Australia (from "A Century of X-Rays and Radioactivity in Medicine: With Emphasis on Photographic Records of the Early Years" R.F. Mould, with permission)

Following Ernest Rutherford's discovery of artificial radioactivity in 1919, Pierre and Marie Curie's daughter, Irène Joliot-Curie and her husband Frédéric Joliot discovered artificial radionuclides such as cobalt-60 (^{60}Co), gold-198 (^{198}Au), and cesium-137 (^{137}Cs). In 1935, they were awarded the Nobel Prize in Chemistry "in recognition of their synthesis of new radioactive elements." These new radionuclides found their way into clinical application in 1958, when Ulrich Henschke first used the artificial nuclide iridium-192 for a brachytherapy treatment at the Memorial Sloan Kettering Cancer Center (New York, USA). It was also Henschke who further reduced radiation exposure of the medical staff in the 1960s, with the development of a remote-controlled afterloading system, which allowed the radiation source to be delivered automatically from a shielded safe through connecting tubes. This reduced the risk of unnecessary exposure of staff and patients to radiation, and it minimized side effects—especially for the medical staff [9, 10]. Today, iridium-192 is one of the most widely used sources for brachytherapy [11, 12]. An example of a modern afterloader is shown in Fig. 2.4.

Thanks to further advances in three-dimensional imaging modalities, computerized treatment planning systems and remote delivery devices, brachytherapy is now a safe and effective treatment option for many types of cancer. As the radiation sources can be precisely positioned within the tumor, brachytherapy makes it possible to apply high doses of radiation while minimizing radiation exposure of nearby organs at risk. It also allows a high level of conformity to be achieved. In recent years, there have been major advances in oncology, but the field of modern brachytherapy has also evolved. Reactor- and cyclotron-produced radionuclides, with higher specific activity and lower γ-ray/photon energy, have expanded their

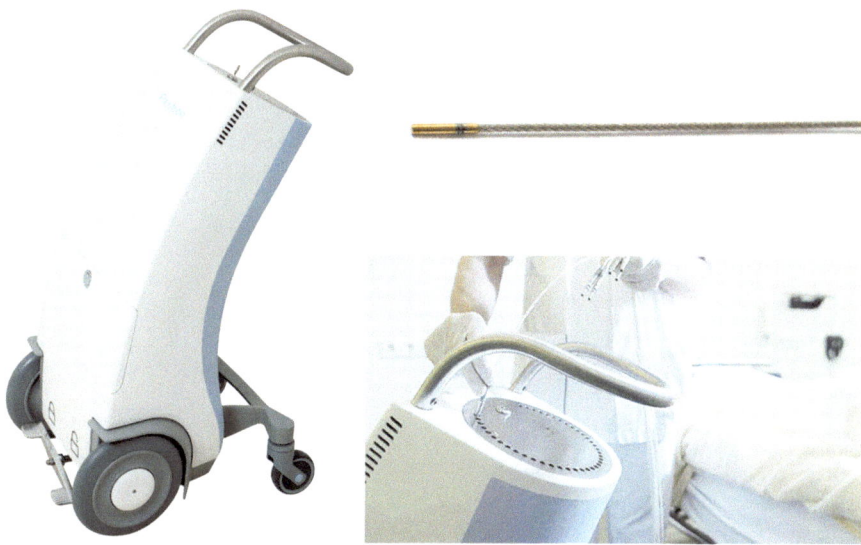

Fig. 2.4 Example of a modern remote afterloading system (Flexitron, Elekta AB, Stockholm, Sweden, left image). When the brachytherapy catheters are correctly positioned within the patient, they are connected to the afterloader via connecting tubes (image lower right). The radiation source (top right image) will only move out of the shielded safe when the medical staff are outside the treatment room. This provides optimum protection from radiation exposure for healthcare professionals in modern brachytherapy

applicability and improved patient safety. Furthermore, computer-based dosimetry has enhanced the therapeutic ratio, and remote afterloading systems have eliminated radiation exposure of personnel.

Imaging Techniques

On November 8, 1895, the physicist Wilhelm Conrad Röntgen discovered X-rays in his laboratory at the University of Würzburg, Germany. Röntgen's discovery occurred accidentally: he was testing whether cathode radiation could pass through the glass, when he noticed a faint light originating from a nearby chemically coated light-sensitive paper screen. He named the new rays that caused this light "X-rays" because of their unknown nature. X-rays are electromagnetic energy waves that act similarly to light rays, but at wavelengths that are approximately 1000 times shorter than those of light. Röntgen conducted a series of experiments to understand his discovery better. He learned that X-rays penetrate human soft tissues, but not substances of higher density such as bone or lead (see example in Fig. 2.5). Röntgen's discovery was considered a medical miracle, and X-rays soon became an important diagnostic tool in medicine, as they allowed doctors to examine the human body's interior, without any surgery. In 1901, Röntgen was awarded the Nobel Prize in Physics "in recognition of the extraordinary services he has rendered by the discovery of the remarkable rays subsequently named after him."

Fig. 2.5 Early X-ray image of the hand of Mrs. Röntgen (from "A Century of X-Rays and Radioactivity in Medicine: With Emphasis on Photographic Records of the Early Years" R.F. Mould, with permission)

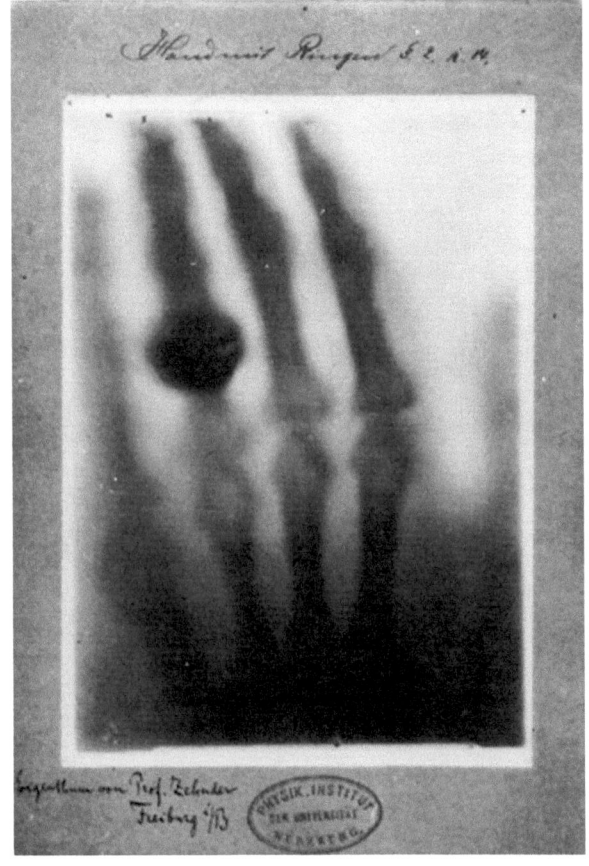

Scientists quickly realized the advantages of X-rays, and X-ray therapy was introduced soon after its discovery. The first treatment was performed in 1896 in Vienna and was the basis of external-beam radiotherapy. However, early adopters of this also discovered some harmful effects of radiation, as several cases of epilation, erythema, burns, and skin damage after exposure to X-rays were reported. Therefore, the British Röntgen Society appointed a committee in April 1898 to collect data on the adverse biological effects of X-rays. However, the risks of X-rays were not fully understood at that time and the radiation protection facilities for many pioneer physicians and technicians remained rudimentary or nonexistent for many years [13, 14].

As far as progress in imaging is concerned, the Austrian mathematician Johann Radon laid the foundation for all current tomographic procedures as early as 1917, with the formulation of the Radon transform and its inverse transform. He showed that a function can be reconstructed by an infinite set of projections [15]. An example of the practical realization of the Radon transform is shown in Fig. 2.6.

Several decades passed until 1972, when Godfrey Hounsfield and Allan Cormack developed the first computed tomography scanner. Hounsfield developed a device in which clusters of X-ray beams sent through the body from different angles were registered after they passed through the body. Advanced computer calculations based on the measured data made it possible to create images of different cross-sections of the body. Cormack developed the necessary calculation methods. In addition to cross-sections of the body, computed tomography also provided the basis for modern three-dimensional imaging. Hounsfield and Cormack were jointly awarded the Nobel Prize in Physiology or Medicine in 1979 "for the development of computer assisted tomography." The Hounsfield scale, a quantitative measure of radiodensity in CT scans, was also named after him [16].

In 1952, Felix Bloch and Edward Purcell received the Nobel Prize in Physics for their development of nuclear magnetic resonance, a basic principle behind magnetic resonance imaging (MRI) [17]. Decades later, Paul Lauterbur used this discovery to create MRI images of the body [18]. Peter Mansfield developed the technique further so that MRI scans with better resolution could be acquired within seconds rather than hours.

CT and MRI are two imaging techniques widely used in modern radiotherapy today, and they are also increasingly being applied in brachytherapy. Owing to the

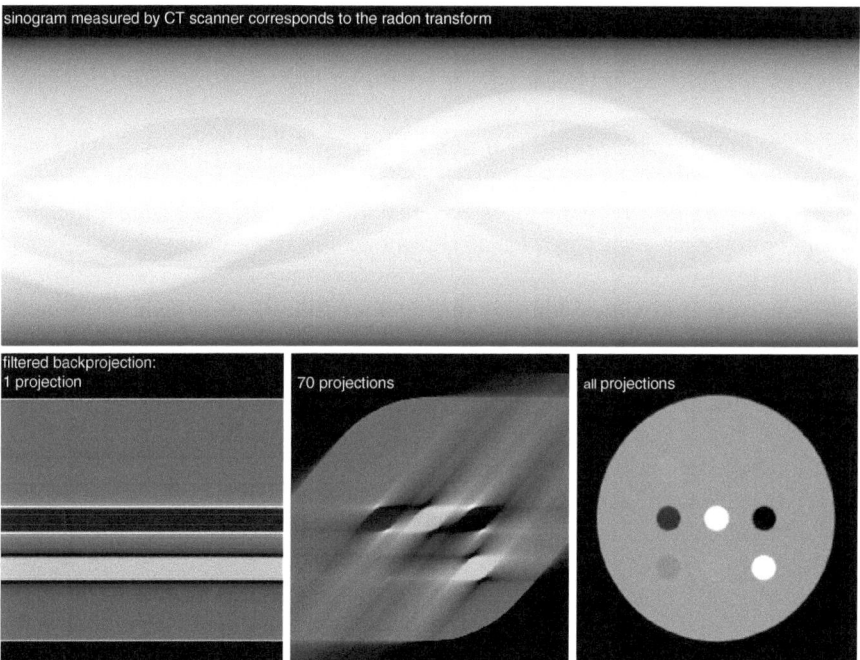

Fig. 2.6 An example of application of the radon transform: CT image reconstruction from a sinogram using filtered back-projection (courtesy of Prof. Guillaume Landry, Department of Radiation Oncology, LMU Munich, Germany)

physical differences in image acquisition, each technique has its advantages and disadvantages. Magnetic resonance imaging provides better information on soft tissue, with excellent spatial resolution, offering a truly multiplanar capability for imaging in any oblique plane; while computed tomography offers very accurate spatial resolution and electron-density information for dosimetry. From the patient's perspective, a CT scan is very fast and has the potential to reduce motion artifacts. However, X-rays are used for CT acquisition and, unlike in MRI, patients are exposed to ionizing radiation. On the other hand, MRI scans can be a problem for patients suffering from claustrophobia because of the smaller gantry size and longer scanning times. Moreover, metal implants or devices in the patient's body may be a contraindication for MRI [19].

Parallel to the development of tomographic imaging during the twentieth century, enormous progress was made in the field of computer technology. The advances in semiconductor development (e.g., transistors, miniaturization, integrated circuits) during recent decades have laid down the basis for the development of highly integrated hardware components (e.g., central processing units, field-programmable gate arrays). This in turn has provided high-speed computational power for processing large amounts of digitalized data by signal-processing algorithms, practically in real-time. Taken together, all these developments have led to the development of modern high-end CT and especially MRI devices for clinical practice [20].

Image-Guided Brachytherapy Treatment Using Modern Imaging Techniques

Beside the implantation of brachytherapy catheters, one of the main working steps in brachytherapy is computer-aided treatment planning. In modern brachytherapy, it is now standard of care to use cross-sectional images as the basis for 3D treatment planning for a large number of indications (see Fig. 2.7). On the cross-sectional images, target volumes are defined and organs at risk are identified before the catheters are reconstructed and the dose distributions optimized by medical physicists. Recently, support from artificial intelligence (AI) has also been increasingly evolving. For example, algorithms for automatic contouring based on AI can pre-contour organs at risk and reconstruct brachytherapy catheters within a few seconds. This approach may in future further reduce the human workload.

The effectiveness of brachytherapy is based on a very high radiation dose, which is applied precisely and directly in the tumor. To spare nearby organs at risk, brachytherapy uses its natural characteristic that dose decreases very steeply with increasing distance from the radiation source. Compared with external-beam radiotherapy, the dose gradient is much steeper, which makes it possible to apply very high doses in one or a few fractions and to reduce significantly the overall treatment time. However, a disadvantage of brachytherapy compared with external-beam radiotherapy is that brachytherapy requires, in most cases, the invasive implantation of the applicators. This is often carried out in close cooperation with colleagues of the

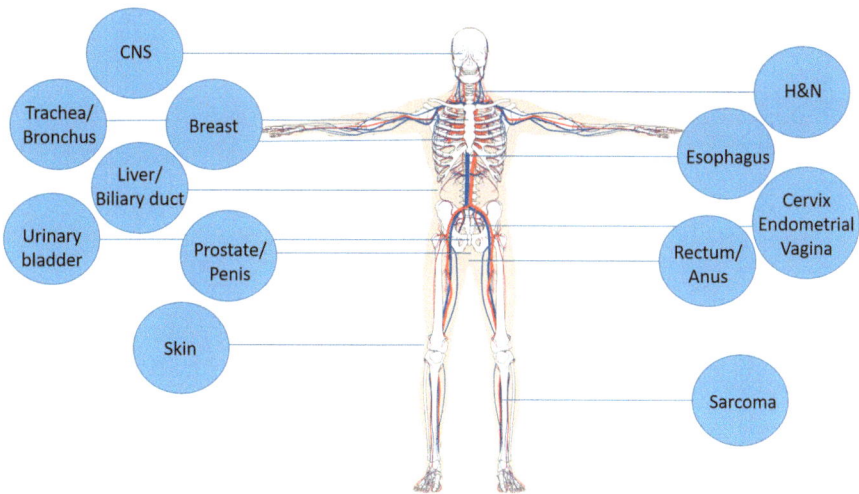

Fig. 2.7 Application areas of modern brachytherapy

corresponding specialist departments (e.g., gynecology, interventional radiology, surgery, gastroenterology, pulmonology, urology, ENT, neurosurgery), as the implantation procedures are sometimes very complex and require appropriate expertise (see Fig. 2.7). This multidisciplinary approach is particularly needed for target volumes that are not accessible without implantation by the special intervention (e.g., internal organs), by surgery (e.g., CNS), or by endoscopy (e.g., bronchus, esophagus, bile ducts) [21]. In this context, image-guidance is used not only for treatment planning but also for the catheter implantation itself. Imaging techniques available for brachytherapy implantation include ultrasound, X-ray, CT, and MRI. An example of a dedicated mobile CT system for interventional brachytherapy is shown in Fig. 2.8.

Example of Image-Guided Brachytherapy in Liver Tumors

In primary or secondary liver malignancies (e.g., hepatocellular carcinoma, cholangiocellular carcinoma, oligometastatic disease) the placement of the brachytherapy catheters can be CT-guided (fluoroscopic), ultrasound-guided, or MR-guided. All these imaging techniques are well suited for image-guidance during catheter placement. Usually, a contrast-enhanced planning CT is acquired for treatment planning. However, since most treatment-planning systems in brachytherapy do not take into account different electron densities, the planning of brachytherapy could also be performed directly on MR images. High-dose-rate brachytherapy is performed by using an afterloading technique, where the treatment time depends on the size of the lesion, the number of catheters, the dwell position, and the activity of the source. An overview of the workflow is depicted in Fig. 2.9.

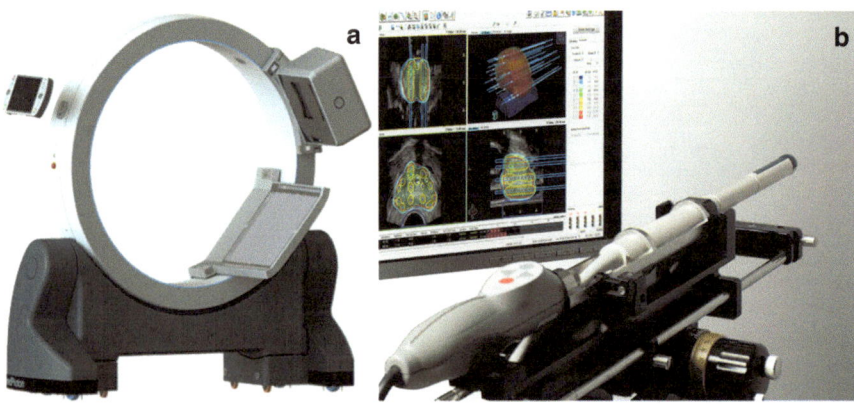

Fig. 2.8 Example of imaging modalities for brachytherapy interventions. (**a**) Dedicated mobile CT imaging device for interventional brachytherapy (Imaging Ring, MedPhoton, Salzburg, Austria). (**b**) Dedicated ultrasound system for prostate brachytherapy interventions with real-time workflow for needle insertion, needle reconstruction, contouring, and dose planning (Ultrasound system with OncoSelect Stepper and Endocavity rotational mover, Elekta AB, Stockholm, Sweden)

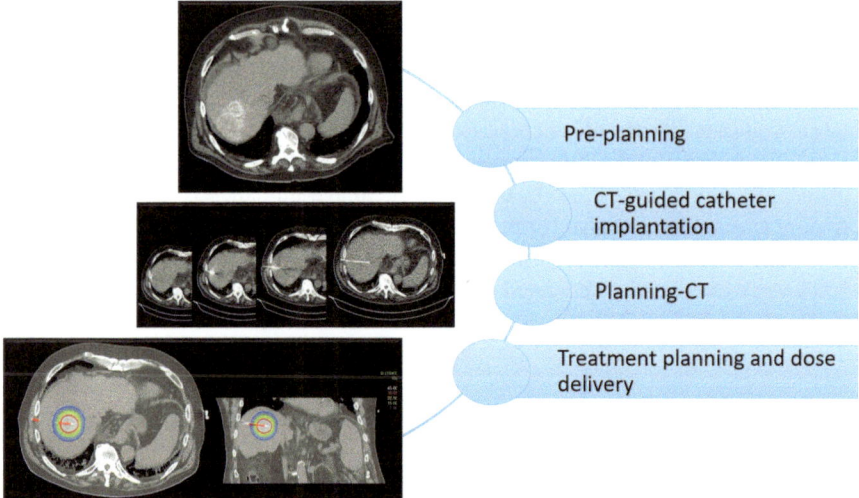

Fig. 2.9 Computed-tomography-guided catheter implantation and brachytherapy-planning workflow for a liver lesion

Brachytherapy allows the treatment of liver lesions with single doses of 15–25 Gy (depending on histology) and results in excellent local control rates even for large primary or secondary liver lesions [22, 23]. In addition, it offers an effective treatment option for centrally located liver lesions near large vessels, in contrast to thermoablative treatment approaches (RFA). In addition, it is less affected by respiratory-dependent movement uncertainties than are most SBRT techniques, as the implanted catheters are fixed in the tumor. Another advantage of brachytherapy is the possibility of a repetitive approach, whereby a hypofractionated fractionation scheme with two or three fractions can be used to spare better the organs at risk or to treat very large tumors [24].

Other Examples of Image-Guided Brachytherapy

The development of transrectal ultrasound and the availability of sophisticated treatment-planning systems have together produced a reliable system for treating prostate-cancer patients by brachytherapy, either as a boost or as monotherapy. Moreover, recent advances in the field of molecular imaging (PET/CT) and contrast-enhanced ultrasound appear promising for the location of intraprostatic lesions [25].

Similarly, image guidance using MRI was introduced in the brachytherapy treatment-planning process for patients with locally advanced cervical cancer. MRI-guided brachytherapy is based on an adaptive target concept, which takes into account the topography of the primary tumor at diagnosis, as well as the regression observed during external-beam radiotherapy [26]. There is now a large body of literature demonstrating that image-guided adaptive brachytherapy (IGABT) leads to better tumor control, increased survival, and decreased treatment toxicity [27].

Key Points
- The first known oncological treatments with brachytherapy were performed shortly after the discovery of radium in 1898.
- To solve the problem of radiation exposure of medical staff due to the manually applied radioactive sources, remote-controlled afterloading systems using artificial radionuclides (e.g., iridium-192) were introduced into clinical practice in the 1960s.
- In modern brachytherapy, it has become standard of care to use cross-sectional images (X-ray, CT, MRT, ultrasound) as the basis for catheter implantation and for 3D treatment planning for a large number of indications.

References

1. Thompson MK, Poortmans P, Chalmers AJ, et al. Practice-changing radiation therapy trials for the treatment of cancer: where are we 150 years after the birth of Marie Curie? Br J Cancer. 2018;119(4):389–407.
2. NobelPrize.org. Marie and Pierre Curie and the discovery of polonium and radium. https://www.nobelprize.org/prizes/themes/marie-and-pierre-curie-and-the-discovery-of-polonium-and-radium/. Accessed 20 Nov 2020.
3. American Brachytherapy Society. History of brachytherapy. https://www.americanbrachytherapy.org/resources/for-patients/history-of-brachytherapy/. Accessed 20 Nov 2020.
4. Gerbaulet A, Pötter R, Mazeron J-J, editors. The GEC ESTRO handbook of brachytherapy. Leuven: ACCO; 2002.

5. Mould RF, editor. Brachytherapy from radium to optimization. Veenendaal: Nucletron Internat. B. V. [u.a.]; 1994.
6. Wikipedia. Brachytherapy. https://en.wikipedia.org/w/index.php?title=Brachytherapy&oldid=988981728. Accessed 20 Nov 2020.
7. IAEA. STI/PUB/1196. http://www-naweb.iaea.org/nahu/DMRP/documents/Chapter13.pdf. Accessed 3 Dec 2020.
8. Aronowitz JN. The "Golden Age" of prostate brachytherapy: a cautionary tale. Brachytherapy. 2008;7(1):55–9.
9. Gupta VK. Brachytherapy—past, present and future. J Med Phys. 1995;20(2):31–5. http://inis.iaea.org/search/search.aspx?orig_q=RN:28030553.
10. Goldstein N. Radon seed implants. Arch Dermatol. 1975;111(6):757.
11. Kemikler G. History of brachytherapy. Turk J Oncol. 2019;34(Suppl 1):1–10.
12. Winston P. Carcinoma of the trachea treated by radon seed implantation. J Laryngol Otol. 1958;72(6):496–9.
13. Mould R. Century of X-rays and radioactivity in medicine: with emphasis on photographic records of the… early years. [S.l.]: CRC Press; 2019.
14. Editors H. German scientist discovers X-rays. https://www.history.com/this-day-in-history/german-scientist-discovers-x-rays. Accessed 20 Nov 2020.
15. Radon J. Über die Bestimmung von Funktionen durch ihre Integralwerte längs gewisser Mannigfaltigkeiten. Ber. Saechsische Akad. Wiss.; 1917.
16. NobelPrize.org. The Nobel Prize in Physiology or Medicine 1979. https://www.nobelprize.org/prizes/medicine/1979/summary/. Accessed 20 Nov 2020.
17. NobelPrize.org. The Nobel Prize in Physics 1952. https://www.nobelprize.org/prizes/physics/1952/bloch/lecture/. Accessed 20 Nov 2020.
18. Lauterbur PC. Image formation by induced local interactions: examples employing nuclear magnetic resonance. Nature. 1973;242(5394):190–1.
19. Lecchi M, Fossati P, Elisei F, et al. Current concepts on imaging in radiotherapy. Eur J Nucl Med Mol Imaging. 2008;35(4):821–37.
20. IEEE Xplore: IEEE Annals of the History of Computing. https://ieeexplore.ieee.org/xpl/RecentIssue.jsp?punumber=85. Accessed 20 Nov 2020.
21. Chargari C, Deutsch E, Blanchard P, et al. Brachytherapy: an overview for clinicians. CA Cancer J Clin. 2019;69(5):386–401.
22. Hass P, Mohnike K, Kropf S, et al. Comparative analysis between interstitial brachytherapy and stereotactic body irradiation for local ablation in liver malignancies. Brachytherapy. 2019;18(6):823–8.
23. Mohnike K, Steffen IG, Seidensticker M, et al. Radioablation by image-guided (HDR) brachytherapy and transarterial chemoembolization in hepatocellular carcinoma: a randomized phase II trial. Cardiovasc Intervent Radiol. 2019;42(2):239–49.
24. Ricke J, Wust P. Computed tomography-guided brachytherapy for liver cancer. Semin Radiat Oncol. 2011;21(4):287–93.
25. Banerjee S, Kataria T, Gupta D, et al. Use of ultrasound in image-guided high-dose-rate brachytherapy: enumerations and arguments. J Contemp Brachytherapy. 2017;9(2):146–50.
26. Haie-Meder C, Pötter R, van Limbergen E, et al. Recommendations from Gynaecological (GYN) GEC-ESTRO Working Group (I): concepts and terms in 3D image based 3D treatment planning in cervix cancer brachytherapy with emphasis on MRI assessment of GTV and CTV. Radiother Oncol. 2005;74(3):235–45.
27. Sturdza A, Pötter R, Fokdal LU, et al. Image guided brachytherapy in locally advanced cervical cancer: improved pelvic control and survival in RetroEMBRACE, a multicenter cohort study. Radiother Oncol. 2016;120(3):428–33.

Radiotherapeutic Fundamentals of Image-Guided HDR Brachytherapy

3

Peter Wust, Oliver Neumann, and Pirus Ghadjar

Introduction

Image-guided high-dose-rate (HDR) brachytherapy (iBT) requires an iridium-192 source of <1 mm size, which is moved in the implanted catheter array according to a treatment plan in order to generate an optimum individual dose distribution for a specified target volume while sparing adjacent organs at risk. Thermoablative approaches, such as radiofrequency ablation (RFA) or laser treatment are widely used, but their application has some general restrictions; these include danger to thermosensitive structures, limitations in treating lesions close to large vessels due to cooling, ineffectiveness in treating lesions with increased arterial tumor perfusion, such as hepatocellular carcinoma or neuroendocrine tumors, and limited local control of lesions >3 cm in size [1–3]. Meanwhile, a variety of modern external radiation techniques are available that compete with iBT, a method that is relatively accurate but invasive. Therefore, the radiation oncologist has to decide which radiotherapy technique is the best for a given target volume, embedded in an individual anatomy and with certain organs at risk or regions of interest (ROI).

Image-guided HDR brachytherapy competes with external radiotherapy techniques such as stereotactic ablative radiotherapy using a dedicated linear accelerator (e.g., Cyberknife) or IMRT (intensity-modulation radiotherapy) techniques such as VMAT (volume-modulated arc therapy) or Tomotherapy.

Before radiotherapy, the target volume is defined according to macroscopic tumor, clinical target volume (CTV), and planning target volume (PTV), as illustrated by Fig. 3.1. The macroscopic tumor has a maximum tumor cell density of 10^8–10^9 cells per mL, if the cells have a size of 10 μm and are more or less tightly

P. Wust (✉) · O. Neumann · P. Ghadjar
Department of Radiation Oncology, Charité – Universitätsmedizin Berlin, Berlin, Germany
e-mail: peter.wust@charite.de; oliver.neumann@charite.de; pirus.ghadjar@charite.de

21

Fig. 3.1 Illustration of CTV and PTV, assuming lesions within organs or regions of interest (ROI) such as liver, lung, or kidney (green). In the CTV we distinguish between the macroscopic tumor (with $\geq 10^8$ cells/mL) and microscopically involved parts of the target (with $< 10^8$ cells/mL)

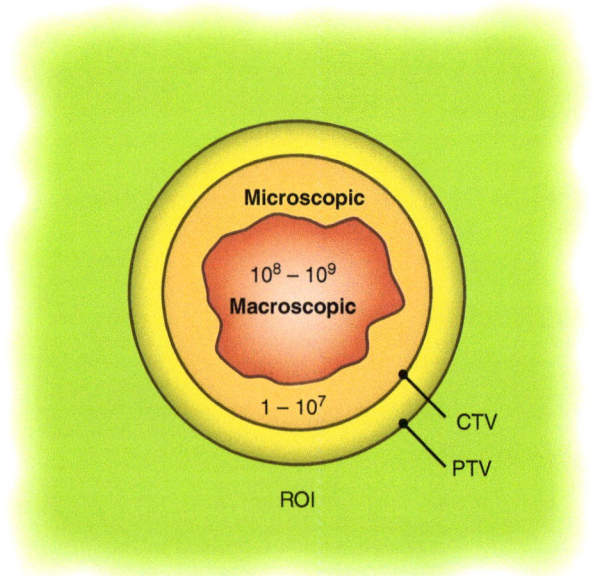

packed. The cell density might be lower because of the tumor stroma; it would then amount to between 10^7 and 10^8 per mL. The CTV contains the macroscopic tumor(s) and should ideally include all tumor cells existing in the patient. There is a gradient of cell density from 10^9 cancer cells per mL down to zero at the boundary of the CTV. Optimum delineation of the CTV in a three-dimensional image dataset demands a high level of clinical experience and as much information as possible: e.g., multimodal imaging, histopathological report (with resection margins), operative report, etc. Finally, the PTV surrounds the CTV and should take account of all possible inaccuracies in dose planning and delivery. Specification of the PTV is a tool to shape the dose distribution such that an adequate dose is delivered to all parts of the CTV with a clinically acceptable probability. Therefore, delineation of the PTV is a complex optimization problem. Radiation oncologists tend to determine PTVs larger than necessary, which increases toxicity. On the other hand, if the PTV is too small, the tumor control may decrease.

All external radiotherapy techniques benefit from the modern image-guided radiotherapy (IGRT) techniques using portal imaging (PI), cone-beam CT (CBCT), mega-voltage CT (MVCT), or most advanced fluoroscopy-based on-line tracking (Cyberknife), all of which decreases the PTV. The final goal of the radiation oncologist is the achievement of a tumor-control probability (TCP) that is as high as possible but with a minimum of long-term side effects or normal-tissue complication probabilities (NTCP).

In this chapter, we will develop criteria to estimate TCP and NTCP for certain indications in order to assess the eligibility of iBT in each case.

Radiation Effects on Tumor Lesions

The biological endpoint of therapeutic radiation against tumor cells is *reproductive cell death* or *mitotic death*. This means that the genome of the irradiated cell is damaged in such a way that cell division is impossible. The cells are either sterilized, i.e., they are no longer able to proliferate, or they die during cell division, or else their daughter cells cannot survive because their DNA content is incomplete. Chromosomal aberrations in a karyogram of a cell sample indicate severe DNA damage and are correlated with reproductive cell death. For in vitro studies the clonogenic assay is the gold standard to determine dose effect (survival) curves. Survival of a cell is then the ability to form a colony excluding any cells that suffer reproductive cell death.

The linear-quadratic (LQ) model is an accepted approach to describe survival curves of various cell lines. It introduces two parameters, α [Gy^{-1}] and β [Gy^{-2}] and also the ratio α/β [Gy] according to Fig. 3.2 [4]. For the survival fraction SF we obtain SF as a function of the intensity D_s [Gy] of a single dose:

$$\text{SF} = \exp\left(-\alpha \times D_s - \beta \times D_s^2\right) \tag{3.1}$$

The parameters α and β depend on the particular cell line; they are highly variable and fundamentally unknown for a given tumor. Experiments to determine α and β are time-consuming and are not possible for an individual tumor, for various reasons (see below). Typical values are listed in Table 3.1. We classify tumors as *radiation-sensitive* ($\alpha \approx 0.3$ Gy^{-1}) down to *radiation-resistant* ($\alpha \approx 0.1$ Gy^{-1}).

Two useful rules of thumb can be derived from Table 3.1 together with Fig. 3.2. First, SF$_2$ (the survival fraction for 2 Gy) is above 0.5 for tumors known as radioresistant (e.g., glioblastoma) and typically near 0.5 or even below 0.5 for radiosensitive cancer diseases (e.g., lymphoma, small-cell lung cancer).

Second, the ratio α/β [Gy], known as the *critical dose*, is an important parameter that characterizes the *fractionation sensitivity* of a tumor or tissue and must be carefully considered [5]. Note that in Fig. 3.2 the two curves have the same SF$_2$ = 0.3, but their courses are very different if the critical dose α/β changes from a value of 10 Gy to a value of 2 Gy. For radiation doses less than 2 Gy, the curve with $\alpha/\beta = 2$ Gy is flatter, which corresponds to greater repair capacity (formation of a shoulder), but the difference is slight. However, above the critical dose of 2 Gy, the slopes diverge dramatically in the semilogarithmic plot. For a single dose of 4 Gy the radiation effect for $\alpha/\beta = 2$ is more than doubled in comparison with $\alpha/\beta = 10$. If the single dose distinctly exceeds the critical dose for a cell type, considerable radiation effects can be expected.

It is easier to estimate this ratio α/β than to determine individual values for α and β. For rapidly proliferating tumors α/β is near 10 Gy, but it might be lower (around 5 Gy) for certain tumors (see Table 3.1). A lower α/β had been assumed for melanoma and prostate carcinoma, which is reflected in practical fractionation schemes

Fig. 3.2 Examples of cell survival curves parameterized by the LQ model for $\alpha/\beta = 2$ Gy (blue) and $\alpha/\beta = 10$ Gy (red). Both curves lead to the same SF_2 of 0.4. For single doses d of >2 Gy (critical dose) the curves rapidly diverge, but they are quite similar for $d < 2$ Gy

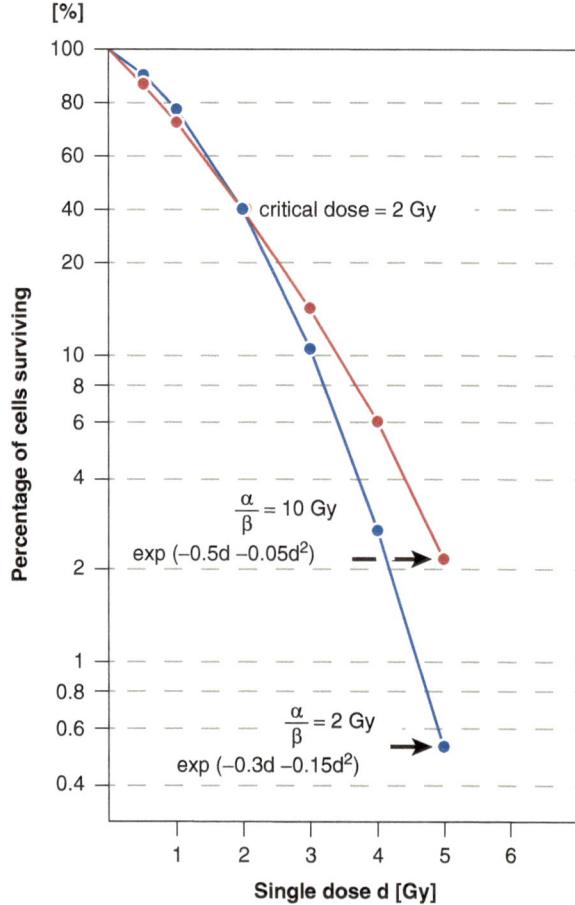

Table 3.1 Parameters α and β for some tumor cell lines allowing calculation of survival curves according to the LQ model

Tumor	α [Gy^{-1}]	β [Gy^{-2}]	SF_2	α/β [Gy]
Glioblastoma	0.24	0.029	0.58	8.3
Melanoma	0.26	0.053	0.51	4.9
Squamous-cell carcinoma	0.27	0.045	0.49	6.0
Adenocarcinoma	0.31	0.055	0.48	5.6
Lymphoma	0.45	0.051	0.34	8.8
Small-cell lung cancer	0.65	0.081	0.22	8.0

(with higher single doses). Skillful evaluation of clinical studies with different fractionation schemes and defined clinical endpoints has made it possible to estimate α/β for tumors and tissues. There is agreement among radiation oncologists that for tumors wide variation of α and β as well as of α/β is possible.

Determining the single dose D_s for tumor control is a standard task in radiation oncology. A TCP of 90% for a lesion with 10^8 tumor cells/mL (according to Fig. 3.1) requires a cell kill of nine decades. According to the LQ model (Eq. 3.1) we assume $SF(D_s) = 10^{-9}$.

Using $\exp(-20.7) = 10^{-9}$ we obtain a quadratic equation $D_s^2 + (\alpha/\beta) D_s = 20.7/\beta$, yielding

$$D_s = \left\{20.7/\beta + (\alpha/2\beta)^2\right\}^{1/2} - (\alpha/2\beta) \tag{3.2}$$

Table 3.2 shows single tumor-control doses for different radiation sensitivities α and critical doses α/β. Typical single doses applied in stereotactic radiotherapy of 20–25 Gy are sufficient for radiation-sensitive tumors (with $\alpha = 0.2$–0.3 Gy^{-1} and $\alpha/\beta < 10$ Gy). For decreasing α/β, the tumor-control dose declines sharply. However, radioresistant tumors (with $\alpha < 0.2$ Gy^{-1} and $\alpha/\beta > 5$ Gy) would often be missed with radiation doses below 25 Gy. Therefore, doses higher than the prescribed standard doses in stereotactic ablative radiotherapy might be desirable under certain conditions.

If we divide the target/tumor V_T into $i = 1,...,N$ volume elements ΔV_i (with $\sum_i \Delta V_i = V_T$) and allocate the dose D_i to each element, we can calculate the tumor-control probability (TCP) according to

$$TCP(\text{target}) = \prod_{i=1...N} \left[1 - SF(D_i)\right] \tag{3.3}$$

A higher D_i in ΔV_i increases TCP of the entire target, which is the clinical objective. Therefore, an inhomogeneous dose distribution (with dose excesses) in the target can increase the TCP and is preferable, if the target consists of macroscopic tumor alone and contains no organ at risk. This condition is fulfilled for liver or lung metastases, but not, e.g., for the prostate, which contains in its central part the urethra as an organ at risk.

If we intend to destroy a tumor lesion with unknown radiosensitivity α and β, the doses in every part of the tumor must be as high as possible. Single doses above 20 Gy are required for a typical radiosensitive tumor with $\alpha = 0.3$ Gy^{-1} and $\alpha/\beta = 10$ Gy, but higher doses are in any case desirable for reliable long-term local control.

Table 3.2 Tumor control with single doses $D_s = \{20.7/\beta + (\alpha/2\beta)^2\}^{1/2} - (\alpha/2\beta)$ depending on α and α/β. For doses of ~50 Gy tumor control is nearly always achieved

	Radiation sensitive	Intermediate	Radiation resistant
α/β [Gy]	$\alpha = 0.3$ Gy^{-1}	$\alpha = 0.2$ Gy^{-1}	$\alpha = 0.1$ Gy^{-1}
20	28	37	55
10	22	28	41
5	16	20	30
2	11	13	19

Radiation Effects of on Normal Tissues

While for tumor cells *clonogenicity* is the common biological endpoint, for normal tissues there are various endpoints for *toxicity*. For rapidly proliferating tissues, e.g., mucosae or skin, endpoints for acute toxicity such as mucositis or dermatitis are associated with $\alpha/\beta = 10$ Gy. Therefore, rapidly regenerating normal tissues and tumors behave in a radiobiologically similar manner. Every tissue can also suffer late effects (e.g., mucosae ulcer or ulceration, subcutaneous fibrosis, telangiectasia of the skin), if the *tolerance dose* in a certain volume is exceeded. Long-term toxicity is more likely for lower α/β, if single doses exceed the critical doses.

Other normal tissues with a slow (liver, kidney, lung) or nearly no (connective tissue, spinal cord, nerves) turnover undergo mainly late effects and are equally well described by lower α/β. Here a conservative value of $\alpha/\beta = 2$ Gy, and estimations of tolerance doses [6] are utilized in clinical practice to avoid toxicity.

The LKB (Lyman–Kutcher–Brown) model is useful to estimate normal-tissue complication probabilities (NTCP) for most organs/tissues and clinical endpoints [7–10]. Parameters of the LKB model for the relevant tissues are listed in Table 3.3. We start with an estimated *tolerance dose* $TD_{50/5}$ for a certain tissue or organ with a defined clinical endpoint (complication). $TD_{50/5}$ leads to the complication in question in 50% of patients within 5 years after irradiation of the *entire organ*, or a large part of its tissue, with this dose. In the LKB model $TD_{50/5}$ is the mean dose of a *Gaussian distribution* of tolerance doses (as a standard, normally distributed random variable) with standard deviation $\sigma = m \times TD_{50/5}$. Integration over this probability function yields the cumulative distribution function, indicating a sigmoid NTCP-curve, as shown in Fig. 3.3. Note that $TD_{5/5}$ (mean dose inducing the complication in 5% of patients within 5 years) is slightly above $TD_{50/5} - 2 \times \sigma$. The parameter m, ranging from 0.1 to 0.4, characterizes the gradient of the NTCP curve and has the value 0.25 for the liver (Table 3.3).

Another crucial parameter is the volume V_i, which is part of the entire volume of the organ V_0 and defines the partial volume i as $v_i = V_i/V_0$. The tolerance dose $TD_{50/5}(v_i)$ of the partial volume is larger than $TD_{50/5}(v_0 = 1)$ and is given by the volume parameter n according to

$$TD_{50/5}\left(V_i\right) = TD_{50/5}\left(V_0\right) / v_i^{\,n} \tag{3.4}$$

Then the NTCP-curve for v_i shifts to higher doses, as shown for the liver in Fig. 3.3 using the parameters of Table 3.3 and a partial volume of ~30% ($v_i = 1/3$), yielding $TD_{50/5}(1/3) = 80$ Gy.

Let D_0 be the dose administered to V_0 indicating a given $NTCP(D_0)$. Then the partial volume v, which has the same complication level for a maximum dose D_{max}, is calculated by reformulation of Eq. 3.4:

$$v = \left(D_0 / D_{max}\right)^{1/n} \tag{3.5a}$$

For example, irradiation of the whole liver with $D_0 = 25$ Gy is equivalent to irradiation of $(25/50)^{1/0.6} \approx 1/3$—i.e., one-third of the liver—with 50 Gy.

Table 3.3 Normal tissue parameters n, m according to the LKB model, α/β-ratios and tolerance doses

Organ tissue	$TD_{5/5}(1)$ [Gy]	$TD_{5/5}(1/3)$ [Gy]	$TD_{50/5}(1)$ [Gy]	$TD_{50/5}(1/3)$ [Gy]	σ [Gy] (1)	σ [Gy] (1/3)	n (volume)	m (slope)	α/β [Gy]	Clinical endpoint
Liver	25	50	40	80	10	20	0.6	0.25	1.5	Radioinduced liver disease (RILD)
Lung	18	45	25	74	12	15	0.9	0.2	2.5	Pulmonary dysfunction
Kidney	23	50	28	65	3	6.5	0.7	0.1	0.5–4	Nephropathy Renal failure
Small bowel	40	50	55	70	10	14	0.1–0.2	0.2	3–5	Obstruction Perforation
Stomach	45	54	60	76	10	11	0.1–0.2	0.15	5	Bleeds/ulcer
Brain	45	60	60	86	12	17	0.2–0.3	0.2	2	Necrosis Cognitive dysfunction
Heart	15	18	29	35	12	14	0.16	0.4	3	Cardiac mortality
Skin	55	65	65	79	6.5	8	0.16	0.1	1–4	Fibrosis/ulcer Telangiectasia
Spinal cord	47	50	70	74	14	15	0.05	0.2	2.5–5	Myelopathy
Nerves Plexus	60	62	100	104	30	31	0.03	0.3	1–3.5	Neuropathy Plexopathy

Abbreviations: $TD_{5/5}$ mean dose leading to a complication rate of 5% within 5 years after irradiation of the entire organ (1) or one-third of it (1/3), $TD_{50/5}$ mean dose leading to a complication rate of 50% within 5 years after irradiation of the entire organ (1) or one-third of it (1/3); $\sigma = m \times TD_{50/5}$

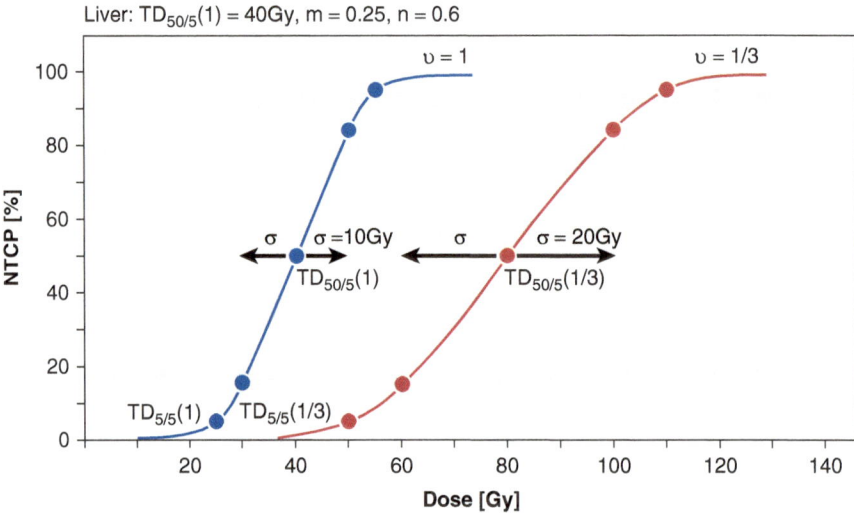

Fig. 3.3 NTCP curves for the liver for the clinical endpoint RILD, obtained by using the parameters m and n of Table 3.3 (see text). Note that $\sigma = m \times \mathrm{TD}_{50/5}$. The NTCP curve is shifted to considerably higher doses if only 1/3 of the liver is exposed. We assume that the total dose is applied by a conventional scheme (5 × 2 Gy per week). Conversion to single doses is possible by Eq. 3.6a

If we have a given dose distribution $D_i < D_{\max}$, $i = 1,...,N$, administered to the partial volumes v_i as quantified by the dose–volume histogram (DVH), then we define an effective volume as weighted average

$$v_{\mathrm{eff}} = \sum_i v_i \times \left(D_i / D_{\max} \right)^{1/n} \tag{3.5b}$$

We can then estimate the actual NTCP(DVH) for this DVH as $\mathrm{NTCP}v_{\mathrm{eff}}\,(D_{\max})$.

We differentiate between two types of normal tissue as classified in Table 3.3. The first type is the *series organ*, which behaves like a *chain*. If a single link in a chain snaps, then the entire chain breaks as well. Such a tissue might suffer an undesirable complication if the radiation dose in a *small volume* has overrun. Then the question arises of how we specify a "small volume." Prototypes of these tissues are *spinal cord* and *nerves*, with the possible adverse effects *myelopathy* or *plexopathy* [11]. For safety reasons we specify for these tissues 0.1 mL as the "small volume"— i.e., only in 0.1 mL is the dose allowed to exceed the tolerance dose, while the reference volume is 3 mL [4]. Thus, employing Eq. 3.4, we can estimate a tolerance dose of 66 Gy in 0.1 mL, if the tolerance dose in 3 mL amounts to 47 Gy and $n = 0.05$ (Table 3.3).

Mucosae and skin also show chain-like behavior, with ulcers or necroses as possible complications. For these tissues, e.g., stomach or intestine, we recommend a slightly higher "small volume" value of 1–3 mL, so as to accept a dose overrun [12, 13].

Series organs are characterized by small n values (0.03–0.2), providing a small volume effect (Table 3.3). In series organs, the *maximum dose* is correlated with toxicity.

The second tissue type is the *parallel organ*, which behaves like a "rope" consisting of a multitude of monofilaments. Such tissues undergo a complication if a large tissue volume or a considerable percentage of the organ is irradiated (corresponding to damage to many filaments). The tolerance dose can then be slight, and much care is required if large volumes, or even the whole organ, are irradiated.

This is illustrated in Fig. 3.3 for the liver [14], which is the organ most commonly treated by iBT [15–17]. While the $TD_{5/5}(v = 1/3) \approx 50$ Gy and $TD_{50/5}(v = 1/3) \approx 80$ Gy for irradiation of the partial liver (here one-third) are rather high and are further increased for even smaller volumes (e.g., $TD_{5/5} \approx 100$ Gy for $v = 0.1$), an unexpectedly low $TD_{5/5}(1) = 25$ Gy must be taken into account for irradiation of the whole liver. Lung, kidneys, and heart are likewise sensitive toward irradiation of the entire organ [18–20].

These parallel organs are characterized by $n \geq 0.6$, providing this considerable volume effect according to Eq. 3.4 (Table 3.3). In parallel organs the *mean dose* is correlated with toxicity.

We note that various organs with n between 0.1 and 0.3 might undergo complications arising from a dose exceedance either in a small volume (e.g., a few mL) or in the whole organ (or a large part of it). In the case of the *small intestine,* we have a $TD_{5/5}$(some mL) of 50 Gy irradiating some mL potentially causing long-term local obstruction or perforation. For volumes above 150 mL the $TD_{5/5}(>150$ mL$) = 15$ Gy is much lower as regards the risk of acute Grade 2 toxicity [12]. In case of the *brain* the $TD_{5/5}$(some 10 mL) of 60 Gy or even higher for smaller volumes can cause local radiation necroses as clinical endpoint [21]. However, the tolerance dose for whole-brain irradiation as regards the risk of cognitive dysfunction is much lower and is probably below 10–20 Gy.

Note that Table 3.3 and Fig. 3.3 show tolerance doses TD for conventionally fractionated regimens (5×2 Gy per week). Therefore, we used the linear-quadratic model to calculate biologically equivalent doses BEQ_{2Gy} (assuming conventional fractionation with $d = 2$ Gy), iso-effective with single doses D_S for tissues with different α/β values [4], in order better to compare the abovementioned techniques in which high single doses are applied to circumscribed lesions (Table 3.4):

$$BEQ_{2Gy} = \left[(\alpha/\beta + D_S)/(\alpha/\beta + 2)\right] \times D_S \qquad (3.6a)$$

In the last column of Table 3.4, for $\alpha/\beta = 10$ Gy, we have added the iso-effective biologically effective doses BED (assuming a low-dose-rate regimen with $d \rightarrow 0$), for easier comparison with published data (see Discussion):

$$BED = \left[(\alpha/\beta + D_S)/\alpha/\beta\right] \times D_S \qquad (3.6b)$$

Table 3.4 shows such $BEQ_{2Gy}(\alpha/\beta)$ equivalent to single doses D_S for some relevant tissues/organs with different α/β values (see Table 3.3). Single doses up to

Table 3.4 Biologically effective doses applied by conventionally fractionated regimens BEQ_{2Gy} (5×2 Gy per week with $d = 2$ Gy) in dependence on α/β that are iso-effective with a single dose D_S. For comparison BED (for $d \to 0$) are shown for $\alpha/\beta = 10$ Gy

D_S [Gy]	BEQ_{2Gy} [Gy] $\alpha/\beta = 1.5$ Gy	BEQ_{2Gy} [Gy] $\alpha/\beta = 2$ Gy	BEQ_{2Gy} [Gy] $\alpha/\beta = 3$ Gy	BEQ_{2Gy} [Gy] $\alpha/\beta = 5$ Gy	BEQ_{2Gy}/BED [Gy] $\alpha/\beta = 10$ Gy
5	10	9	7	5	3/8
8	23	20	16	11	7/14
10	34	30	24	17	10/20
12	48	42	34	24	14/26
15	73	64	51	36	21/38
18	103	90	72	51	30/50
20	126	110	88	63	37/60
25	189	169	140	107	73/88
30	274	225	192	137	80/120
35	365	324	266	200	131/158

Abbreviations: D_s single dose, BEQ_{2Gy} biologically equivalent dose for conventionally fractionated regimens of 5×2 Gy per week, BED biologically effective dose for a low-dose rate regimen with $d \to 0$

12 Gy appear safe even for normal tissues with $\alpha/\beta = 2$ Gy, with increasing risk for single doses beyond 15 Gy. We note that the liver is particularly sensitive to large single doses because of its low α/β of 1.5 Gy. In consequence, only two fractions of 5 Gy to the entire liver that are iso-effective with 20 Gy in conventional fractionation might induce a RILD in 2% of patients, a non-negligible proportion, according to Fig. 3.3.

On the other hand, for proliferating tumors with $\alpha/\beta = 10$ Gy single doses of >25 Gy appear necessary. However, the treatment-limiting α/β values in tumors are unknown and might be variable, in particular considering radioresistant, so-called "quiescent," cells [22].

Normal tissues such as liver, lung, and kidneys benefit strongly from lowering the volume with low doses of radiation. Conversely, these tissues tolerate rather high doses in a limited volume. Thus, image-guided HDR brachytherapy appears ideally suited to treating single or oligotopic tumor lesions in these organs.

Radiotherapy Techniques for Radio-Ablation with Single Doses

Various ablative radiation techniques are available to treat tumor lesions adjacent to normal tissues. The ratio TCP/NTCP (see above) measures the *therapeutic ratio* and is useful to compare radiation techniques.

Image-guided HDR brachytherapy generates high doses around the catheters in parts of the target, which elevates the TCP (see Eq. 3.3). Likewise, a steep dose gradient spares the surrounding tissues, reducing the NTCP of adjacent tissues. Both features favor iBT in particular for intrahepatic, intrapulmonal, or intrarenal metastases or tumors, because precisely these organs (liver, lung, kidney) are sensitive to high-volume radiation exposure with low or medium radiation doses ($n > 0.6$ in Table 3.3).

Dose–volume histograms (DVH) are cumulative distribution functions of the dose distributions in the regions of interest (ROI) and depict the relationship between the percentage X of volume V_X of the specified ROI and the minimum radiation dose D_X deposited in V_X. Then the doses related to V_0 and V_{100} are respectively the maximum dose D_{max} and the minimum dose D_{min} administered to the ROI.

Figure 3.4 shows idealized DVHs favorable for a target that contains a lot of normal tissue (blue), a target that consists only of the macroscopic tumor (red), and an ROI adjacent to the target (green), e.g., the liver.

The blue curve characterizes adjuvant radiotherapy with a microscopic tumor disease. A homogeneous dose distribution is adequate (ideally resulting in a rectangular box), if the tumor cell load (microscopic disease) is interspersed at a constant level throughout the CTV. We note that modern radiation technology utilizing intensity-modulated radiotherapy (IMRT) allows a risk-adapted dose distribution to be attained if the cell load (see Fig. 3.1) varies. Especially for the histopathological R1 finding after resection (indicating a positive resection margin) a higher dose is required because the number of tumor cells per mL is probably greater adjacent to the R1 area than near the R0 margins (risk area in Fig. 3.4).

The red curve shows a typical iBT situation, in which, e.g., a liver metastasis is treated. Higher doses in the interior of the target (PTV) increase the TCP but do not burden any organ. Inspecting Table 3.4 we estimate a single dose of 30 Gy, equivalent to a conventionally fractionated radiation with 80 Gy for $\alpha/\beta = 10$ Gy, instead of the standard dose of 20 Gy. Table 3.2 shows that required single doses can be even higher for reliable local control (maximizing the TCP).

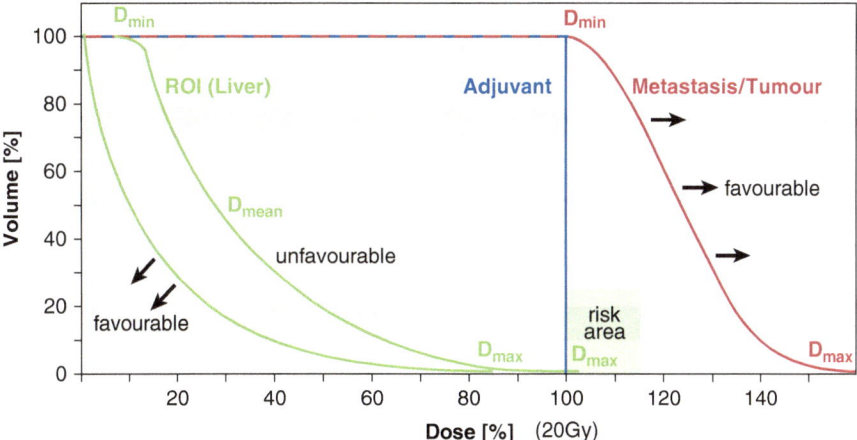

Fig. 3.4 Schematic DVH curves for certain indications: For the adjuvant radiotherapy the DVH of the PTV is ideally rectangular (blue curve) with some dose escalation in risk areas (depending on tumor cell density). For the radiotherapy of a solid tumor the dose in the PTV should be as high as possible (red curve). In the surrounding ROI (e.g., liver) the DVH (green curve) should be shifted to zero and is characterized by D_{min} and D_{mean}, both as small as possible

The green curves describe the ROI outside the PTV, such as the liver, which tolerates high doses in small volumes, but is sensitive to lower doses in large volumes. Under ideal conditions, the green curve should approach the zero line as quickly as possible. The minimum dose delivered to the whole organ (in Fig. 3.4, about 10% for the outer green curve) might result in a long-term risk, which is particularly relevant for younger patients. The maximum dose D_{max} approaches the prescribed target dose (here 20 Gy), but the volume exposed to doses near D_{max} should be as small as possible.

To compare iBT with radiosurgery technologies, we analyzed a series of spherical liver metastases in a peripheral location with diameters from 1 to 5 cm and segmented adjacent ROI (liver, right/left kidney, stomach, heart, right lung) as shown in Fig. 3.5. We ascertained the intralesional dose distributions delivered (estimating the TCPs) and the burden to the adjacent organs (estimating the corresponding NTCPs), and we compared four advanced radiation techniques suitable for radio-ablation that are briefly described below. Older techniques such as fixed-field IMRT or 3D-conformal radiotherapy were excluded from the comparison.

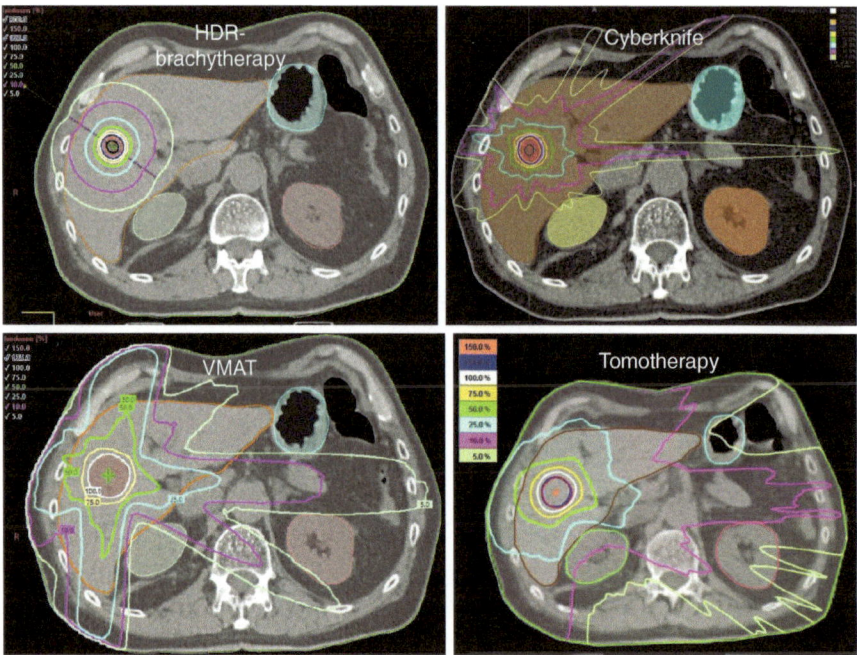

Fig. 3.5 Dose distributions comparing the four radiotherapy techniques, if the standard single dose of 20 Gy is administered to a 2 cm lesion. The isodoses range from 150% (30 Gy, orange), 125% (25 Gy, dark blue) through 100% (20 Gy, white), 75% (15 Gy, yellow), 50% (green, 10 Gy), 25% (5 Gy, light blue), and 10% (2 Gy, purple) to 5% (1 Gy, light green), as shown in the inserted scales. The ROIs are also shown, such as liver (brown), stomach (blue), and kidneys (green, red). For this small lesion HDR brachytherapy is clearly superior in comparison with the external techniques

VMAT (volume-modulated arc therapy): This is the standard of care, using common linear accelerators (Siemens/Varian Medical Systems Inc., Palo Alto, 94304 CA, USA and Electa AB, SE-103 93 Stockholm, Sweden). VMAT employs one or more arcs rotating around the iso-center typically located in the lesion, with variable speed, intensity, and multileaf collimator (MLC) setup. The leaves have a thickness of 0.5 cm in the center (10×10 cm). To account for breathing-induced movement of the liver the diameter was enlarged by only 1 cm to form the PTV. To restrict the safety margin to 5 mm we assumed patient compliance to control respiratory motion, either with shallow breathing or by breath-hold techniques. Optimization of dose specifications for the PTV and the ROI (limiting $V_{X\%}$, volume with doses $\geq$ X%) is performed by use of the planning system Eclipse®.

Tomotherapy: This is a competitive technology using a binary (on/off) collimator of 1 cm thickness that allows full intensity modulation, slice by slice, in a dedicated linear accelerator (Accuray Inc., Sunnyvale, CA 94089, USA). Tomotherapy shows greater superiority for complex target volumes and complicated constraints [23], but it is theoretically nearly equivalent to VMAT for simple, e.g., spherical, targets. Again, the diameter of the CTV was enlarged by only 1 cm to form the PTV, assuming adequate control of respiratory motion. The planning system Tomoplan® calculated optimized dose distributions taking into account the selected restrictions.

Cyberknife: This radiosurgery system uses a compact linear accelerator on a robotic manipulator that can radiate from a large spherical angle using standard circular collimators of selected diameter. Its principal advantages are full three-dimensional performance and the integrated image-guidance system that allows online tracking during radiation. Almost perfect tracking is implemented for Cyberknife by using gold-marker implants. Their implantation is an image-guided invasive procedure similar to the catheter implantation for brachytherapy, but less critical in terms of accuracy. The PTV and CTV were set to be equal. An inverse planning algorithm is available.

Image-guided HDR brachytherapy: We assumed one or five accurately implanted catheters in the lesion and used the planning system Brachyvision®. The quality of iBT depends critically upon the precise placing of the catheters.

We must regard iBT and Cyberknife as being, or requiring, invasive procedures, if we compare them with noninvasive external radiation methods (VMAT, Tomotherapy). Thus, for iBT and Cyberknife we can set PTV and CTV to be equal because catheters do not move relative to the lesion and almost perfect tracking is performed. For any noninvasive radiation technique, respiratory movement of the liver or lung typically results in a PTV margin of 0.5 cm when there is hypoventilation. Therefore, we compared dose distributions of iBT and Cyberknife for lesions of diameter d with lesions of diameter $d + 1$ [cm] for the external radiation techniques referenced.

We optimized the dose distributions, aiming for mean doses as high as possible inside the lesions, ensuring a 20 Gy target coverage above 95% and minimum burden to the liver comparing V_{10Gy}, V_{5Gy}, V_{2Gy}, and V_{1Gy}. Figure 3.5 shows examples of dose distributions for these treatment techniques applied to a lesion with a diameter of $d = 2$ cm. Important DVH parameters for the lesions and the ROI liver, right kidney, and stomach are listed in Table 3.5 for lesion sizes $d = 1, 2, 3,$ and 5 cm.

Image-guided HDR brachytherapy is by far the most effective, yielding mean intralesional doses $D_{mean} > 55$ Gy, whereby increasing the number of catheters (5 versus 1 catheter) homogenizes the intralesional dose distribution and lowers D_{mean}. We achieved a much lower D_{mean} of approximately 30 Gy by Cyberknife and Tomotherapy and only 22 Gy by VMAT. For lesion sizes above 3 cm the rather high TCP is combined with improved conformality in the high-dose range around 10 Gy, with sparing of the liver in the low-dose range (around 1–2 Gy), and with low exposure of the other surrounding organs (e.g., right kidney, stomach), in comparison with all external radiation techniques. For lesions of >3 cm, D_{mean} is still superior for iBT, but dose reduction in the liver and surrounding tissues declines continuously with increasing size. For lesions of >3 cm diameter the liver volume with the low dose of 1–2 Gy is even larger for iBT in comparison with all external techniques, but the liver volume exposed with 5 Gy is still less or equal and the strikingly high dose to the tumor remains unchanged. Interestingly, the use of more catheters (5 versus 1 catheter) considerably increases toxicity, but it fails to improve either the effectiveness of treatment or the sparing of surroundings.

Image-guided HDR brachytherapy achieves the highest conformality for small lesions, which is also reflected in the dose distribution (Table 3.5, Fig. 3.5). For example, for the 1 cm lesion only 0.5 mL healthy liver is exposed to >10 Gy, compared with 1.3 mL for Cyberknife and around 20 mL for VMAT/Tomotherapy. Moreover, the sparing of the liver in the low-dose range is excellent, e.g., for the 1 cm lesion only 70 mL healthy liver is exposed to 1 Gy, compared with 200–400 mL with external techniques. We emphasize that these advantages require nearly perfect positioning of the catheter(s). For all lesion sizes the conformality of the Cyberknife lies between that of iBT and that of VMAT/Tomotherapy, but low-dose exposures (volume > 1–2 Gy) are in the same range for all external techniques and higher than for interstitial techniques.

The VMAT technique, standard in modern linear accelerators, performs with lower intralesional mean doses of ~22 Gy accompanied by the lowest liver exposure at 1 Gy for lesions sized ≥3 cm. Tomotherapy achieves higher intralesional mean doses of ~30 Gy but with an accordingly larger load to the surroundings. The isodoses for higher doses (5–10 Gy) are visually more compact for Tomotherapy than for VMAT (Fig. 3.2).

For better comparison we calculated therapeutic ratios using the terms

$$D_{mean}\left(\text{lesion } d\right) / \left(\% \text{ liver} > 10\,\text{Gy}\right)$$

quantifying TCP versus high-dose exposure (conformality) and

$$D_{mean}\left(\text{lesion } d\right) / \left(\% \text{ liver} > 1\,\text{Gy}\right)$$

quantifying TCP versus low-dose exposure (long-term risk). We plotted the therapeutic ratios for each radiotherapy technique in dependence upon lesion sizes in

Table 3.5 DVH parameters of hepatic spherical lesions of 1–5 cm diameter irradiated with a single dose of 20 Gy (>95% coverage) comparing HDR brachytherapy with current external radiation techniques. Note the relationship between CTV and PTV (upper line)

Technique	HDR brachytherapy (CTV ≡ PTV)	Cyberknife (CTV ≡ PTV)	VMAT (d_{HDR} + 1 cm)	Tomotherapy (d_{HDR} + 1 cm)
Lesion ∅ 1 cm/2 cm (0.7 mL/5.2 mL)	1 catheter			
Irradiation time [min]	0.9/3.2	72/51	2.6/2.3	3.0/4.2
D_{mean} [Gy]	56.3/58.1	28.6/34.2	23.9/22.8	25.5/28.2
Coverage 20 Gy [%]	100/98	99.6/99	100/98	100/100
Liver mean dose [Gy]	0.3/1.1	0.7/1.2	1.0/1.7	1.4/2.5
Volume > 10 Gy [mL (%)]	0.5 (0.04)/6 (0.45)	1.3 (0.1)/9.4 (0.7)	17.5 (1.3)/54 (4)	25 (1.9)/77 (5.8)
Volume > 5 Gy [mL (%)]	2 (0.2)/18 (1.3)	8.4 (0.6)/62 (4.6)	94 (7.0)/165 (12)	100 (7.5)/236 (17.7)
Volume > 2 Gy [mL (%)]	24 (1.8)/161 (12)	58 (4)/248 (19)	187 (14)/282 (21)	360 (27)/466 (35)
Volume > 1 Gy [mL (%)]	71 (5)/417 (31)	220 (16)/444 (33)	269 (20)/376 (28)	413 (31)/560 (42)
Kidney right D_{max} [Gy]	0.4/1.2	1.1/3.4	2.6/3.7	3.0/4.6
Stomach D_{max} [Gy]	0.1/0.2	0.8/1.4	0.5/1.4	1.3/2.1
∅ 3 cm lesion (16.5 mL)	1/5 catheters			
Irradiation time [min]	6.9/6.4	64	2.1	5.1
D_{mean} [Gy]	58.2/50.1	31.7	21.5	32.5
Coverage 20 Gy [%]	98/96	97.5	93	99
Liver mean dose [Gy]	2.1/2.0	2.0	2.3	4.4
Volume > 10 Gy [mL (%)]	24 (1.8)/22 (1.6)	24 (1.8)	81 (6.0)	187 (14)
Volume > 5 Gy [mL (%)]	59 (4.4)/54 (4.0)	138 (10.5)	207 (15.4)	373 (28)
Volume > 2 Gy [mL (%)]	443 (33)/416 (31)	460 (35)	403 (30)	600 (45)
Volume > 1 Gy [mL (%)]	887 (66)/860 (64)	657 (50)	598 (40)	733 (55)
Kidney right D_{max} [Gy]	2.7/2.5	3.9	8.5	6.4
Stomach D_{max} [Gy]	0.5/0.5	2.2	0.9	3.1
∅ 5 cm lesion (75.9 mL)	1/5 catheters			
Irradiation time [min]	18.8/17.4	53	1.8	6.1
D_{mean} [Gy]	58.7/46.3	34.2	22.1	31.3
Coverage 20 Gy [%]	98/98	99.4	97	99
Liver mean dose [Gy]	4.7/4.6	4.4	4.1	5.2
Volume > 10 Gy [mL (%)]	128 (9.5)/120 (9.0)	126 (10)	159 (12)	253 (19)
Volume > 5 Gy [mL (%)]	443 (33)/416 (31)	446 (36)	417 (31)	653 (49)
Volume > 2 Gy [mL (%)]	1102 (82)/1048 (78)	791 (63)	712 (53)	773 (58)
Volume > 1 Gy [mL (%)]	1304 (97)/1290 (96)	937 (75)	874 (65)	959 (72)
Kidney right D_{max} [Gy]	2.7/2.5	3.9	9.2	8.9
Stomach D_{max} [Gy]	0.5/0.5	2.8	2.9	2.7

Abbreviations: *CTV* clinical target volume, *PTV* planning target volume, D_{max} maximum dose, D_{mean} mean dose, *HDR* high-dose-rate, *VMAT* volumetric-modulated arc technique

Fig. 3.6. Image-guided HDR brachytherapy always performed better, but these advantages declined with increasing lesion size. The Cyberknife came second and the external standard techniques (VMAT, Tomotherapy) came third. While for a lesion of $d = 1$ cm the therapeutic ratios were far apart, by two decades (high dose) or one decade (low dose), for $d = 5$ cm the ratios differed only by a factor of 2–3.

The performance of the (typically invasive) Cyberknife lay between those of iBT and VMAT/Tomotherapy, but again the advantage declined with increasing lesion size.

VMAT showed a slight advantage over Tomotherapy for small lesions, mainly because of finer leaves in the center (0.5 cm versus 1 cm), while Tomotherapy performed better for large and complex target volumes (as illustrated in Fig. 3.6, right).

Table 3.5 also shows relevant differences in irradiation times that might influence the treatment decision. Each Cyberknife treatment session takes about 1 h, in comparison with only 2 min for VMAT and 3–6 min for Tomotherapy. In iBT the treatment time is quite short for small lesions and increases considerably with lesion size, e.g., around 20 min for lesions of 5 cm (assuming recent renewal of the iridium source) and up to 40 min if the source has not been renewed for some time (typically up to 2 months).

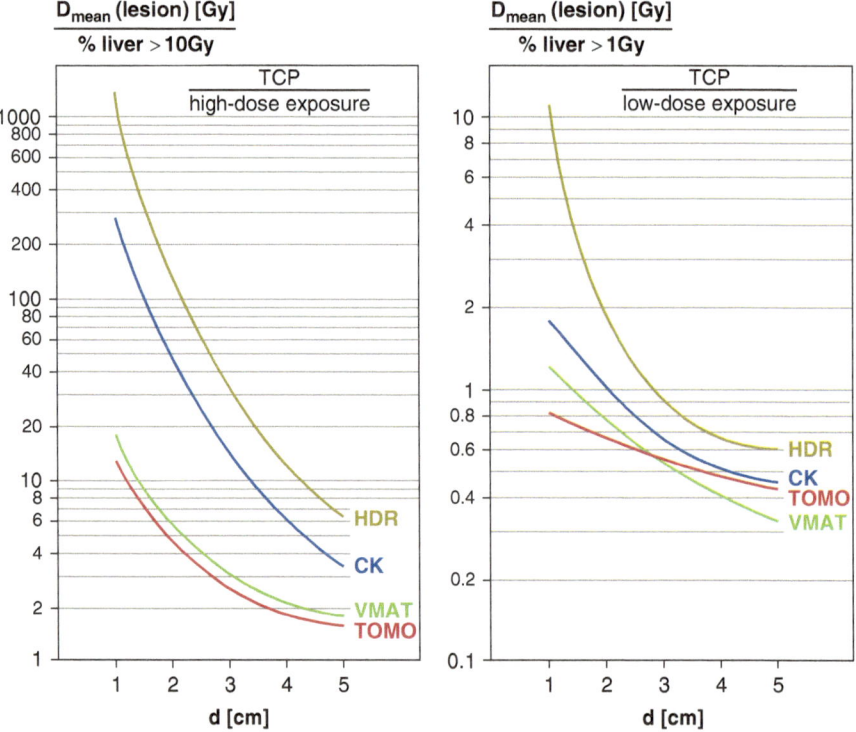

Fig. 3.6 Therapeutic ratios as functions of lesion size for all the four radiation techniques were calculated by the ratio TCP (quantified by mean dose to the lesion) over high-dose exposure (conformality, left) or low-dose exposure (long-term risks, right) of the liver

In addition, in making a treatment decision we must consider that the feasibility, the invasiveness, and the risks of these techniques differ greatly.

In summary, iBT is by far the most effective technique for single dose radio-ablation, even for larger lesions, but sparing of the surroundings declines with increasing lesion size and finally approaches the benchmarks associated with external-beam radiosurgical techniques.

Comparison of Image-Guided HDR Brachytherapy with Fractionated Radiotherapy

A dose-escalation study by Ricke et al. [16] revealed long-term local control (>3 years) in 95% of lesions for a single dose of 25 Gy (BED = 88 Gy) and only 65% for 20 Gy (BED = 60 Gy). We have listed BEDs (α/β = 10 Gy) for easier comparison with published studies (Table 3.4, Eq. 3.6b). Local control was also correlated with D_{min} (>20.5 Gy), indicating that coverage is important because of the steep dose gradient at the tumor margin.

Herfarth et al. [24] achieved for liver tumors/metastases a lower local control rate of 80% for 22–26 Gy single fractions at the reference point (80% enclosing the PTV).

Numerous clinical trials with various fractionation schemes were recently reviewed [25]. Generally, a BED(α/β = 10 Gy) > 100 Gy was found to achieve satisfactory long-term local control. In a careful evaluation [26] a BED of 138 Gy was estimated for long-term (>1 year) local control of 90% for colorectal cancer, which turned out to be the most resistant cancer type. Such high BEDs require single doses above 30 Gy (Table 3.4), which in our analysis are most likely to be attained by iBT.

To achieve intralesional BED of above 100 Gy, fractionated stereotactic ablative radiotherapy (SABR) is commonly used [25]. An optimum SABR schedule of 3×16 Gy was suggested [27] yielding BED = 125 Gy (for α/β = 10 Gy). Klement [26] recommended 3×17 Gy for colorectal cancer metastases, to achieve a BED of 138 Gy.

The possibility of fractionated SABR is an important asset of external radiotherapy techniques, in particular for larger lesions. However, treatment of a few circumscribed lesions in a single session appears attractive as well. The choice between the various options might finally depend on patient preferences.

Key Points
- Image-guided HDR brachytherapy (iBT) is an attractive therapeutic option for lesions of the liver, kidney, or lung, which competes with other *radio-surgical* techniques (Cyberknife, VMAT, Tomotherapy) as well as *fractionated* stereotactic ablative radiotherapy.
- Single doses over 30 Gy in tumor lesions are required to ensure a reliable local control and are easiest achieved by the use of iBT.

- Radioinduced toxicity is divided into *high-dose exposure of small volumes* (e.g., %liver >10 Gy) and *low-dose exposure of large volumes* (e.g., %liver >1 Gy). Organs at risk such as liver, kidney, and lung are particularly sensitive to radiation exposure of large volumes, even if the radiation doses are low (e.g., some Gy).
- High-dose, as well as low-dose exposures, are incomparably low if iBT is used on small lesions (≤3 cm diameter), but approach and exceed the values of the competing radiosurgical methods with increasing lesion sizes.
- If we compare iBT with the competing radiation methods, we have to weigh radioinduced risks against the risks associated with the implantation procedure, which are especially relevant for the lung. Noninvasiveness is a big plus point for external radiation techniques, but the final recommendation depends on numerous aspects, including individual patient preferences.

References

1. Ricke J, Wust P, Wieners G, Beck A, Cho CH, Seidensticker M, Pech M, Werk M, Rosner C, Hänninen EL, Freund T, Felix R. Liver malignancies: CT-guided interstitial brachytherapy in patients with unfavorable lesions for thermal ablation. J Vasc Interv Radiol. 2004;15:1279–86.
2. Ricke J, Wust P. Computed tomography–guided brachytherapy for liver cancer. Semin Radiat Oncol. 2011;21:287–93.
3. Wong SL, Mangu PB, Choti MA, et al. American Society of Clinical Oncology 2009 clinical evidence review on radiofrequency ablation of hepatic metastases from colorectal cancer. J Clin Oncol. 2010;28:493–508.
4. Hall EJ, Giaccia AJ. Radiobiology for the radiologist. 8th ed. Philadelphia: Wolters Kluwer; 2019.
5. Thames HD, Hendry JH. Fractionation in radiotherapy. London: Taylor & Francis; 1987.
6. Emami B, Lyman JT, Brown A, et al. Tolerance of normal tissue to therapeutic irradiation. Int J Radiat Oncol Biol Phys. 1991;21(1):109–22.
7. Burman C, Kutcher GJ, Emami B, Goitein M. Fitting of normal tissue tolerance data to an analytic function. Int J Radiat Oncol Biol Phys. 1991;21(1):123–35.
8. Kutcher GJ, Burman C, Brewster L, Goitein M, Mohan R. Histogram reduction method for calculating complication probabilities for three-dimensional treatment planning evaluations. Int J Radiat Oncol Biol Phys. 1991;21(1):137–46.
9. Lyman JT. Complication probability as assessed from dose-volume histograms. Radiat Res. 1985;104(2s):S13–9.
10. Marks LB, Yorke ED, Jackson A, et al. Use of normal tissue complication probability models in the clinic. Int J Radiat Oncol Biol Phys. 2010;76(3):S10–9.
11. Kirkpatrick JP, van der Kogel AJ, Schultheiss TE. Radiation dose–volume effects in the spinal cord. Int J Radiat Oncol Biol Phys. 2010;76(3):S42–9.
12. Kavanagh BD, Pan CC, Dawson LA, Das SK, et al. Radiation dose–volume effects in the stomach and small bowel. Int J Radiat Oncol Biol Phys. 2010;76(3):S101–7.
13. Streitparth F, Pech M, Böhmig M, Rühl R, Peters N, Wieners G, Steinberg J, Lopez-Haenninen E, Felix R, Wust P, Ricke J. In vivo assessment of the gastric mucosal tolerance dose after single fraction, small volume irradiation of liver malignancies by computed tomography–guided, high-dose-rate brachytherapy. Int J Radiat Oncol Biol Phys. 2006;65(5):1479–86.

14. Pan CC, Kavanagh BD, Dawson LA, Li XA, et al. Radiation-associated liver injury. Int J Radiat Oncol Biol Phys. 2010;76(3):S94–S100.
15. Ricke J, Seidensticker M, Lüdemann L, Pech M, Wieners G, Hengst S, Mohnike K, Cho CH, Hänninen EL, Al-Abadi H, Wust P. In vivo assessment of the tolerance dose of small liver volumes after single-fraction HDR irradiation. Int J Radiat Oncol Biol Phys. 2005;62(3):776–84.
16. Ricke J, Mohnike K, Pech M, Seidensticker M, Rühl R, Wieners G, Gaffke G, Kropf S, Felix R, Wust P. Local response and impact on survival after local ablation of liver metastases from colorectal carcinoma by computed tomography–guided high-dose-rate brachytherapy. Int J Radiat Oncol Biol Phys. 2010;78(2):479–85.
17. Rühl R, Lüdemann L, Streitparth F, Seidensticker M, Mohnike K, Pech M, Wust P, Ricke J. Radiobiological restrictions and tolerance doses of repeated single-fraction HDR irradiation of intersecting small liver volumes for recurrent hepatic metastases. Radiat Oncol. 2010;5(1):44.
18. Dawson LA, Kavanagh BD, Paulino AC, et al. Radiation-associated kidney injury. Int J Radiat Oncol Biol Phys. 2010;76(3):S108–15.
19. Gagliardi G, Constine LS, Moiseenko V, et al. Radiation dose–volume effects in the heart. Int J Radiat Oncol Biol Phys. 2010;76(3):S77–85.
20. Marks LB, Bentzen SM, Deasy JO, et al. Radiation dose–volume effects in the lung. Int J Radiat Oncol Biol Phys. 2010;76(3):S70–6.
21. Lawrence YR, Li XA, El Naqa I, et al. Radiation dose–volume effects in the brain. Int J Radiat Oncol Biol Phys. 2010;76(3):S20–7.
22. Fletcher GH, Nervi C, Withers HR, editors. Biological bases and clinical implications of tumor radioresistance. New York: Masson Publishing; 1983.
23. Bortfeld T, Webb S. Single-arc IMRT? Phys Med Biol. 2008;54(1):N9.
24. Herfarth KK, Debus J, Lohr F, Bahner ML, Rhein B, Fritz P, Höss A, Schlegel W, Wannenmacher MF. Stereotactic single-dose radiation therapy of liver tumors: results of a phase I/II trial. J Clin Oncol. 2001;19:164–70.
25. Romesser PB, Neal BP, Crane CH. External beam radiation therapy for liver metastases. Surg Oncol Clin N Am. 2021;30:159–73.
26. Klement RJ. Radiobiological parameters of liver and lung metastases derived from tumor control data of 3719 metastases. Radiother Oncol. 2017;123:218–26.
27. Robin TP, Raben D, Schefter TE. A contemporary update on the role of stereotactic body radiation therapy (SBRT) for liver metastases in the evolving landscape of oligometastatic disease management. Semin Radiat Oncol. 2018;28:288–94.

A Physicist's View

4

Justus Well, Lukas Nierer, and Guillaume Landry

Introduction

The treatment-planning situation in image-guided brachytherapy (iBT) is challenging for the responsible physicist. Owing to the time-critical nature of this technique, all tasks need to be performed swiftly in a safe and structured manner. The main tasks are preplanning, reconstruction of catheters, dose optimization, plan quality assurance, and treatment delivery. For the successful performance of all of these tasks in the given setting, a high level of expertise and confidence on the part of the planning physicist is essential. Dose optimization can be challenging, especially when adjacent radiosensitive organs at risk make it difficult to achieve complete dose coverage, even if there was sufficient time for dose optimization. There are also a number of other rare occurrences that the physicist may encounter. For example, a catheter could retract slightly from the patient between the interventional catheter placement and the beginning of dose delivery. Similarly, two catheters that are located very close to each other might not be accurately distinguishable on the planning image dataset. Therefore, thorough preparation is a key factor in overcoming minor and major challenges in the time-critical setting of iBT.

Preplanning

Before the actual treatment planning, when it becomes clear that the dose-planning will be particularly challenging because of complex target lesions or proximity to OARs, it can be helpful to provide a preplan before catheter implantation. This is

J. Well (✉) · L. Nierer · G. Landry
Department of Radiation Oncology, Ludwig Maximilian University (LMU) Hospital Munich, Munich, Germany
e-mail: justus.well@med.uni-muenchen.de; lukas.nierer@med.uni-muenchen.de; guillaume.landry@med.uni-muenchen.de

based on 3D imaging. The planning target volume (PTV), and organs at risk (OAR) are delineated by a physician. Thereafter, a proposal for the number and placement of catheters can be developed. In principle, catheters should be positioned in parallel, as this configuration provides a good and reproducible dose coverage of the PTV. If more than one catheter is used, the catheters should be placed close to the boundary of the PTV. In this way, the planning physicist has more flexibility in terms of sparing OARs and optimizing dose coverage, and the center of the PTV will consequently receive a sufficient dose. If the shape of the PTV differs considerably from a convex volume, any major bulge should be covered by an additional catheter. Ideally, catheters should be positioned very close to OARs, as the steepest dose gradient is found near the catheter. Thus, a sufficient PTV dose coverage close to the OAR will be easiest attainable with dwell positions nearby.

Practical aspects must also be taken into account. The proposed positioning of the catheters must follow practically accessible paths. Therefore, preplanning should be done in close collaboration with the interventional radiologist. Finally, the proposed placement of the catheters should be able to provide a dose distribution that is robust toward minor deviations during catheter placement. Parallel placement of the catheters best guarantees this robustness.

Reconstruction of Catheters

After catheter placement by the interventional radiologist, computed tomography (CT) acquisition and PTV and OAR delineation with all catheters in place, the next step is the reconstruction of catheters in the treatment planning system (TPS). Each catheter must be correctly identified and the first dwell position in each catheter must be marked. As an alternative to marking the first dwell position, a reference mark with a known offset can be used. However, this offset must be taken into account during treatment planning.

Even if the interventional radiologist labels the catheters and the respective PTVs on CT printouts or clinical drawings, the most reliable strategy for mapping the catheters in the TPS is to reconstruct the numbering from the surface of the patient, as this allows direct visual validation of correct catheter numbering and connection of transfer tubes. It may be helpful to make a schematic drawing of how the catheters exit through the skin of the patient (see Fig. 4.1). When two or more adjacent

Fig. 4.1 The correct numbering of the catheters in the CT can be determined from this sketch of the catheters as they exit the surface of the patient

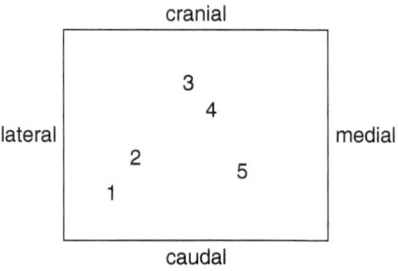

catheters cross each other inside the patient, the notes or drawings provided by the interventional radiologist are usually helpful as a second validation. In addition, if catheter insertion is performed by the Seldinger technique, and the brachytherapy catheter is placed inside an angiography sheath, then the excess end of the brachytherapy catheter from the angiography sheath can be measured outside the patient as a second validation (see Fig. 4.2). Using this information, the internal excess length of the brachytherapy catheter can be calculated. The distance from the end of the angiography sheath to the tip of the brachytherapy catheter can also be measured in the CT slices (see Fig. 4.3). This information can serve as additional confirmation that the assignment of the catheter numbering was correct for adjacent catheters. If it is not possible to resolve all doubts, an imaging procedure with distinct CT markers in one or more catheters is required. Unfortunately, this is only an option if the brachytherapy catheter extends, inside the patient, beyond the radio-opaque angiography sheath. Furthermore, it could be helpful to analyze the sequence of catheter placement, documented by the fluoroscopic CT series. However, this method is only safe if the numbering performed by the interventional radiologist corresponds to the sequence of catheter placement.

After successful catheter reconstruction, the 3D view of catheters and regions of interest of the TPS should be used, to verify the correct reconstruction of catheters (e.g., no kinks visible) and to gain a better understanding of the spatial orientation and location of target volumes and organs at risk.

As mentioned above, the first dwell position in each catheter must be determined carefully. In case of an error, all dwell positions of the affected catheter will be shifted and the real dose distribution will differ greatly from the dose distribution as calculated by the TPS. Even worse, such mistakes might remain unnoticed until the effects of under- or overdosage become clinically manifest during follow-up. Therefore, it is of the utmost importance to determine the correlation of the treatment unit length indexer with the dwell positions in the catheter, as part of the quality assurance program for all catheters and markers, before the patient's first

Fig. 4.2 The excess end of the brachytherapy catheter to the angiography sheath outside the patient can be measured

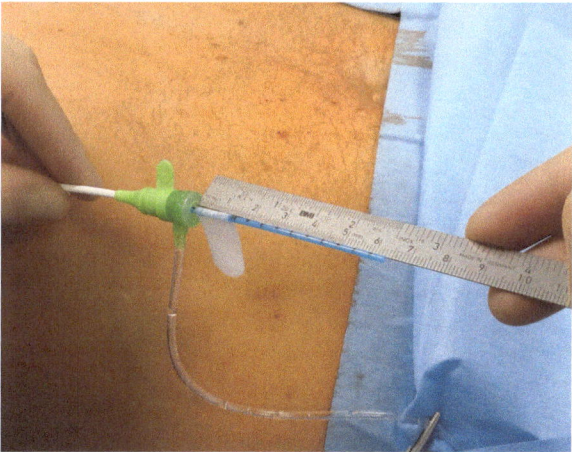

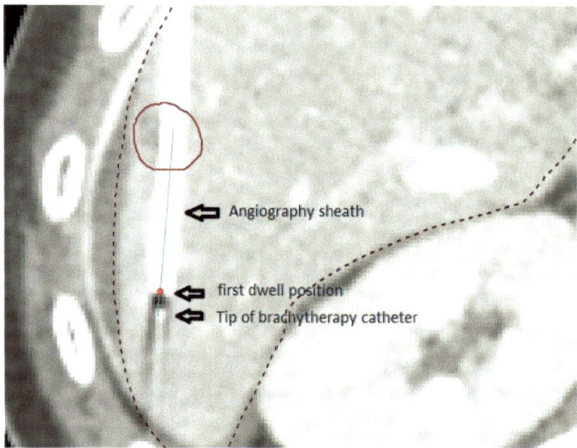

Fig. 4.3 The excess of the brachytherapy catheter to the angiography sheath inside the patient can be calculated from the finding outside of the patient. This can be checked against the finding from the CT inside the patient and can thus help, in case of doubt, to identify the catheters inside correctly

treatment. Usually, the radiodense tip of the brachytherapy catheter is easily visible on the CT (Fig. 4.4a). The angiography sheath can be seen with great reliability, as it is highly radio-opaque.

The distance (offset) between the radiodense tip of the brachytherapy catheter and the first dwell position must be measured in preparation for starting this method. This requires an autoradiograph with several equidistant dwell positions, for example, every 20 mm, to ensure that the source cable is not compressed at the first dwell position (see Fig. 4.4b). If the brachytherapy catheters do not have a fixed length, owing to their production process, every single brachytherapy catheter must be measured before use. The result of this measurement allows the calculation of the distance from the afterloader to the first dwell position.

From a physicist's point of view, a CT slice thickness of 2 mm is a good compromise between exact catheter imaging and acquisition time, dose exposure, and data volume. At a slice thickness of 3 mm, the catheter tip may disappear between two slices and the reconstruction will be less accurate.

Dose Optimization

When optimizing the dose, as a first step one should follow the strategy of trying to achieve full coverage of the PTV with the prescribed dose. In the following steps, the reduction of overall dwell time and sparing of OARs will take place.

In the first step, the constraints upon dose administered to the OARs may be exceeded. The following optimization should result in a plan that provides the best dose coverage with the shortest overall dwell time while meeting all OAR constraints. Since the method for optimizing the dose distribution depends very much on the specific case, the planner should be familiar with all methods provided by the TPS. Familiarity with all the display options provided by the TPS, such as 3D viewing or rotation of reconstructed slices, is mandatory for the optimization process and

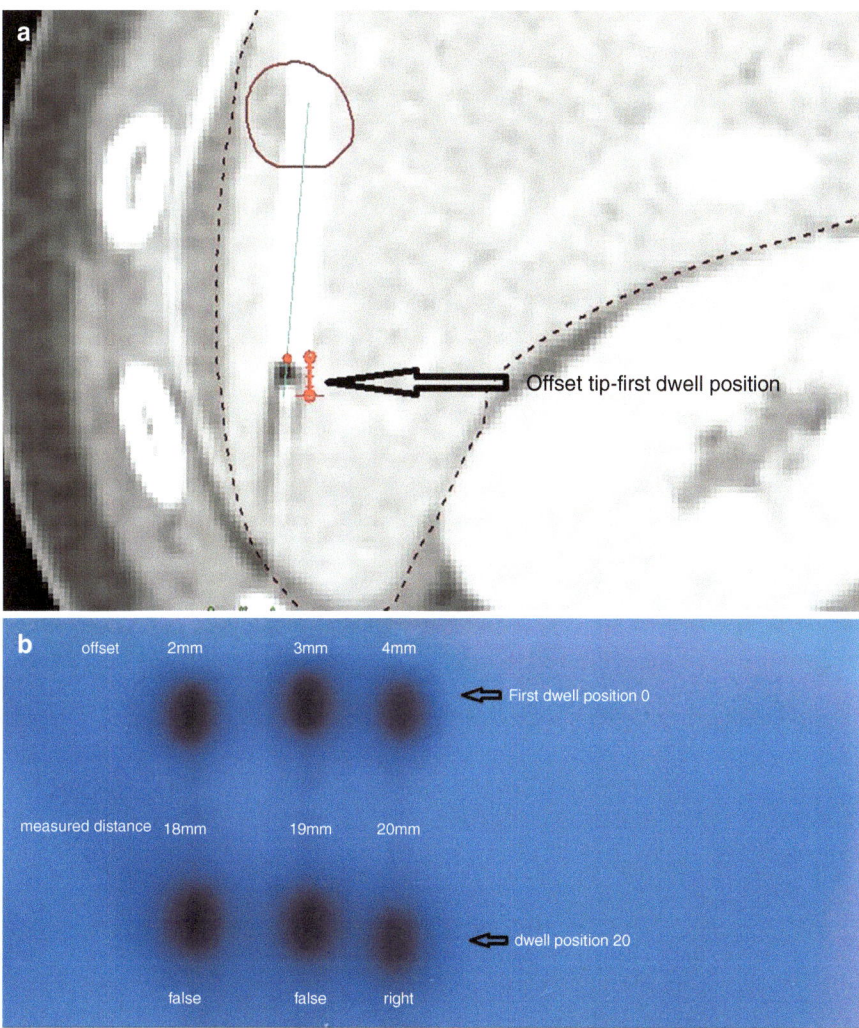

Fig. 4.4 (**a**) Brachytherapy catheter with offset from tip to first accessible dwell position. (**b**) Autoradiography of the first dwell position and a second one at a defined distance (20 mm). If the measured distance between the two positions is less than the defined one, the offset has been chosen too small and the source cable will be compressed when trying to reach an inaccessible position

assessment of the dose distribution. Especially, reconstructed slices parallel and vertical to a brachytherapy catheter or to the dose gradient between PTV and OAR are very helpful. When catheters and small PTVs are mapped one-to-one, the manual adjustment of dwell times is often the fastest strategy to achieve full dose coverage. Similarly, if the dose distributions of several PTVs overlap (see Fig. 4.5), the balancing adjustments can be quickly performed manually. If one PTV is covered by more than one catheter (see Fig. 4.6), semiautomatic dose optimizers such as

Fig. 4.5 In case of overlapping dose distributions of PTVs positioned close to each other, the balancing adjustment is rapidly made by manual manipulation of dwell times

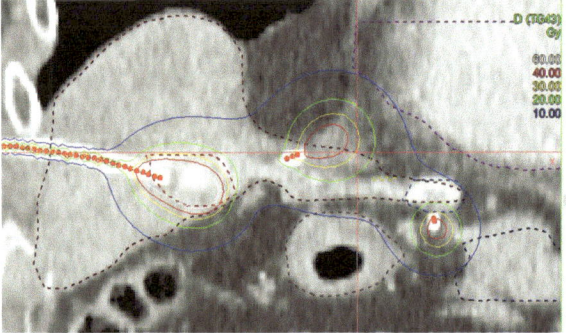

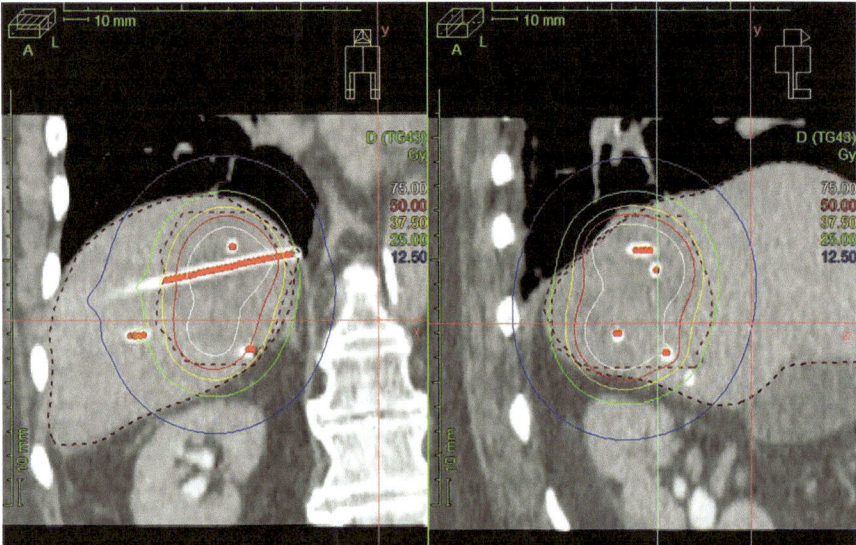

Fig. 4.6 A first guess for the distribution of dwell times on several catheters in one PTV can be obtained by automatic optimization procedures such as HIPO (hybrid inverse planning and optimization, Elekta AB, Sweden) or IPSA (inverse planning simulated annealing, Elekta AB, Sweden)

HIPO [1] (hybrid inverse planning and optimization, Elekta AB, Sweden) or IPSA [2] (inverse planning simulated annealing, Elekta AB, Sweden) can be useful to obtain an initial dose distribution. Based on this, the graphical dwell time adjustment (some TPSs provide intuitive and practical graphical tools) is a good method to complete the optimization, especially if small parts of the PTV were initially not sufficiently covered.

To reduce the dose to OARs, graphical dwell time adjustment is often tricky, because it preferentially reduces the dwell times near the OAR to zero, even though these dwell positions are important for homogeneous coverage of the PTV and frequently do not expose the OAR to a high dose, thanks to the steep gradient. Sparing of OARs requires a sophisticated balance between reducing near and far dwell times equally.

For sparing of OARs, in most cases, the optimized plan with the lowest overall dwell time is the best solution. However, in special cases, it may be necessary to shift dwell times that are needed to cover a specific region of the PTV to dwell positions farther from the OAR, to reduce dose exposure adequately. This shifting is best accomplished by manual adjustment of the dwell times. If sufficient dose coverage of the PTV and acceptable sparing of the OAR cannot be achieved simultaneously, a more inhomogeneous dose distribution in the PTV has to be accepted. The trade-off between the loss of full dose coverage and efficacy of the treatment or the acceptance of possible higher risks for side effects must be evaluated in close collaboration with the physician in each specific case. However, as a rule, the sparing of OARs always has priority over full dose coverage.

In most cases, irradiation of the puncture tract can be performed to prevent tumor seeding along the puncture tract. However, results from the literature [3] are inconclusive on whether this is mandatory. The puncture tract irradiation is usually planned after an acceptable treatment plan has been achieved. The impact on dose to PTV and OARs should be considered, and the dose report should not be completed before activation of dwell positions along the puncture tract up to the skin. Therefore, a slight reduction of dwell times in the PTV might be necessary. The dose at the surface of the catheter should be at least 5 Gy. In any case, dwell positions should not be activated too close to the skin and a small margin should be left to reduce the skin dose.

Overall, owing to the reduced time frame for plan optimization, the goal should generally not be the theoretically best plan, but the plan that is best practically achievable within a reasonable time interval.

Plan Approval and Verification

The principle of double verification should also be applied to the brachytherapy workflow wherever possible. After the responsible physician has accepted the treatment plan, based on the dose distribution and dose–volume histogram (DVH), it is the responsibility of the medical physicist to verify the overall integrity of the treatment plan and the correctness of all technical plan parameters. Since a thorough dosimetric verification of the treatment plan is not possible before the treatment application, because of the nature of the technique, optional quality assurance checks need to be carried out. Plan parameters, such as the correct catheter offset length or the correct channel mapping should be double-checked and documented by using a checklist. Furthermore, plan integrity should be checked after transfer from the TPS to the afterloading control system or after plan approval, if the TPS and afterloader control system share the same database. Plan integrity checks include the source activity, the correct time/date, a reasonable overall treatment time, etc. All of these parameters should be verified manually. An automated script providing metadata information from the underlying DICOM plan file may provide additional information.

Treatment Delivery

If appropriate hardware is available on site, an in-room imaging device is ideally used to verify independently that no catheter dislocations have occurred between planning CT acquisition and the start of dose application.

Before starting the irradiation, a second person must check the correct assignment of the transfer tubes from the afterloader to the brachytherapy catheters. This should be done by the planning physicist, to ensure that the numbering of the catheters as it appears on the surface of the patient matches the reconstruction performed in the TPS. Before starting the irradiation, an additional dummy run, through all catheters, can be performed in some afterloading systems, to check if all catheters are accessible by the source.

Large PTVs can lead to long overall irradiation times of up to 1 h with irradiation sources at reference strength (370 GBq for iridium-192). Owing to radioactive decay, this strength decreases and the irradiation time increases accordingly. For ^{192}Ir, a source replacement interval of 2 months is desirable, to avoid irradiation times that exceed 2 h for large PTVs. Even this will be difficult to tolerate for some patients.

Emergency Procedures

For each different brachytherapy technique, the emergency procedure must be evaluated. In an emergency, it cannot be decided whether the source cable drive failed or the isotope capsule has separated from the cable. The latter must be considered as a worst-case scenario. With catheter-in-catheter techniques, the emergency procedure is in principle easy to handle. The brachytherapy catheters can be quickly removed from the angiography sheaths. This ensures that there is no longer a radiation source inside the patient. Once the source has been removed, the vault should be evacuated quickly. A hand-held radiation detector can be used to verify that the source was successfully removed from the patient. Possible bleeding complications are to be taken care of by the medical staff.

Future Perspectives

As opposed to many other treatment sites, the impact of model-based dose calculations following the recommendations of the AAPM TG-186 [4] has only recently been investigated for liver brachytherapy [5]. While the liver is a fairly homogeneous organ, and one could assume that the uniform water assumption is a valid approximation for clinical dose calculations, the increased density means that distant isodoses

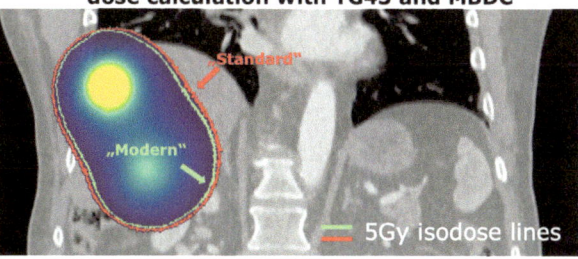

dose calculation with TG43 and MBDC

Liver density 6% higher than water's: *increased attenuation*

Lung density 20%-40% of water's: *decreased backscatter*

ΔV$_{5Gy}$: 6% of liver volume

Standard"

„Modern"

5Gy isodose lines

Fig. 4.7 TG43 dose calculation (labeled as "Standard") compared with MBDC (labeled as "Modern") for an example of a liver brachytherapy case. Higher liver density and lower lung density combine to reduce the liver volume receiving 5 Gy or more by 6%

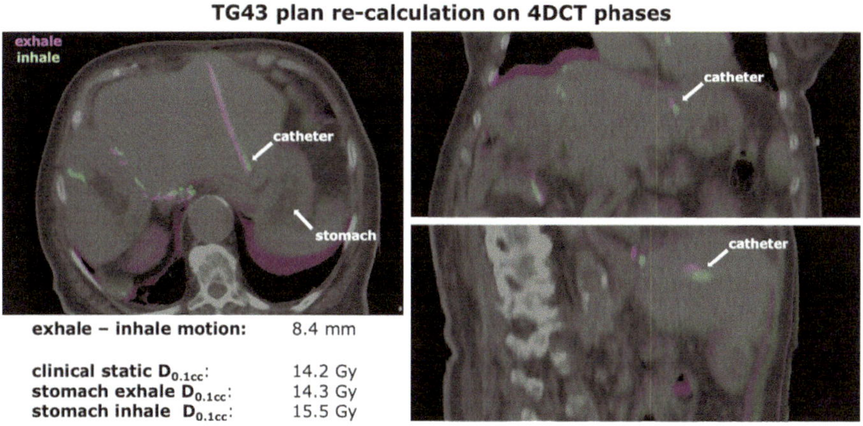

TG43 plan re-calculation on 4DCT phases

exhale inhale

catheter

catheter

catheter

stomach

exhale – inhale motion:	8.4 mm
clinical static D$_{0.1cc}$:	14.2 Gy
stomach exhale D$_{0.1cc}$:	14.3 Gy
stomach inhale D$_{0.1cc}$:	15.5 Gy

Fig. 4.8 Clinical TG43 plan recalculated on exhale and inhale phases of a 4DCT scan by catheter reconstruction on individual phases and copying of planned source dwell times. (Left) axial slice, (top right) coronal slice, and (bottom right) sagittal slice. Dose not shown, to highlight motion better

will differ between TG43 and TG186 calculations. Furthermore, the low density of the lung has an impact on the backscatter situation at the superior lung border. This means that clinical parameters related to liver toxicity such as V_{5Gy} and V_{10Gy} of the lung, which can sometimes restrict the dose to the treated lesion, can be overestimated by TG43 by up to 6% (V_{5Gy}) of the liver volume, which is non-negligible compared with the 66% liver volume limit for V_{5Gy} [5]. This is illustrated in Fig. 4.7. Clinically, these effects may be accounted for by making use of commercial model-based dose calculation algorithms validated against Monte Carlo simulations.

Beyond the use of model-based dose calculations, uncertainties in liver dose delivery may stem from respiratory motion in cases where the catheter may move dynamically inside the liver, or organs at risk come closer to the catheter over the course of the respiratory cycle. It may thus be desirable to be able to compute the dose on the basis of a 4DCT scan where the catheter has been reconstructed on each respiratory phase, along with the delineations of the organs at risk. Figure 4.8 shows an example case where the maximum dose ($D_{0.1cc}$) to the stomach, a dose-limited organ at risk, was shown to vary with the respiratory phase.

Key Points
- The treatment-planning situation in image-guided brachytherapy (iBT) is challenging for the responsible physicist. Owing to the time-critical nature of this technique, all tasks need to be performed swiftly in a safe and structured manner.
- The main tasks are preplanning, reconstruction of catheters, dose optimization, plan quality assurance, and treatment delivery.
- A high level of expertise and confidence on the part of the planning physicist is essential, and thorough preparation is a key factor in overcoming minor and major challenges in the time-critical setting of iBT.

References

1. Lahanas M, et al. A hybrid evolutionary algorithm for multi-objective anatomy-based dose optimization in high-dose-rate brachytherapy. Phys Med Biol. 2003;48(3):399–415.
2. Lachance B, et al. Early clinical experience with anatomy-based inverse planning dose optimization for high-dose-rate boost of the prostate. Int J Radiat Oncol Biol Phys. 2002;54(1):86–100.
3. Büttner L, et al. Tumor seeding along the puncture tract in CT-Guided Interstitial High-Dose-Rate Brachytherapy. J Vasc Interv Radiol. 2020;31(5):720–7. https://doi.org/10.1016/j.jvir.2019.10.006.
4. Beaulieu L, et al. Report of the Task Group 186 on model-based dose calculation methods in brachytherapy beyond the TG-43 formalism: current status and recommendations for clinical implementation. Med Phys. 2012;39(10):6208–36.
5. Duque AS, et al. The dosimetric impact of replacing the TG-43 algorithm by model based dose calculation for liver brachytherapy. Radiat Oncol. 2020;15(1):60.

Image-Guided Brachytherapy: Interventional Setting, Technique, and Peri-interventional Patient Management

5

Maciej Pech, Konrad Mohnike, and Maciej Powerski

General Considerations

The specific, invasive technique of interstitial brachytherapy as a procedure for treatment by irradiation possesses special features that distinguish it from percutaneous, noninvasive radiation therapy and from other invasive, local-ablative procedures such as radio-frequency ablation. The aim of the intervention by image-guided brachytherapy (and the fundamental difference *vis-à-vis* conventional, percutaneous irradiation) is the CT- or MRT-guided implantation, into the target organ, of the catheter through which the radiation source will later be introduced. The real position of the radiation source relative to the tumor therefore corresponds almost exactly (with only minor uncertainties) to the planned one, resulting in an irradiation of the tumor according to the irradiation plan. This is especially advantageous in the treatment of the upper abdomen and the lungs. Even though the concepts of "target-volume definition" and "organ at risk" are defined in the ICRU 50 guideline, it is here that interstitial brachytherapy differs significantly from conventional irradiation procedures [1]. Consistently with this, users of this technique have developed, in the literature, definitions that deviate from the standard ones, for specifying both the target dose and the dose to organs at risk [2–5].

M. Pech · M. Powerski
Department of Radiology and Nuclear Medicine, University Hospital Magdeburg, Magdeburg, Germany
e-mail: Maciej.Pech@med.ovgu.de; maciej.powerski@med.ovgu.de

K. Mohnike (✉)
Department of Diagnostics, Department of Interventional Oncology & Radionuclide Therapy, Diagnostic Therapeutic Center Berlin, Berlin, Germany

Department of Radiology and Nuclear Medicine, University Hospital Magdeburg, Magdeburg, Germany
e-mail: konrad.mohnike@berlin-dtz.de

© The Author(s), under exclusive license to Springer Nature Switzerland AG 2021
K. Mohnike et al. (eds.), *Manual on Image-Guided Brachytherapy of Inner Organs*, https://doi.org/10.1007/978-3-030-78079-1_5

51

Several specific features of interstitial brachytherapy are to be noted:

1. In image-guided HDR brachytherapy, the catheters are fixed securely within the tumor volume, both by pressure from the surrounding tissue and by suture fixation on the skin surface. Consequently, only minimal uncertainty regarding the position of the catheter is caused by movement of organs and specifically by respiratory motion, which—in particular in irradiation of the liver—is of great importance. This represents a substantial advantage of interstitial brachytherapy over percutaneous irradiation.
2. Another major difference between HDR brachytherapy and percutaneous irradiation is the steep decline in dose toward the surroundings, as the radiation source lies directly within the tumor, which is thus irradiated from the inside. It follows from this that in treatment of the liver the organ at greatest risk is the liver itself, and further organs at risk must be in the immediate vicinity for critical doses to be reached. For example, in the treatment of left or central hepatic tumor this can be applied to the stomach or the duodenum; other organs at relevant risk are the hepatic duct and the colon, the kidneys, the skin, and the ribs. For the stomach, the duodenum, and the hepatic duct, limiting doses for brachytherapy have been determined in clinical studies [6–12].
3. After the conclusion of treatment and during removal of the catheter, the puncture tract cannot be coagulated, as is the case with radio-frequency ablation. This is remedied by exploiting the long angiography sheath, which carries the brachytherapy catheter: after removal of the brachytherapy catheter, the angiography sheath is used to introduce appropriately shaped gelatine sponges to "embolize" the puncture tract. For brachytherapy of the lung, a tissue adhesive is used. This can reduce the risk of bleeding complications, but it can only be done when the Seldinger method has been used. In contrast, the other beneficial effect of thermal ablation on the puncture tract—the killing of any tumor cells that were inadvertently carried over by the intervention, and thus the avoidance of puncture-tract metastases—is achieved in interstitial brachytherapy by co-irradiation of the puncture tract [13].

Interventional Setting

For interventions in the upper abdomen or the lung, the catheter should be implanted by an interventional radiologist trained in this, who is familiar with the planned geometry of the catheter placement in the tumor. Implantation should take account of the planned dose, the adjacent organs at risk, and any possible specific complications.

Coordination with a radiotherapeutic iBT expert is a prerequisite for a successful intervention. Prior planning with pre-interventional, digital anticipation of the optimum catheter position can also be helpful, and planning systems for this are currently undergoing trials at various centers. As was hitherto the case, the team comprises an assistant trained in such interventions and a physician who will perform the analgosedation (which in general does not correspond to general anesthesia) and will monitor the patient's vital signs, ideally using an appropriate electronic device. For planning the irradiation itself, after the catheter has been inserted and the planning imaging has been performed, a medical physicist is consulted.

The intervention is conducted under sterile conditions. The safety of the intervention is critically dependent upon the team's awareness of the patient's general state of health, of any comorbidities and comedications, and of the patient's current laboratory values.

The catheter is usually implanted under CT-fluoroscopic guidance; some centers also have the possibility of using guidance by open MRI, which presupposes the availability of MR-compatible materials. Sonographically guided implantation is the exception rather than the rule, and it represents an interesting additional option if the site staff possess the necessary experience; even then however imaging for planning purposes by CT or MRI is necessary afterward (Fig. 5.1).

Materials

The intervention table corresponds to a puncture or angiography table. If the Seldinger technique is chosen, the table carries the materials for skin disinfection, sterile swabs and compresses, a scalpel, a hollow puncture needle, a stiff guidewire, a long 6F angiography sheath, the 6F brachytherapy catheter, suture material for suturing the sheath to the skin and sterile water for moistening and rinsing the instruments on the table (Fig. 5.2).

A side table is used in the removal of the angiography sheaths after the conclusion of the brachytherapy. On this are placed pieces of gelatine sponge, cut out and rolled to "cigars" of about 30 × 1 mm, and also a scalpel, a pair of scissors, forceps, clips, needle holders if required, material for skin disinfection, sterile swabs and compresses (Fig. 5.3).

Implantation Method: Positioning of the Patient

The patient is placed such as to offer the best possible access to the tumor, with account being taken of the intracorporeal distance that the catheter must travel, any possible structures at risk, and the constitution of the patient, who must remain in this position for several hours. For liver and lung interventions, a supine position, if appropriate slightly raised on the right side, is normally chosen, while for interventions in the kidneys, adrenal glands, or lymph nodes, a prone position or a right or left lateral position may be chosen. Normally, the interventional radiologist stands on the patient's right side, and exceptionally on the left. Access for analgosedation is extended to the rear side of the gantry so that from there the analgosedation can be adjusted during the intervention. It is usual to oxygenate the patient peri- and post-interventionally through a nasal tube, because of the depressant effect that the analgosedation has upon respiration (Fig. 5.4).

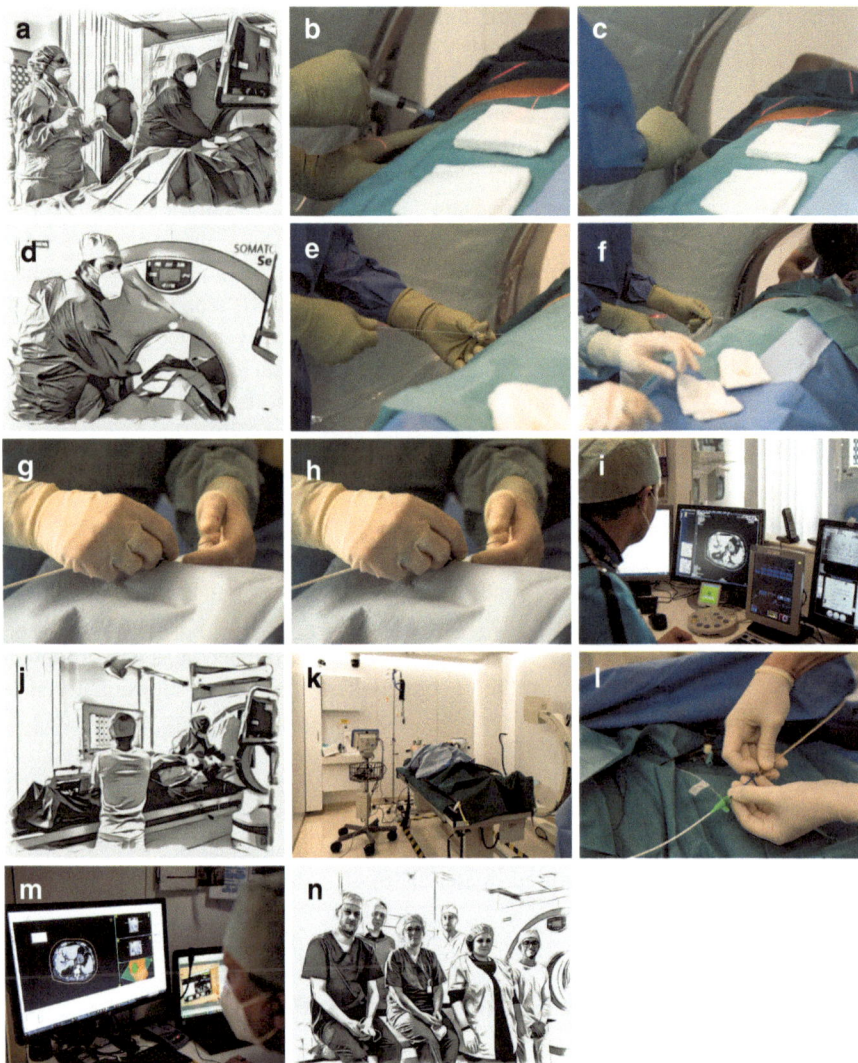

Fig. 5.1 Setting and conduct of an interventional iBT treatment. (**a**) Setting in the CT suite. Specialist for radiation oncology, administering analgosedation during the intervention; nurse, interventional radiologist. (**b**) Local anesthesia. (**c**) Puncture of the tumor with the hollow needle. (**d**) Fluoroscopic control. (**e**) The needle's sheath is being taken out. (**f**) Insertion of the guidewire. (**g**) Insertion of the 6F long angiography sheath. (**h**) Insertion of the 6F brachytherapy catheter. (**i**) Check of the planning-CT. (**j**) Just before transportation of the patient to the afterloading suite. (**k**) Patient in the afterloading suite. (**l**) Connection to the source-sheath. (**m**) Delineation of the planning target volume. (**n**) Team iBT: interventional radiologist, specialist for radiation oncology (and iBT analgosedation), interventional nurse, CT technician, surveillance nurse, medical physicist

Fig. 5.2 Intervention table

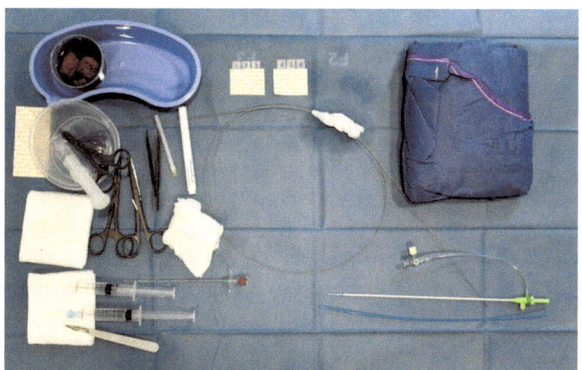

Fig. 5.3 Side table for removal of the angiography sheath

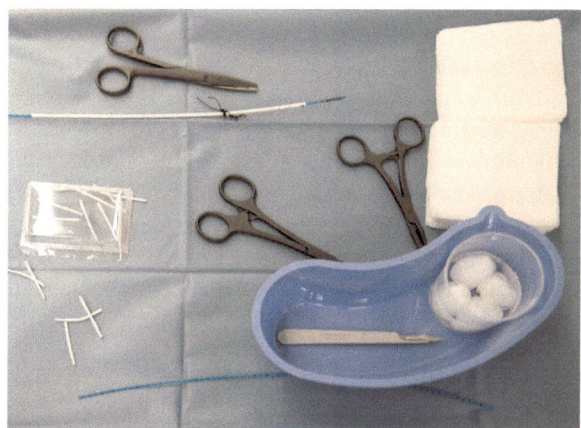

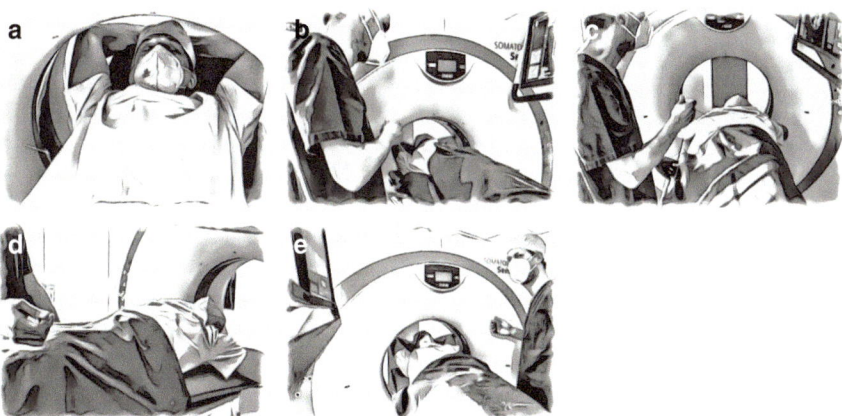

Fig. 5.4 Positioning, interventional radiologist (IR) and patient. (**a**) Supine position of the patient (liver, lung). (**b**) The IR stands on the patient's right side, with the patient slightly raised on the right side (liver, e.g., segment 1 interventions). (**c**) Prone position of the patient for interventions in the kidneys, adrenal glands, or lymph nodes; sometimes also a right or left lateral position may be appropriate. (**d**) Prone position of the patient, contralateral (left) puncture (the IR stands on the right side). (**e**) The IR stands on the left side

Implantation Method: CT

The interstitial introduction of the brachytherapy catheter is usually performed under analgosedation with local anesthesia, and sometimes under general anesthesia. CT fluoroscopy is widely used for implanting long angiography sheaths that will accommodate the brachytherapy catheter [14–17]—at specialized centers MRI guidance is also used. Depending upon the method used, the catheter is removed with or without closure of the puncture tract [2, 3, 18–20]. Fundamental distinction is made between the Seldinger method, described above, and direct puncture, which is preferred at some centers [4, 5]. In some cases, virtual preplanning of the catheter position(s) and the resulting radiation volume(s) is carried out, taking into account the planned dose to the tumor and the surrounding structures at risk.

After the preplanning, a (usually) native planning-CT is acquired and subsequently, under CT fluoroscopy, one or several catheters are introduced into the tumor volume. In the Seldinger procedure, after removal of the needle core a stiff wire (Amplatz, Boston Scientific) is pushed in and, over this, the long 6F angiography sheath (Terumo, Japan) is introduced, which then guides the brachytherapy catheter. The brachytherapy catheter is closed at the tip and is furnished with a millimeter scale, which is needed for correctly bringing the radiation source to the end of the open sheath without fluoroscopy (Fig. 5.1).

Another method, favored by some practitioners on account of its simplicity, is direct puncture using 6F plastic catheters of length 200 mm, with a steel core (Nucletron B.V., Veenendaal, The Netherlands, OncoSmart ProGuide Round Needle) and a closed tip, which however does not allow closure of the puncture tract with the gelatine plugs mentioned above [4, 5]. The number of catheters applied depends upon the size and shape of the tumor under treatment. In general, one catheter is implanted for every 1–2 cm tumor diameter.

Implantation Method: MRI

When the catheter is implanted under open MRI, the interventionist is shown fluoroscopy-like images in all three spatial planes on a radio-frequency-shielded LCD screen in real-time (approximately one image per second). This ensures safe catheter implantation, even in very small lesions. Beforehand, T1-weighted, contrast-enhanced (Gd-EOB-DTPA, Primovist, Bayer, Germany) planning MRI is conducted; here the hepatocytic specificity of Primovist usually prevents uptake in liver tumors, which correspondingly are seen as hypointense regions. The materials used for puncture are a ceramic scalpel (e.g., SLC Ceramic, Germany) for the incision, an 18G MR-compatible puncture needle 150–200 mm long (e.g., Invivo, Germany), and a hydrophilic standard angiography wire (e.g., Terumo, Japan). After insertion of the catheter, a guidewire is inserted into the standard brachytherapy catheter for visualization [17].

Radiation Treatment Planning: Imaging

After implantation of the catheter, a planning-CT, usually with a contrast agent, is performed. If MRI guidance is used, then a T1-weighted, contrast-enhanced (Gd-EOB-DTPA, Primovist, Bayer, Germany) planning MRI is conducted. In both cases, a slice thickness of 3 mm is chosen, in order to achieve exact definition of the target volume and the catheter position. In individual cases, co-registration with PET (positron emission tomography) may be necessary, if for example the administration of contrast agent is impossible or only the PET-positive portions of a partially necrotic lesion are to be defined as target volume. Typically, the irradiation is performed by HDR (high-dose-rate) brachytherapy with an iridium-192 (^{192}Ir) source. The duration of irradiation is determined by the size of the target volume, the number of catheters, the planned dose, and the activity of the source (diminishing with time); typically, it lies between 10 and 60 min. The puncture tract is irradiated at the same time, which is intended to help avoid puncture-tract metastases.

Conclusion of Treatment: Withdrawal of the Brachytherapy Catheter and the Sheath

After the irradiation has ended, first the brachytherapy catheter and then the sheath are removed. During retraction of the sheath, its open end is exploited to insert gelatine-sponge plugs to close the puncture tract thus avoiding complications due to bleeding. In lung interventions, tissue adhesive is used; this is only possible when the Seldinger method has been used for insertion (Fig. 5.5).

This point and the following 2–3 h are critical for the onset of possible complications. Strict bed rest for at least 4–8 h after the intervention is strongly recommended.

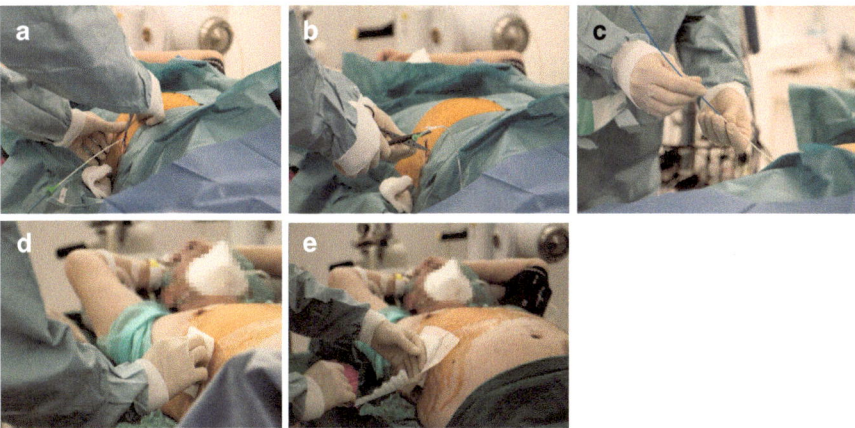

Fig. 5.5 Removal. (**a**) Removal of the suture. (**b**) Cutting of the sheath valve after removal of the brachytherapy catheter. (**c**) Insertion of gelatine "torpedoes" through the sheath. (**d**) Disinfection of the puncture site. (**e**) Skin patch

Intervention-Related Complications and Their Treatment

Immediately after removal of the catheter, attacks of shivering may occur. The cause of this is unclear, but it may be triggered by tumor necrosis factors. The shivering can be treated with midazolam and/or metamizole and generally recedes after 10–30 min. Other possible complications in the hours following the procedure include bleeding complications, meaning that especially frequent electronic and clinical surveillance is required. If there are signs of shock, internal bleeding must be excluded by CT, and immediate intervention is needed if active arterial bleeding is detected. The treatment of choice is angiographic embolization with particles or coils; surgical measures are only rarely needed (Fig. 5.6). Liver abscesses can above all occur in patients with a history of biliodigestive anastomosis, with a latency of weeks to months, and they can be clinically silent. Typically, patients report isolated episodes of shivering and/or fever lasting a few hours or days, which resolve spontaneously. Laboratory values only rarely provide guidance, especially as C-reactive protein is frequently elevated because of the tumor. Not uncommonly, the white-blood-cell count is elevated or depressed, but this does not necessarily indicate the presence of abscess-associated leucocytosis. Evidence of an abscess is obtained by imaging, preferably by contrast-enhanced CT, and the treatment of choice is drainage with culturing, preceded by appropriate initial antibiotic treatment (Fig. 5.7).

During or after lung brachytherapy, minor pneumothorax is regularly observed, which however usually resolves without further treatment and can be monitored by thoracic X-ray examination. Rarely, thoracic suction drainage is required. In isolated cases, fulminant intrapulmonary or intrathoracic hemorrhage occurs. For this reason, when pulmonary iBT is performed, facilities for intubation and rapid access to thoracic surgery are essential [21].

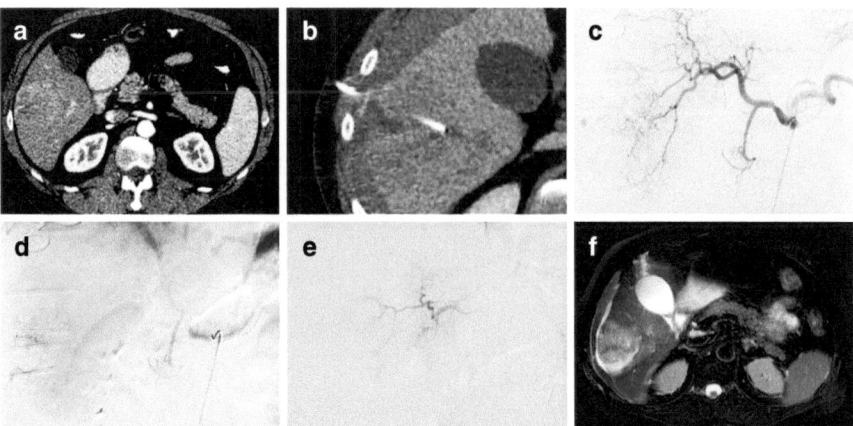

Fig. 5.6 Hemorrhage during catheter placement. (**a**) CT before iBT. (**b**) Subcapsular hematoma and arterial blush supporting active arterial bleeding in the CE-CT. (**c, d**) Subsequent angiography over the A. hepatica with a peripheral bleeding blush corresponding to the CT. (**e**) Angiography after embolization with Gelaspon and coils. (**f**) T2 MRI after embolization

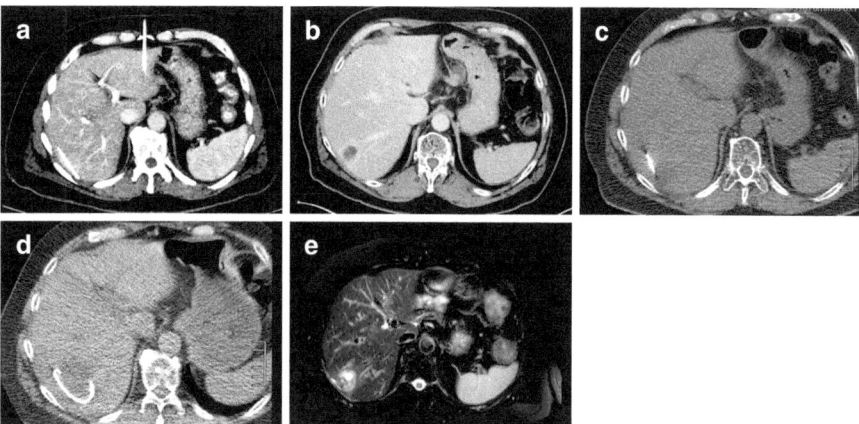

Fig. 5.7 Liver abscess after iBT following a recent papillotomy. (**a**) Implanted catheters. (**b**) CE-CT with the suspicion of abscess formation. CT fluoroscopy, (**c**) puncture and (**d**) subsequent drainage. (**e**) Later examination, T2-weighted MRI

Chapter 17 describes more comprehensively the possible complications following iBT and the factors that promote them.

Clinical Environment Required for Interstitial Brachytherapy

Interstitial brachytherapy of the liver, lung, lymph nodes, kidney, and adrenal glands is usually performed at centers within full-service hospitals on an in-patient basis. This is appropriate, as there is always a possibility that rare complications will occur, requiring emergency management and immediate care of the patient. This applies particularly for arterial hemorrhage, which can occur after iBT of the liver or lung, and also of the kidneys or adrenal glands. The patient should remain in the hospital for 2–3 days, as delayed bleeding and liver laceration have occasionally been observed as late as 24 h after the intervention.

At individual centers, where there is a high degree of expertise, brachytherapy of the liver may also be performed on an out-patient basis with subsequent in-patient stay at a partner hospital. This requires meticulous patient selection. Very simply stated: empirical evidence shows that iBT of colorectal liver metastases and metastases of most primary and small cholangiocellular carcinomas is normally complication-free and is only moderately prone to (acute) complications. In contrast, patients usually require an in-patient hospital stay during the intervention if they have received iBT for hepatocellular carcinomas and have reduced liver function; for hepatocellular carcinomas and cholangiocellular carcinomas at a subcapsular location; for mammary carcinomas with liver metastases after several prior systemic therapies; or for renal cell carcinomas or metastases of the adrenal glands. Anticoagulation that cannot be interrupted because of comorbidities also demands an in-patient setting; see also Chap. 17.

Key Points
- The brachytherapy catheter is usually implanted by the Seldinger method, as a rule under guidance by CT fluoroscopy.
- iBT demands a high degree of cooperation between interventional radiology and radiation therapy, in order to ensure optimum irradiation.
- The 2–3 h following removal of the catheter(s) are critical for the onset of possible complications. Strict bed rest for at least 4–8 h after the intervention is strongly recommended.
- For safety reasons, it is usual to conduct the procedure in an in-patient setting.
- At individual centers, with a high degree of expertise, brachytherapy of the liver may also be performed on an out-patient basis with subsequent in-patient stay at a partner hospital.

References

1. Bethesda M. ICRU 50. Prescribing, recording, and reporting photon beam therapy. Bethesda: International Commission on Radiation Units and Measurements Press; 1993.
2. Ricke J, Mohnike K, Pech M, et al. Local response and impact on survival after local ablation of liver metastases from colorectal carcinoma by computed tomography-guided high-dose-rate brachytherapy. Int J Radiat Oncol Biol Phys. 2010;78:479–85.
3. Ricke J, Wust P, Wieners G, et al. Liver malignancies: CT-guided interstitial brachytherapy in patients with unfavorable lesions for thermal ablation. J Vasc Interv Radiol. 2004;15:1279–86.
4. Tselis N, Chatzikonstantinou G, Kolotas C, et al. Hypofractionated accelerated computed tomography-guided interstitial high-dose-rate brachytherapy for liver malignancies. Brachytherapy. 2012;11:507–14.
5. Tselis N, Chatzikonstantinou G, Kolotas C, Milickovic N, Baltas D, Zamboglou N. Computed tomography-guided interstitial high dose rate brachytherapy for centrally located liver tumours: a single institution study. Eur Radiol. 2013;23:2264–70.
6. Mohnike K, Wolf S, Damm R, et al. Radioablation of liver malignancies with interstitial high-dose-rate brachytherapy : complications and risk factors. Strahlenther Onkol. 2016;192:288–96.
7. Ricke J, Seidensticker M, Ludemann L, et al. In vivo assessment of the tolerance dose of small liver volumes after single-fraction HDR irradiation. Int J Radiat Oncol Biol Phys. 2005;62:776–84.
8. Seidensticker M, Burak M, Kalinski T, et al. Radiation-induced liver damage: correlation of histopathology with hepatobiliary magnetic resonance imaging, a feasibility study. Cardiovasc Intervent Radiol. 2015;38(1):213–21.
9. Seidensticker M, Seidensticker R, Damm R, et al. Prospective randomized trial of enoxaparin, pentoxifylline and ursodeoxycholic acid for prevention of radiation-induced liver toxicity. PLoS One. 2014;9(11):e112731.
10. Seidensticker M, Seidensticker R, Mohnike K, et al. Quantitative in vivo assessment of radiation injury of the liver using Gd-EOB-DTPA enhanced MRI: tolerance dose of small liver volumes. Radiat Oncol. 2011;6:40.
11. Streitparth F, Pech M, Bohmig M, et al. In vivo assessment of the gastric mucosal tolerance dose after single fraction, small volume irradiation of liver malignancies by computed tomography-guided, high-dose-rate brachytherapy. Int J Radiat Oncol Biol Phys. 2006;65:1479–86.

12. Wybranski C, Seidensticker M, Mohnike K, et al. In vivo assessment of dose volume and dose gradient effects on the tolerance dose of small liver volumes after single-fraction high-dose-rate Ir-192 irradiation. Radiat Res. 2009;172:598–606.
13. Damm R, Zorkler I, Rogits B, et al. Needle track seeding in hepatocellular carcinoma after local ablation by high-dose-rate brachytherapy: a retrospective study of 588 catheter placements. J Contemp Brachytherapy. 2018;10:516–21.
14. Fischbach F, Bunke J, Thormann M, et al. MR-guided freehand biopsy of liver lesions with fast continuous imaging using a 1.0-T open MRI scanner: experience in 50 patients. Cardiovasc Intervent Radiol. 2011;34:188–92.
15. Fischbach F, Thormann M, Seidensticker M, Kropf S, Pech M, Ricke J. Assessment of fast dynamic imaging and the use of Gd-EOB-DTPA for MR-guided liver interventions. J Magn Reson Imaging. 2011;34:874–9.
16. Rak M, Konig T, Tonnies KD, Walke M, Ricke J, Wybranski C. Joint deformable liver registration and bias field correction for MR-guided HDR brachytherapy. Int J Comput Assist Radiol Surg. 2017;12:2169–80.
17. Ricke J, Thormann M, Ludewig M, et al. MR-guided liver tumor ablation employing open high-field 1.0T MRI for image-guided brachytherapy. Eur Radiol. 2010;20:1985–93.
18. Ricke J, Wust P. Computed tomography-guided brachytherapy for liver cancer. Semin Radiat Oncol. 2011;21:287–93.
19. Ricke J, Wust P, Stohlmann A, et al. CT-guided interstitial brachytherapy of liver malignancies alone or in combination with thermal ablation: phase I-II results of a novel technique. Int J Radiat Oncol Biol Phys. 2004;58:1496–505.
20. Ricke J, Wust P, Stohlmann A, et al. [CT-Guided brachytherapy. A novel percutaneous technique for interstitial ablation of liver metastases]. Strahlenther Onkol. 2004;180:274–80.
21. Peters N, Wieners G, Pech M, et al. CT-guided interstitial brachytherapy of primary and secondary lung malignancies: results of a prospective phase II trial. Strahlenther Onkol. 2008;184:296–301.

Björn Friebe and Tina Streitparth

Clinical Management

Patient Management in the Outpatient Clinic for Microtherapy and Interventional Radiology

After a detailed presentation and discussion in an interdisciplinary tumor consultation with expert clinicians, the prognostic and oncological treatment plans are drawn up. Coordination and planning of the treatment with a radiation oncology iBT expert is a prerequisite for a successful intervention. Informed consent not only for the intervention by an interventional radiology expert but also for the irradiation itself by a radiation oncology expert, should be obtained at least 24 h beforehand. In order to get a clear impression of the patient's health situation, a personal consultation in an outpatient clinic for microtherapy and interventional radiology is useful and desirable. The basis for the planning is already arranged here, with an exact explanation of the planned intervention using high-dose-rate iBT provided in advance. In addition to the technical, practical process, this naturally includes a detailed explanation of side effects, risks, and alternatives [1]. Exact written documentation is also mandatory. The actual informative discussion, to be documented in writing, takes place 24 h before the intervention and is conducted by the radiological Interventionalist [2]. The radiological-interventional outpatient clinic is where

B. Friebe (✉)
Department of Radiology and Nuclear Medicine, University Hospital Basel,
Basel, Switzerland

Department of Radiology and Nuclear Medicine, University Hospital Magdeburg,
Magdeburg, Germany
e-mail: bjoern.friebe@usb.ch

T. Streitparth
Department of Radiology, Ludwig Maximilian University (LMU) Hospital Munich, Munich,
Germany
e-mail: Tina.streitparth@med.uni-muenchen.de

63

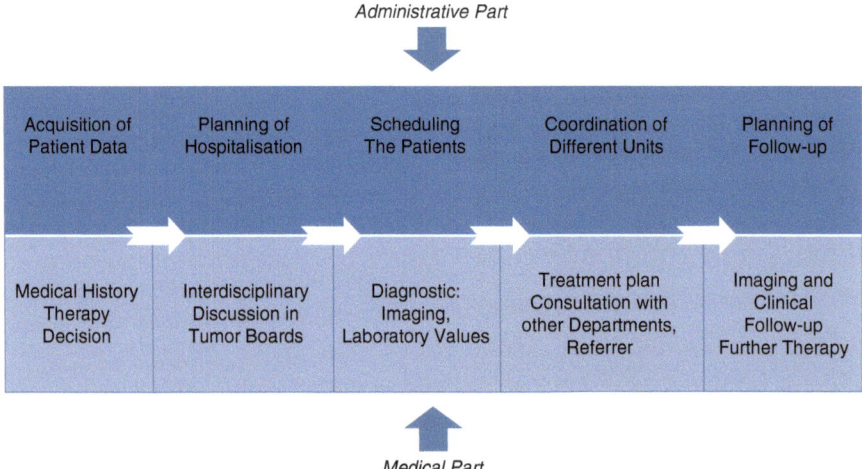

Fig. 6.1 The figure shows the complexity of the entire organization at administrative and medical levels. Exact coordination of the individual planning steps is necessary for an effective process

coordination takes place, at both medical and administrative levels (Fig. 6.1). Figure 6.1 shows the interaction between medical and administrative therapy planning. This unit consists ideally of a team with the medical area headed by colleagues experienced in making therapy decisions and in assessing the response after iBT. A compassionate approach to patients and their relatives is essential and promotes a trusting relationship between doctor and patient, but this must be backed up by well-run logistics and individual organization, which in iBT present a major challenge. From the beginning, the collection of patient data and the coordination of inpatient admission, which includes coordination with various departments, through to the scheduling of regular imaging and laboratory follow-up care, experienced administrative planning is required.

Admission to the Ward and Peri-interventional Standard Procedure

After several years of practical experience in the clinical-inpatient care of interventional radiology patients in our own clinic, our team has worked on an interdisciplinary basis with colleagues from internal medicine, gastroenterology/hepatology, oncology, and infectiology (e.g., *Antibiotic Stewardship*) on standard operation procedures (SOPs). These are updated at regular intervals. They include inpatient preparation, clinical processes conducted by the ward doctor, and inpatient and post-interventional follow-up care. In general, an SOP relates to specific interventions; there are special features within the SOP that deal with the organ systems, and their underlying diseases, that are to be treated.

Normally patients are admitted to our radiological-interventional ward 1 day before therapy for individual preparation, with patients admitted by our clinical team. The pre-therapeutic day is used for a thorough anamnesis, a radiological-internistic overall physical examination, and in particular the recording of previous internal diseases; the latter helps in assessing pre- and post-operative risk. Of course, this also includes a recording of all medications. A detailed explanation of iBT also takes place here. However, a separate explanation of the radiation treatment is given by colleagues in radiation therapy. The procedure itself is carried out under what is known as analgesic sedation with fentanyl and midazolam [3].

For the iBT of the liver, a blood sample with a complete blood count, a differential blood count, clinical chemistry (electrolytes, creatinine and GFR, liver parameters), coagulation values, and, depending on the tumor entity, the determination of special tumor markers as well as thyroid-stimulating hormone are performed. A blood-group determination is definitely a part of the routine, alongside regular electrocardiograms (ECGs). On the day of admission, two large-lumen entrances (G18) are laid. Imaging examinations such as MRI of the liver with hepatocyte-specific contrast media (Primovist®) and multiphase CT thorax and abdomen examinations are usually repeated if the available imaging is older than 6 weeks. Depending on the underlying tumor disease, it may be necessary to supplement further examinations such as lung function.

On the day of the intervention, patients fast, starting at midnight. In consultation with the interventionalist and after a detailed discussion with the team, the necessary medication is taken. Pre- or peri-interventionally, patients receive 1000 mL E 153 or Sterofundin (for patients with renal insufficiency: NaCl 0.9%), 8 mg dexamethasone as a short infusion and 8 mg ondansetron as a short infusion administered through one of the intravenous (IV) accesses already placed.

Anesthesia and Peri-interventional Patient-Monitoring

IBT is usually carried out under analgesic sedation using fentanyl and midazolam IV. For patients with an increased peri-interventional risk due to previous or concomitant disease, or at the patient's own request, general anesthesia or spinal anesthesia can also be carried out after clarification and preparation by colleagues in anesthesia. For legal reasons, information about a planned general anesthetic must be given at least 24 h before the planned procedure [2, 4].

The planned analgesic sedation is described by the clinical interventionalist as part of the information discussion.

Since the interventional radiologist is carrying out the procedure, it has become established in our routine to involve a qualified medical employee, whose task is to administer the medication as well as to monitor and accompany the patient.

If the percutaneous iBT is performed under analgesic sedation and local anesthesia, systemic sedation with a 2.5–10 mg midazolam IV is performed under monitoring (RR, pulse, O_2 saturation) and a 50–200 µg fentanyl IV is used together with local anesthesia, e.g., xylocaine 2% injected locally.

The monitoring of the vital parameters should at least include a three-channel ECG, pulse oximetry, and a noninvasive blood-pressure measurement.

Particularly when respiratory-depressant medication is used, close monitoring of the patient's vital parameters is necessary and must begin before the medication is administered. It may also be necessary to administer additional analgesic medication during the radiation [2, 4, 5].

In our routine, exact, regular documentation of vital parameters and administered medication in a monitoring protocol is necessary and standard. Such a sedation protocol, in which the recorded vital parameters are documented, should be created before the procedure is initiated. All medications administered, including any special incidents or complications, alongside vital parameters, must be recorded in the protocol; this is kept with the patient at all times.

After the iBT, the brachytherapy catheters are removed; during this a hemostatic material (gel foam) is introduced. It is also recommended to administer analgesic medication during the removal [1]. If we are performing CT-guided iBT of primary or secondary lung malignancies, the catheters are removed with fibrin tissue. This takes place in the interventional CT scan, 2 h after the removal, and normally a chest X-ray should be carried out to check for possible complications such as pneumothorax.

After the catheter has been removed, the patient is usually monitored for at least another 30–60 min, followed by a routine ultrasound of the abdomen. If the patient is symptom-free and there is no suspicion of bleeding or other complications during the ultrasound, the patient can finally be taken to the appropriate ward. The decision to move the patient to the ward is made by the medical staff, ideally by the interventionist or the accompanying physician.

Standard Operative Procedures and Follow-Up

After the interventional procedure, intensive monitoring, and completed sonography of the abdomen without any post-interventional complications, patients are taken back to their ward where they must remain in bed for 2–3 h. Patients are allowed to eat and drink 4 h after the intervention. Laboratory and ultrasound checks are repeated on the first and second day after brachytherapy. If there are no complications, our patients can normally be discharged on the third day after the intervention.

We have also developed standardized procedures for the post-interventional course, depending on the location of the iBT. Usually, patients can already be mobilized 4–6 h after the interventional procedure. More often than not, we have patients who receive anticoagulation, and as a rule this can be resumed in the evening or on the following morning.

The peri-interventional use of anticoagulation also requires precise evaluation. Mohnike et al. have analyzed the bleeding and thromboembolic rate after CT- and MRI-guided liver interventions in patients who were under peri-interventional thrombosis prophylaxis [6]. In the study, a total of 781 ablations were performed in

446 patients, of which 669 were iBT and 112 radiofrequency ablations. There were 63 bleeding complications, with significantly more bleeding occurring in the group of patients who received prophylaxis. In contrast, only one thromboembolic event was encountered. Furthermore, there were more bleeding complications in the group of patients who received radiofrequency ablation (RFA) instead of brachytherapy, with serious bleeding complications more frequent in those patients with cirrhosis. After severe bleeding complications, there was an increased 30-day and 90-day mortality rate. Therefore, ablative interventions should preferably be carried out depending on an adequate coagulation status and after an adequate pause in systemic anticoagulation [6].

Particular attention should be paid to tumor manifestations close to the stomach or the small intestine. In a prospective study of 33 patients, we investigated the tolerance dose of the gastric mucosa after iBT in liver metastases in segments II and III. A tolerance dose of 15.5 Gy per 1 mL of organ surface area of the stomach was established for the clinical endpoint of endoscopically proven symptomatic gastric ulcer [1, 7]. As a prophylactic measure, we recommend therapy with proton-pump inhibitors (PPI) when liver lesions near the stomach are treated [1, 7].

Patients with a tumor located centrally in the liver (e.g., segments V/VIII or I), or who have intrahepatic CCCs or very large tumor volumes, are often treated several times. They have an increased risk of developing a liver abscess or a cholangitis after iBT. In such cases, we use peri-interventional antibiosis (e.g., oral ciprofloxacin 500 mg, 1-0-1 for 2 weeks, or IV antibiosis with piperacillin/tazobactam for 10 days).

As already mentioned, large tumor volumes in the liver are often treated several times to protect liver function, and special care must be taken with regard to the possibility of RILD (radiation-induced liver disease). RILD usually develops 4–6 weeks after interstitial radiation of extensive volumes, with resulting ascites and impaired liver function. This typically manifests itself in laboratory changes: increased bilirubin and alkaline phosphatase [8]. It is recommended that a dose of ≥ 10 Gy be applied to a maximum of one-third the liver volume. A liver-protective regimen including enoxaparin, pentoxifylline, and ursodeoxycholic acid has been shown to reduce significantly the rate of RILD over an 8-week period following targeted radiotherapy [8].

Regarding percutaneous brachytherapy of renal masses, special procedures are to be followed, e.g., because of the more severe bleeding complications after CT-guided puncture of the kidney. Each patient is provided with a urinary bladder catheter in advance; this can usually be removed 2 days after the intervention, provided there is no hematuria. In order to check the effect of brachytherapy on healthy kidneys, we monitor the safety of this procedure closely by examining the kidney function pre- and post-interventionally using MAG-3 kidney sequence scintigraphy. After an iBT of renal masses, the renal function was investigated in 16 patients with 20 renal lesions. Follow-up was conducted after a median of 22.5, with one patient requiring permanent hemodialysis 32 months after brachytherapy. No other patient developed a significant worsening in global renal function. The local control rate was 95%, including repeated brachytherapy of two recurrences [9, 10].

Follow-Up and Imaging

Single high-dose-rate iBT of inner organs can be applied in almost every organ and can provide useful oncological options for cancer patients, especially for patients with oligometastatic disease. In contrast to conventional radiation therapy, iBT offers the advantage of applying very high local radiation doses to tumors while sparing radiation-sensitive tissues, and it can be repeated many times for different tumor sites and organs if necessary. In order to evaluate treatment-response imaging, follow-up is crucial. Regarding iBT, some general aspects of treatment response of local and locoregional treatments and some special aspects of iBT have to be considered; they are addressed in the following sections.

General Aspects of Treatment Response of Locoregional Therapies

In order to objectify therapy response of cancer patients, especially in clinical trials, the WHO criteria were introduced in the early 1980s [11]. According to these criteria, the sum of the two largest perpendicular diameters of all lesions of a patient is calculated, and thresholds for complete remission, partial remission, stable, and progressive disease were defined for the first time. Later on, the RECIST criteria [12] were developed; these were much easier to apply and seemed to have the same accuracy in evaluating response to therapy [13], which is why they are nowadays standard for most tumor types. In the latest version of RECIST, the sum of the longest diameters of at most five lesions defines a patient's therapy response [14]. Although the RECIST criteria have proved their ability to offer accurate and reproducible assessment of tumor burden in many studies, they have one persistent, major limitation: they only assess morphology and do not consider special treatment-related effects that can occur in certain local or locoregional therapies. Thus, a tumor response to therapy might not necessarily be reflected by tumor shrinkage so that a tumor response can be mistaken for a lack of response.

This limitation moved increasingly into the foreground with the introduction of new therapies, such as immune-modulating therapies. In the field of immune-modulating therapies, a so-called pseudoprogression can mimic a real progression. This finally led to the development of the immune-related RECIST criteria (irRE-CIST) [15], which at least partly overcome this problem, one that was unknown before the era of immune-modulating therapies.

As in immune-modulating therapies, the dynamic and emerging field of local and locoregional therapies quickly revealed limitations of RECIST. Unlike in systemic therapies, the major goal of local or locoregional therapies is not tumor shrinkage (or disappearance) but the induction of tumor necrosis. In order to detect tumor necrosis after ablation or locoregional treatment, physicians worldwide are working on new image-based markers. Koda et al., for instance, were successful in predicting local tumor progression rates of hepatocellular carcinomas treated by

RFA, by application of a new ablation margin assessment immediately after RFA [16].

These observations are also partly reflected in new response assessment guidelines such as mRECIST [17] or the EASL [18] guidelines for the evaluation of therapy response of hepatocellular carcinoma. Nevertheless, the question of optimum tumor response assessment to a local or locoregional treatment is the subject of an ongoing debate that will presumably continue with the development of new local and locoregional therapies.

Special Aspects of Response Assessment in iBT

As in other local ablative techniques, the basis of image-based therapy such as iBT is always the task of identifying the patients who are likely to profit most from local ablation. Usually, this is done best by MRI with Gd-EOB-DTPA. By performing MRI with Gd-EOB-DTPA before local ablative therapy, several goals can be achieved that are crucial for a good response to these therapies. First of all, MRI can identify patients with oligometastatic disease. The concept of oligometastatic disease includes patients with few metastases in not more than two or three organs. Although the definition of the relatively new concept of oligometastatic disease allows some variation (more metastasis in more than three organs), the best response rates are described in patients where oligometastatic disease is limited to one organ. In these case series, long-term survival, and in 20–50% even cure, could be achieved [19].

Secondly, the therapy applied should be validated by imaging. This means that it has to be checked whether the lesion that was treated is fully ablated at baseline. In RFA or other thermal techniques, this can be done by CT or MRI directly after therapy. In cases of full ablation, a non-enhancing thermonecrosis should be visualized that, ideally, is greater than the lesion itself. Post-therapeutic hemorrhage can be misleading, but it is usually well excluded by subtraction images. In a fully ablated lesion no contrast enhancement should be seen. In iBT, complete coverage of the lesion can be ensured by the use of radiation-planning software. In order to cover all the lesions, there needs to be a sufficient number of catheters to cover the lesion geometrically. Thereby, irregular tumor volumes can receive a sufficiently large radiation dose to induce necrosis. Although the radiation dose applied in iBT falls very steeply from the lesion to the periphery, and therefore spares surrounding organs, it nonetheless induces some damage in the surrounding healthy tissue, as is already well known from percutaneous radiation [20].

These effects on healthy liver tissue can be displayed very well in MRI with Gd-EOB-DTPA, by a diminished uptake of Gd-EOB-DTPA. It can be seen as early as 3 days after ablation with a maximum extent observed 6 weeks after therapy. These areas of reduced or lost liver function correlate well with the magnitude of the radiation dose applied [21] (Fig. 6.2), and these areas can be depicted in Gd-EOB-DTPA precisely according to the doses applied around the lesions.

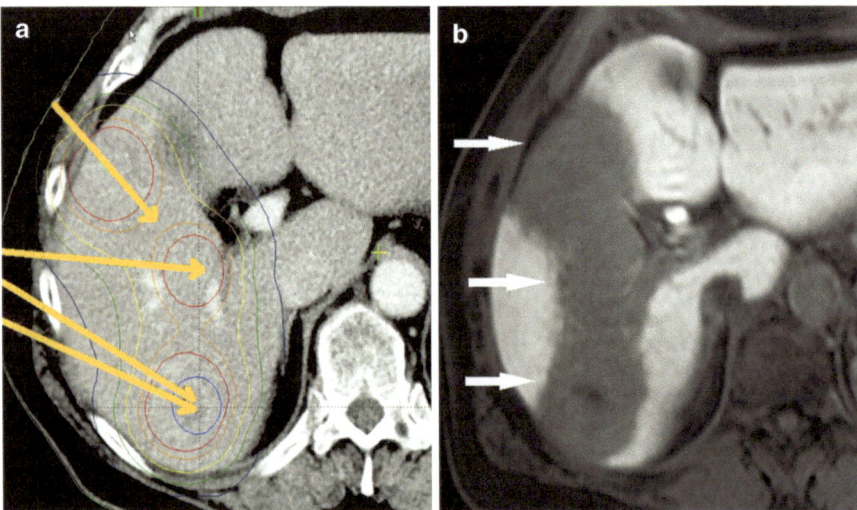

Fig. 6.2 (**a**) Radiation planning with isodose lines and preceding location of catheters (yellow arrows). (**b**) Gd-EOB-DTPA MRI after iBT displays areas of diminished uptake of contrast media by hepatocytes (dark areas) that correspond to temporary dysfunctional liver parenchyma around the ablated lesions

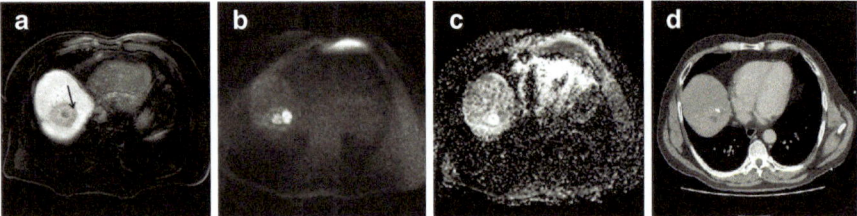

Fig. 6.3 (**a**) Follow-up Gd-EOB-DTPA MRI after iBT shows areas of focal dysfunctional liver parenchyma around a darker central necrosis. In the medial zone of the dysfunctional liver, parenchyma can be seen as a slightly focal dark area (arrow). (**b**) This area can be clearly diagnosed as a new lesion at the edge of the treated zone (high signal intensity with high b value ($b = 800$). (**c**) ADC-map of B. (**d**) The lesion was treated again by CT-guided iBT (CT of pretreatment planning with catheter, white)

The reader of a follow-up-MRI after iBT has to be aware of these changes, to prevent misinterpretation of these findings as progressive disease. In the further course of follow-up, it has been observed that the areas of reduced liver function are usually repaired by the liver within 6 months. Thus, during early follow-up it can be difficult to detect a new lesion within a zone of reduced liver function that might not have received the full radiation dose. In such cases diffusion-weighted imaging can usually give decisive hints, although sometimes one can also see dark, irregular focal areas of contrast-sparing at hepatobiliary phase; these areas are even darker than those revealing reduced liver function (Fig. 6.3).

Normally a follow-up interval of 3 months after therapy is adequate for response assessment of one or more tumors. Tumor response needs to be assessed not only in a defined tumor but also in the patient as a whole; his/her whole oncological situation must be reevaluated. In order to meet this requirement, physicians need to decide when is the best time to change the therapy, to repeat the therapy or also to stop a therapy, for instance, if a patient wishes to stop the therapy (see also the section "Clinical Management"). These decisions have to be made in a multidisciplinary team of oncologists, radiologists, and radiation physicists.

In the case of new or recurrent lesions, iBT offers the possibility of repeated treatment, even at the same site, without the risk of RILD, as in conformal radiation therapy [22, 23]. Thus, if new or recurrent lesions are present, ablative therapy should be planned if the patient is still oligometastatic. In cases of progression to polymetastatic disease, at distant or local tumor sites, locoregional options and systemic options should be checked.

If there is progression but the patient still has oligometastatic disease, iBT can be repeated many times, even to the point where the patient may finally become untreatable. The ultimate goal of ablation is indeed survival—not local control. In this sense, physicians treating their patients by local ablation methods should try to prolong to time to untreatable progression (TTUP) as much as possible. The relatively new concept of TTUP is supported by data that show that quite a substantial proportion of patients with (for instance) initially unresectable liver metastases can show long-term survival with chronic metastatic disease and will therefore profit greatly from local ablation [24].

In summary, it can be stated that, in cases of progression, iBT can be repeated, or combined with other techniques, or adapted to the extent of progression, as long as the progression does not exceed the technical possibilities of local ablation and as long as the progression is not polymetastatic. In the cases of polymetastatic disease, systemic options should be checked.

Key Points
- An interventional radiology outpatient clinic with competent medical and administrative staff is the key for patient acquisition and adequate organization.
- Coordination and planning of the treatment with a radiation oncology iBT expert is a prerequisite for a successful intervention.
- A radiological ward allows intensive patient care and interdisciplinary communication with other clinical disciplines.
- Single high dose iBT of inner organs can be applied in almost every organ, and repeatedly, until untreatable progression sets in; patients with oligometastatic disease seem to profit most from iBT.

- Image-guided validation of complete ablation of lesions at baseline is crucial for differentiating between local recurrence and initial incomplete
  ablation and in order to predict response in future treatments.
- Physicians assessing follow-up imaging of iBT need to be aware of special
  treatment-related effects of iBT and different treatment-related response
  criteria in order to assess tumor response correctly and thus guide the
  patient to appropriate further treatment options.

References

1. Bretschneider T, Ricke J, Gebauer B, Streitparth F. Image-guided high-dose-rate brachytherapy of malignancies in various inner organs—technique, indications and perspectives. J
   Contemp Brachytherapy. 2016;8(3):253–63.
2. Mahnken AH, Thomas Ch. Interventionelle Radiologie, Kapitel: Perkutane Interventionen.
   Thieme Verlag; 2019.
3. Romagnoli S, Fanelli F, Barbani F, Uberoi R, Esteban E, Lee MJ, Nielsen PT, Mahnken AH,
   Morgan R. CIRSE standards of practice on analgesia and sedation for interventional radiology
   in adults. Cardiovasc Intervent Radiol. 2020;43:1251–60.
4. Wiggermann P, Beyer L, Schicho A. Perkutane Tumorablation der Leber: Streitparth F, Gäble
   A. 5. Technische Grundlagen und Materialien der Mikrowellenablation (MWA). Breitenseher
   Publisher; 2019.
5. Strnad V, Pötter R, Kovacs G et al. Praktisches Handbuch der Brachytherapie 2. Auflage—
   Bremen; Uni-Med Verlag; 2010. ISBN 978-3-8374-1205-5.
6. Mohnike K, Sauerland H, Seidensticker M, Hass P, Kropf S, Seidensticker R, Friebe B,
   Fischbach F, Fischbach K, Powerski M, Pech M, Grosser OS, Kettner E, Ricke J. Haemorrhagic
   complications and symptomatic venous thromboembolism in interventional tumour ablations: the impact of per-interventional thrombosis prophylaxis. Cardiovasc Intervent Radiol.
   2016;39:1716–21.
7. Streitparth F, Pech M, Böhmig M, Ruehl R, Peters N, Wieners G, Steinberg J, Lopez-Haenninen
   E, Felix R, Wust P, Ricke J. In vivo assessment of the gastric mucosal tolerance dose after single fraction, small volume irradiation of liver malignancies by computed tomography-guided,
   high-dose-rate brachytherapy. Int J Radiat Oncol Biol Phys. 2006;65:1479–86.
8. Seidensticker M, Seidensticker R, Damm R, Mohnike K, Pech M, Sangro B, Hass P, Wust
   P, Kropf S, Gademann G, Ricke J. Prospective randomized trial of enoxaparin, pentoxifylline and ursodeoxycholic acid for prevention of radiation-induced liver toxicity. PLoS One.
   2014;9(11):e112731.
9. Friebe B, Bretschneider T, Ricke J, Liehr UB, Wendler JJ, Klingler HC, Susani M, Sevcenco
   S. Kapitel 2: Alternative Verfahren beim Nierenzellkarzinom. 2.1: Lokalablative, bildge-
   führte Verfahren bei Nierentumoren. Alternative operative Therapien in der Uroonkologie.
   Operationen, Interventionelle Techniken, Radiochemotherapie. Schostak Martin, Blana
   Andreas. Berlin Heidelberg: Springer; 2016.
10. Damm R, Streitparth T, Hass P, Seidensticker M, Heinze C, Powerski M, Wendler JJ, Liehr
    UB, Mohnike K, Pech M, Ricke J. Prospective evaluation of CT-guided HDR brachytherapy
    as a local ablative treatment for renal masses: a single-arm pilot trial. Strahlenther Onkol.
    2019;195(11):982–90.
11. Miller AB, Hoogstraten B, Staquet M, Winkler A. Reporting results of cancer treatment.
    Cancer. 1981;47:207–14.

12. Therasse P, Arbuck SG, Eisenhauer EA, Wanders J, Kaplan RS, Rubinstein L, Verweij J, Van Glabbeke M, van Oosterom AT, Christian MC, Gwyther SG. New guidelines to evaluate the response to treatment in solid tumors. European Organization for Research and Treatment of Cancer, National Cancer Institute of the United States, National Cancer Institute of Canada. J Natl Cancer Inst. 2000;92(3):205–16. https://doi.org/10.1093/jnci/92.3.205.
13. Choi J-H, Ahn M-J, Rhim H-C, Kim J-W, Lee G-H, Lee Y-Y, Kim I-S. REcist 1.1. Comparison of WHO and RECIST criteria for response in metastatic colorectal carcinoma. Cancer Res Treat. 2005;37(5):290–3.
14. Eisenhauer EA, Therasse P, Bogaerts J, et al. New response evaluation criteria in solid tumours: revised RECIST guideline (version 1.1). Eur J Cancer. 2009;45:228–47.
15. Wolchok JD, Hoos A, O'Day S, Weber JS, Hamid O, Lebbé C, et al. Guidelines for the evaluation of immune therapy activity in solid tumors: immune-related response criteria. Clin Cancer Res. 2009;15:7412–20. https://doi.org/10.1158/1078-0432.CCR-09-1624.
16. Koda M, Tokunaga S, Okamoto T. Clinical usefulness of the ablative margin assessed by magnetic resonance imaging with Gd-EOB-DTPA for radiofrequency ablation of hepatocellular carcinoma. J Hepatol. 2015;63(6):1360–7.
17. Lencioni R, Llovet JM. Modified RECIST (mRECIST) assessment for hepatocellular carcinoma. Semin Liver Dis. 2010;30:52–60.
18. Forner A, Ayuso C, Varela M. Evaluation of tumor response after locoregional therapies in hepatocellular carcinoma: are response evaluation criteria in solid tumors reliable? Cancer. 2009;115(3):616–23.
19. Weiser MR, Jarnagin WR, Saltz LB. Colorectal cancer patients with oligometastatic liver disease: what is the optimal approach? Oncology (Williston Park). 2013;27:1074–8.
20. Doi H, Shiomi H, Masai N, et al. Threshold doses and prediction of visually apparent liver dysfunction after stereotactic body radiation therapy in cirrhotic and normal livers using magnetic resonance imaging. J Radiat Res. 2016;57:294–300.
21. Seidensticker M, Seidensticker R, Mohnike K. Quantitative in vivo assessment of radiation injury of the liver using Gd-EOB-DTPA enhanced MRI: tolerance dose of small liver volumes. Radiat Oncol. 2011;6:40.
22. Rühl R, Lüdemann L, Czarnecka A. Biological restrictions and tolerance doses of repeated single-fraction hdr-irradiation of intersecting small liver volumes for recurrent hepatic metastases. Radiat Oncol. 2010;5:44.
23. Toesca DA, Osmundson EC, Eyben RV, et al. Central liver toxicity after SBRT: an expanded analysis and predictive nomogram. Radiother Oncol. 2017;122:130–6.
24. Adam R, Wicherts DA, de Haas RJ. Patients with initially unresectable colorectal liver metastases: is there a possibility of cure? J Clin Oncol. 2009;27(11):1829–35.

Image-Guided Brachytherapy in Oligometastasis: Criteria for Patient Selection from an Oncological Perspective

Kerstin Schütte and Christian Schulz

Introduction

Treatment of cancer is stage-specific; in the curative setting it aims at long-term disease-free survival and in the palliative setting it aims at prolongation of survival while maintaining quality of life. Distant metastases are widely regarded as manifestations of a systemic malignant disease, mostly indicating palliative treatment. In this setting, treatment of local or regional disease is supposed not to affect survival [1]. However, concepts have evolved that apply a more comprehensive and personalized view of patients with metastatic malignant disease, and that follow the hypothesis that metastasis-directed treatments are potentially curative in some patients [2]. This chapter is intended (1) to provide insights into the concept and biology of oligometastasis, (2) to summarize the current evidence supporting the use of ablative therapies including local ablative interventional treatments and surgical approaches in these selected patients, and (3) to offer criteria for identifying patients with metastatic cancer who have the potential to benefit from local therapies.

K. Schütte (✉)
Department of Internal Medicine and Gastroenterology, Niels-Stensen-Kliniken
Marienhospital Osnabrück, Osnabrück, Germany
e-mail: kerstin.schuette@niels-stensen-kliniken.de

C. Schulz
Medical Department II, Ludwig Maximilian University (LMU) Hospital Munich, Munich, Germany
e-mail: Chr.Schulz@med.uni-muenchen.de

© The Author(s), under exclusive license to Springer Nature
Switzerland AG 2021
K. Mohnike et al. (eds.), *Manual on Image-Guided Brachytherapy of Inner Organs*, https://doi.org/10.1007/978-3-030-78079-1_7

Concept of Oligometastasis

One of the hallmarks of cancer is its ability to generate cells that move out of the primary tumor, invade adjacent tissues, and are transferred to distant sites where they potentially succeed in colonization [3, 4]. This invasion–metastasis cascade is a complex, multistep process depending on an interplay between host factors and intrinsic characteristics of tumor cells [5–7]. The metastatic potential of cells within a single neoplasm is heterogeneous, and only a few cells within a primary tumor are able to give rise to metastasis. Metastases are genetically very unstable and are clonal in origin, which leads to high biological heterogeneity within and among metastases [7]. This is one of the causes of intra-patient differences between metastases in response to tumor-directed therapies.

Distant metastases are the leading cause of cancer-related death and account for at least 2/3 of deaths among patients with solid tumors [8].

In the nineteenth century, Halsted proposed a theory of cancer spread; he regarded it as a contiguous process from the primary tumor through the lymphatics to the lymph nodes and then to distant organs [1, 9]. This is the basis of modern radical *en bloc* surgery. In the mid-twentieth century, a further theory was discussed that classifies clinically apparent cancer as a systemic disease with potentially multiple and widely spread metastases that might also take the form of undetected (occult) micrometastases [1, 10]. Metastatic cancer is generally considered incurable, and treatment aims at the prolongation of survival and palliation of symptoms. Long-term survivors and complete response to therapy are exceptional in patients with metastasized solid tumors. However, more than 50 years ago, a debate already arose on the question of whether curative treatment of metastatic disease is an option. This debate initially focused on solitary metastases [2, 11]. In this context, the terms "metachronous metastases" (developing sometime after treatment of the primary neoplasm) and "synchronous metastases" (diagnosed at the same time as the primary neoplasm) were introduced [11].

The hypothesis of oligometastasis was first presented by Samuel Hellman and Ralph R. Weichselbaum in 1995 [1]. In a landmark editorial in the *Journal of Clinical Oncology,* they discussed the contiguous and systemic theories of cancer and endorsed consequences of a third paradigm that classifies cancer disease on a biological spectrum ranging from localized to systemic disease, with many intermediate states.

Weichselbaum and Hellmann proposed a differentiated synthesis of the above-mentioned theories. They argued that the metastatic capacity of a tumor evolves during tumor progression, and is influenced by tumor size and progression. In their view, the likelihood, number, and sites of metastases represent a state of tumor development, with the consequent possibility of intermediate tumor stages between localized primary disease and diffuse systemic disease. They hypothesized that, for certain tumors, metastases might be limited to a single or limited number of organs (oligometastasis) and that the malignant disease in these patients will not necessarily progress to widespread distribution of cancer [1, 12]. They emphasize that this oligometastatic state is based on a state of limited metastatic capacity and is a characteristic of many tumors during their clinical evolution [1]. They differentiate between two groups of patients with oligometastatic disease: first, "tumors early in the chain of progression may have metastases limited in number and location because the facility for metastatic growth has not been fully developed and the site for such growth is restricted," and second, "patients who had widespread metastases that were mostly eradicated by systemic agents, the chemotherapy having failed to destroy those remaining because of the number of tumor cells, the presence of drug-resistant cells, or the tumor foci being located in some pharmacologically privileged site" [1]. Although these scenarios may look identical in imaging, they require a comprehensive view as they differ significantly in their clinical outcome.

Definition of Oligometastatic Disease

Within the 25 years since the introduction of the concept of an oligometastatic state, there has been much debate on how to define it. There is a lack of biomarkers that distinguish clearly between patients with oligometastatic disease and those with a poorer prognosis because of widespread, possibly undetected metastases; consequently, identification of patients in the respective groups frequently relies on imaging. Guidelines endorsed by various professional societies differ in their definition of oligometastatic disease (OMD) in respect of number of tumor manifestations and number of sites affected. This hampers comparison of reports on local treatments and their outcomes in metastatic cancer. In 2020, a consensus recommendation of the European Society for Radiotherapy and Oncology (ESTRO) and the European Organisation for Research and Treatment of Cancer (EORTC) was published [13]. The authors agreed to use "oligometastatic disease" as an umbrella term and further subclassify this state by applying clinical and tumor-related information. They identified five factors as the basis for a classification system for oligometastatic disease. This system comprises nine distinct states of oligometastatic disease. Key distinctions in differentiation are (1) between an induced oligometastatic state (where the patient has a history of polymetastatic disease and has responded to therapy) and a genuine oligometastatic state (where the patient has no history of polymetastatic disease); (2) between de novo (freshly diagnosed) and repeated (previously treated) oligometastatic disease; (3) whether the interval between diagnosis of the primary tumor and the metastases was shorter or longer than 6 months, (4) whether the metastases developed while the patient was under active systemic treatment or during a treatment-free interval; and (5) in patients with repeated oligometastatic disease, whether current imaging reveals any lesions to be progressive. The authors' aim was to judge the prognostic value of these criteria and to assess their acceptance and compliance in routine practice within a prospective cohort trial (OligoCare).

   Another recent consensus paper by experts from ESTRO (European Society for Radiotherapy and Oncology) and ASTRO (American Society for Radiation Oncology) aims at standardization of definitions and outcome reports [14]. Although they detected significant heterogeneity in current definitions of oligometastatic disease (OMD) in their systematic literature review, they agreed to define OMD as 1–5 lesions with all metastatic sites being safely treatable. A controlled primary tumor may or may not be present [14].

Possible Effects of Radical Treatment in Oligometastatic Disease

In recent decades, alternatives and adjuncts to systemic treatments for patients with limited metastatic cancer have been explored with the aim of prolonging patients' overall or progression-free survival. These have included surgery, stereotactic body radiation therapy (SBRT), catheter-based (interstitial) high-dose-rate brachytherapy (iBT), and other local ablative techniques—for example, radiofrequency ablation (RFA), microwave ablation (MWA), and irreversible electroporation (IRE).

A positive effect beyond prolongation of survival by treatment of OMD, either by surgery or by local ablative techniques, is the possibility to defer the initiation or the switch of systemic therapy and thereby to postpone systemic side effects of therapy [12].

Systemic targeted treatments and immunotherapy come to the fore in several tumor entities, especially in malignant melanoma, renal cell carcinoma, non-small-cell lung cancer, breast cancer, and hepatocellular carcinoma. Abscopal effects on other metastases following radiotherapy, hyperthermia, or surgery with antitumor action have been reported; these are probably immune-mediated. First reports on the combination of radiotherapy with systemic immune checkpoint inhibitors, leading to impressive clinical responses, have been published. On this basis, early prospective clinical trials combining radiotherapy with immune checkpoint blockage in several tumor entities have been initiated [12, 15, 16].

Imaging Before Local Treatment in Oligometastatic Disease

A critical point in the identification of patients who might benefit from metastasis-directed therapy in OMD is, inevitably, the sensitivity of the imaging modality used to detect further metastatic disease. Staging should therefore include a comprehensive workup with sensitive imaging of all sites of common metastases of the primary tumor and its histology, in order to detect small lesions. The authors of the ESTRO-ASTRO OMD consensus paper, after diligent review of published studies, do not define specific imaging modalities as a requirement, but they recommend PET/CT, contrast-enhanced CT scans of chest, abdomen, and pelvis and/or MR brain or spine (when indicated) for diagnostic evaluation [14]. Prognostic scores based on disease-burden biomarkers (number, size, and distribution of metastases) have been developed to identify patients with metastatic cancer who might benefit from radical treatment [17]. As the majority of clinical scoring systems have been developed on the basis of historical imaging strategies that might have missed micrometastases, with an impact on survival, the need for more a comprehensive workup of patients, using novel imaging and also molecular biomarkers, has been expressed. Functional tumor imaging aiming at quantification of aspects of tumor morphology and behavior (e.g., vessel density, metabolic imaging, assessment of tumor heterogeneity) might be incorporated into clinical scenarios in the future [17]. Further integrated approaches will potentially combine clinical with molecular staging in oncological risk stratification [18], leading to subtyping of metastases with respect to microRNA expression patterns and genomic profiling in combination with imaging data [19].

Evidence for Metastasis-Directed Therapy in Oligometastatic Tumors

Most of the published studies are either early-stage clinical studies or retrospective in nature. Only a very limited number of prospective, randomized, controlled clinical studies on this topic have been published. Therefore, it is not clear whether the unexpected excellent clinical outcome in patients treated for OMD with local therapies is an effect of metastasis-directed therapy or an effect of selection of favorable tumor biology [20]. Hence, it is a clinical challenge to define a subgroup of patients with metastatic cancer who would experience major benefit from metastasis-directed interventions without the intervention's side effects outweighing its benefit (according to the principle *primum non nocere*).

Only a few prospective phase II and III studies on the effect of local treatment in OMD have been published so far. A selection of these is summarized in Table 7.1.

For several tumor entities, local ablative therapies in OMD are addressed in current national and international guidelines on the basis of these findings.

Table 7.2 gives an overview of selected guideline statements on this issue.

The Integrated View

Local ablative therapies, including iBT, achieve high local control rates and are associated with low mortality and low rates of major complications. However, several aspects need to be taken into account if local therapy of OMD by surgery, locoregional therapy, or a combination of both is under consideration. These include the patient (especially his/her general performance status, comorbidities, and personal preferences), tumor-related factors (sites and size of target lesions), history of disease (tumor biology), and technical aspects (local expertise with certain local ablative techniques, secure treatability of all target lesions). The most important factors are summarized in Fig. 7.1. The patient's prognosis in OMD depends on the risks of harm from metastasis-directed therapies, the probability of achieving complete tumor ablation, and the probability of survival in case of complete elimination of the cancer manifestations that are assumed to be driving the disease [21]. Each patient should undergo individual assessment and discussion, at an experienced tumor center, in a multidisciplinary tumor board that includes experts from surgery, pathology, oncology, radiology, interventional radiology, and radiation oncology.

Table 7.1 Selection of published prospective, randomized, controlled phase II or III trials on the benefit of metastasis-directed therapy in OMD; adopted from [22]

Author, year	Primary location	N, criteria	CT phase	Comparators	Results	Ref.
Palma et al., 2019	Various	99 Controlled primary tumor, 1–5 metastatic lesions	II	Palliative standard of care vs. palliative standard of care combined with SABR	Median OS 28 months in the control arm (95%CI 18–39 months) vs. 50 months in the SABR arm (95%CI 29–83 months); $p = 0.006$; HR = 0.47 with 95%CI 0.27–0.81 Five-year OS rates were 17.7% (95%CI 6–34%) vs. 42.3% (95%CI, 28–56%); $p = 0.006$	[23, 24]
Ruers et al., 2012	CRC	119 Hepatic metastases <10, no extrahepatic disease	II	Systemic treatment vs. systemic treatment combined with RFA (± resection)	Difference in OS in favor of the combined modality arm (HR = 0.58 with 95%CI, 0.38–0.88, $p = 0.01$) Median OS was 45.6 months (95%CI 30.3–67.8 months) in the combined modality arm vs. 40.5 months (95%CI 27.5–47.7 months) in the systemic-treatment-only arm	[25, 26]

(continued)

Table 7.1 (continued)

Author, year	Primary location	N, criteria	CT phase	Comparators	Results	Ref.
Gomez et al., 2016	NSCLC	49 Stage IV NSCLC, three or fewer metastatic disease lesions after first-line systemic therapy, ECOG 2 or less, after standard first-line systemic therapy, and with no disease progression before randomization	II	Local consolidative therapy (LCT; (chemo) radiotherapy or resection of all lesions) with or without subsequent maintenance treatment or maintenance treatment alone, which could be observation only (MT/O)	Median follow-up time 38.8 months (range 28.3–61.4 months) PFS benefit: median 14.2 months (95%CI 7.4–23.1 months) with LCT vs. 4.4 months (95%CI 2.2–8.3 months) with MT/O; $p = 0.022$ OS benefit in the LCT arm, median 41.2 months (lower 95%CL 18.9 months, upper CL not reached) vs. 17.0 months (95%CI 10.1–39.8 months) with MT/O; $p = 0.017$	[27, 28]

(continued)

Table 7.1 (continued)

Author, year	Primary location	N, criteria	CT phase	Comparators	Results	Ref.
Lyengar et al., 2018	NSCLC	29 Patients with limited metastatic NSCLC (primary plus up to five metastatic sites) whose tumors did not possess EGFR-targetable or ALK-targetable mutations but did achieve partial response or stable disease after induction chemotherapy	II	Maintenance chemotherapy alone vs. SABR followed by maintenance chemotherapy	Significant improvement in PFS in the SABR-plus-maintenance-chemotherapy arm of 9.7 months vs. 3.5 months in the maintenance chemotherapy alone arm ($p = 0.01$)	[29]
Gore et al., 2017	ED-SCLC	86 One to four extracranial metastases after a complete response or partial response to chemotherapy	II	Prophylactic cranial irradiation (PCI) or PCI plus consolidative radiation therapy (PCI + cRT) to intrathoracic disease and extracranial metastases for extensive-disease SCLC	1-year OS did not differ between the groups: 60.1% (95%CI 41.2–74.7) for PCI and 50.8% (95%CI 34.0–65.3) for PCI + cRT ($p = 0.21$) The 3- and 12-month rates of progression were 53.3% and 79.6% for PCI and 14.5% and 75% for PCI + cRT Time to progression favored PCI + cRT (HR = 0.53, 95%CI 0.32–0.87, $p = 0.01$)	[30]

(continued)

Table 7.1 (continued)

Author, year	Primary location	N, criteria	CT phase	Comparators	Results	Ref.
Phillips et al., 2020	Prostate	54 Recurrent hormone-sensitive prostate cancer and 1–3 metastases detectable by conventional imaging; patients had not received ADT; within 6 months of enrolment or 3 or more years total	II	SABR or observation	Treatment with SABR improved median progression-free survival ("median not reached" vs. 5.8 months; HR 0.30; 95%CI 0.11–0.81; $p = 0.002$) Total consolidation of PSMA radiotracer-avid disease decreased the risk of new lesions at 6 months (16% vs. 63%; $p = 0.006$)	[31]
Ost et al., 2018	Prostate	62 Asymptomatic PCa were eligible if the patient had had biochemical recurrence after primary PCa treatment with curative intent, three or fewer extracranial metastatic lesions detected by choline positron-emission tomography/ computed tomography, and serum testosterone level was >50 ng/mL	II	Surveillance or MDT of all detected lesions (surgery or stereotactic body radiotherapy)	Median ADT-free survival was 13 months (80%CI 12–17 months) for the surveillance group and 21 months (80%CI 14–29 months) for the MDT group (hazard ratio 0.60 with 80%CI 0.40–0.90; log-rank $p = 0.11$)	[32]

(continued)

Table 7.1 (continued)

Author, year	Primary location	N, criteria	CT phase	Comparators	Results	Ref.
Boevé et al., 2019	Prostate	432 Prostate-specific antigen; (PSA) > 20 ng/mL and primary bone mPCa found on bone scan	III	ADT with EBRT or ADT alone	No significant difference was found in OS (HR 0.90 with 95%CI 0.70–1.14; $p = 0.4$) Median time to PSA progression in the radiotherapy group was 15 months (95%CI 11.8–18.2), compared with 12 months (95%CI 10.6–13.4) in the control group The crude HR (0.78; 95%CI 0.63–0.97) was statistically significant ($p = 0.02$)	[33]

(continued)

Table 7.1 (continued)

Author, year	Primary location	N, criteria	CT phase	Comparators	Results	Ref.
Parker et al., 2018	Prostate	2061 Newly diagnosed metastatic prostate cancer	III	Standard of care (control group) or standard of care and radiotherapy (radiotherapy group)	Radiotherapy improved failure-free survival (HR 0.76 with 95%CI 0.68–0.84; $p < 0.0001$) but not overall survival (HR 0.92 with 95%CI 0.80–1.06; $p = 0.266$) Failure-free survival was improved in patients with low metastatic burden at baseline who were allocated radiotherapy (HR 0.59 with 95%CI 0.49–0.72; $p < 0.0001$)	[34]
Your et al., 2020	Nasopharynx	126 Biopsy-proven mNPC; patients demonstrated complete or partial response following 3 cycles of cisplatin; and fluorouracil chemotherapy	III	Chemotherapy plus radiotherapy or chemotherapy alone	Improved OS (stratified HR 0.42 with 95%CI 0.23–0.77; $p = 0.004$) in favor of combination Progression-free survival was also improved (stratified HR 0.36 with 95%CI 0.23–0.57)	[35]

Abbreviations: *SABR* stereotactic ablative radiotherapy, *CRC* colorectal cancer, *ED-SCLC* extensive-disease small-cell lung cancer, *EBRT* external-beam radiation therapy, *ADT* androgen-deprivation therapy, *OS* overall survival, *HR* hazard ratio, *CI* confidence interval, *CL* confidence limit, *NSCLC* non-small-cell lung cancer, *LCT* local consolidative therapy, *MT* maintenance treatment, *PFS* progression-free survival, *MDT* metastasis-directed therapy, *PCa* prostate cancer

Table 7.2 Current European consensus guidelines on treatment of OMD in selected cancer entities

Tumor entity	Guideline	Key points	Reference
Colorectal cancer	ESMO	• OMD may be characterized by the existence of metastases at up to two or occasionally three sites and five or sometimes more lesions, predominantly visceral and occasionally lymph-nodal • For patients with OMD, systemic therapy is the standard of care and should be considered as the initial part of every treatment strategy (exception: patients with single/few liver or lung lesions) • The best local treatment should be selected from a "toolbox" of procedures according to disease location, treatment goal ("the more curative, the more surgery"/higher importance of local/complete control), treatment-related morbidity, and patient-related factors such as comorbidity/-ies and age • In patients with unresectable liver metastases only, or OMD, local ablation techniques such as thermal ablation or highly conformal radiation techniques (e.g., SBRT, HDR-brachytherapy (iBT) can be considered. The decision should be taken by a multidisciplinary tumor board and be based on local experience, tumor characteristics, and patient preference	[36]
NSCLC	ESMO	• Stage IV patients with limited synchronous metastases at diagnosis may experience long-term disease-free survival (DFS) following systemic therapy and local consolidative therapy (LCT: high-dose RT including stereotactic ablative body RT (SABR) or surgery) • There are no published data on the impact of LCT on OS or long-term toxicity • Stage IV patients with limited metachronous metastases may be treated with a local treatment, as some may experience long-term DFS	[37]
Breast cancer	ESMO	• Oligometastatic disease is defined as low-volume metastatic disease with a limited number and size of metastatic lesions (up to five and not necessarily in the same organ), potentially amenable to local treatment aimed at achieving a complete remission status • A small but very important subset of patients with advanced breast cancer, for example, those with oligometastatic disease or low-volume metastatic disease that is highly sensitive to systemic therapy can achieve complete remission and long survival. A multimodal approach, including locoregional treatments with curative intent, should be considered for these selected patients. A prospective clinical trial addressing this specific situation is needed	[38]
Prostate cancer	ESMO	• Earlier visualization of recurrence makes it technically possible to selectively ablate metastases. Hypothetically, this would slow down progression and improve survival • Phase II trials have paved the way for larger confirmatory phase III trials, but they should not be regarded as conclusive evidence in favor of offering metastasis-directed therapy	[39]

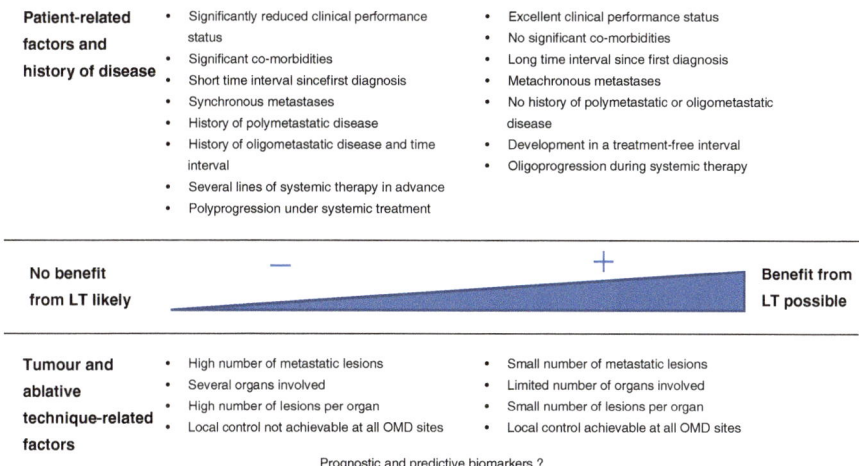

Fig. 7.1 Overview of relevant factors influencing the decision to offer local therapies (LT) to patients with OMD

Decisions should rely on published evidence and guideline recommendations. Patients need to be fully informed on the advantages and disadvantages of local treatment, as well as the scientific uncertainties, in a well-balanced way. If possible, local treatment of OMD should take place within a clinical trial.

Key Points
- Diligent workup of the patient's medical history, his/her general status, and the history of malignant disease are essential before treatment of OMD can be considered.
- Imaging in advance of any decision to offer local treatment to OMD should be comprehensive and sensitive, and should address all sites of common metastases for the primary tumor and its histology, in order to detect small lesions.
- Each patient with OMD should undergo individual assessment and review in a multidisciplinary tumor board.
- Patients need to be fully informed on the advantages and disadvantages of local treatment, as well as on the scientific uncertainties, in a well-balanced way.

References

1. Hellman S, Weichselbaum RR. Oligometastases. J Clin Oncol. 1995;13(1):8–10.
2. Milano MT, Biswas T, Simone CB 2nd, Lo SS. Oligometastases: history of a hypothesis. Ann Palliat Med. 2021;10(5):5923–30. https://doi.org/10.21037/apm.2020.03.31.
3. Hanahan D, Weinberg RA. The hallmarks of cancer. Cell. 2000;100(1):57–70.
4. Hanahan D, Weinberg RA. Hallmarks of cancer: the next generation. Cell. 2011;144(5):646–74.
5. Talmadge JE, Fidler IJ. AACR centennial series: the biology of cancer metastasis: historical perspective. Cancer Res. 2010;70(14):5649–69.
6. Fidler IJ. Tumor heterogeneity and the biology of cancer invasion and metastasis. Cancer Res. 1978;38(9):2651–60.
7. Fidler IJ. Commentary on "tumor heterogeneity and the biology of cancer invasion and metastasis". Cancer Res. 2016;76(12):3441–2.
8. Dillekas H, Rogers MS, Straume O. Are 90% of deaths from cancer caused by metastases? Cancer Med. 2019;8(12):5574–6.
9. Halsted WS. I. The results of operations for the cure of cancer of the breast performed at the Johns Hopkins Hospital from June, 1889, to January, 1894. Ann Surg. 1894;20(5):497–555.
10. Fisher B. Laboratory and clinical research in breast cancer—a personal adventure: the David A. Karnofsky memorial lecture. Cancer Res. 1980;40(11):3863–74.
11. Rubin P. Comment: are metastases curable? JAMA. 1968;204(7):612–3.
12. Palma DA, Salama JK, Lo SS, Senan S, Treasure T, Govindan R, et al. The oligometastatic state—separating truth from wishful thinking. Nat Rev Clin Oncol. 2014;11(9):549–57.
13. Guckenberger M, Lievens Y, Bouma AB, Collette L, Dekker A, deSouza NM, et al. Characterisation and classification of oligometastatic disease: a European Society for Radiotherapy and Oncology and European Organisation for Research and Treatment of Cancer consensus recommendation. Lancet Oncol. 2020;21(1):e18–28.
14. Lievens Y, Guckenberger M, Gomez D, Hoyer M, Iyengar P, Kindts I, et al. Defining oligometastatic disease from a radiation oncology perspective: an ESTRO-ASTRO consensus document. Radiother Oncol. 2020;148:157–66.
15. Postow MA, Callahan MK, Barker CA, Yamada Y, Yuan J, Kitano S, et al. Immunologic correlates of the abscopal effect in a patient with melanoma. N Engl J Med. 2012;366(10):925–31.
16. Hiniker SM, Chen DS, Knox SJ. Abscopal effect in a patient with melanoma. N Engl J Med. 2012;366(21):2035; author reply 2035–6.
17. Franklin JM, Sharma RA, Harris AL, Gleeson FV. Imaging oligometastatic cancer before local treatment. Lancet Oncol. 2016;17(9):e406–14.
18. Foster CC, Pitroda SP, Weichselbaum RR. Staging the metastatic spectrum through integration of clinical and molecular features. J Clin Oncol. 2019;37(15):1270–6.
19. Pitroda SP, Khodarev NN, Huang L, Uppal A, Wightman SC, Ganai S, et al. Integrated molecular subtyping defines a curable oligometastatic state in colorectal liver metastasis. Nat Commun. 2018;9(1):1793.
20. Haussmann J, Matuschek C, Bolke E, Orth K, Ghadjar P, Budach W. The role of local treatment in oligometastatic and oligoprogressive cancer. Dtsch Arztebl Int. 2019;116(50):849–56.
21. Boffa DJ. Local option: the rational use of local therapy in patients at high risk to die of metastatic progression. J Oncol Pract. 2018;14(6):344–9.
22. Scarborough JA, Tom MC, Scott JG. Revisiting a null hypothesis: exploring the parameters of oligometastasis treatment. Int J Radiat Oncol Biol Phys. 2021;110(2):371–81. https://doi.org/10.1016/j.ijrobp.2020.12.044.
23. Palma DA, Olson R, Harrow S, Gaede S, Louie AV, Haasbeek C, et al. Stereotactic ablative radiotherapy versus standard of care palliative treatment in patients with oligometastatic cancers (SABR-COMET): a randomised, phase 2, open-label trial. Lancet. 2019;393(10185):2051–8.
24. Palma DA, Olson R, Harrow S, Gaede S, Louie AV, Haasbeek C, et al. Stereotactic ablative radiotherapy for the comprehensive treatment of oligometastatic cancers: long-term results of the SABR-COMET phase II randomized trial. J Clin Oncol. 2020;38(25):2830–8.

25. Ruers T, Punt C, Van Coevorden F, Pierie J, Borel-Rinkes I, Ledermann JA, et al. Radiofrequency ablation combined with systemic treatment versus systemic treatment alone in patients with non-resectable colorectal liver metastases: a randomized EORTC Intergroup phase II study (EORTC 40004). Ann Oncol. 2012;23(10):2619–26.

26. Ruers T, Van Coevorden F, Punt CJ, Pierie JE, Borel-Rinkes I, Ledermann JA, et al. Local treatment of unresectable colorectal liver metastases: results of a randomized phase II trial. J Natl Cancer Inst. 2017;109(9):djx015.

27. Gomez DR, Blumenschein GR Jr, Lee JJ, Hernandez M, Ye R, Camidge DR, et al. Local consolidative therapy versus maintenance therapy or observation for patients with oligometastatic non-small-cell lung cancer without progression after first-line systemic therapy: a multicentre, randomised, controlled, phase 2 study. Lancet Oncol. 2016;17(12):1672–82.

28. Gomez DR, Tang C, Zhang J, Blumenschein GR Jr, Hernandez M, Lee JJ, et al. Local consolidative therapy vs. maintenance therapy or observation for patients with oligometastatic non-small-cell lung cancer: long-term results of a multi-institutional, phase II, randomized study. J Clin Oncol. 2019;37(18):1558–65.

29. Iyengar P, Wardak Z, Gerber DE, Tumati V, Ahn C, Hughes RS, et al. Consolidative radiotherapy for limited metastatic non-small-cell lung cancer: a phase 2 randomized clinical trial. JAMA Oncol. 2018;4(1):e173501.

30. Gore EM, Hu C, Sun AY, Grimm DF, Ramalingam SS, Dunlap NE, et al. Randomized phase II study comparing prophylactic cranial irradiation alone to prophylactic cranial irradiation and consolidative extracranial irradiation for extensive-disease small cell lung cancer (ED SCLC): NRG oncology RTOG 0937. J Thorac Oncol. 2017;12(10):1561–70.

31. Phillips R, Shi WY, Deek M, Radwan N, Lim SJ, Antonarakis ES, et al. Outcomes of observation vs stereotactic ablative radiation for oligometastatic prostate cancer: the ORIOLE phase 2 randomized clinical trial. JAMA Oncol. 2020;6(5):650–9.

32. Ost P, Reynders D, Decaestecker K, Fonteyne V, Lumen N, De Bruycker A, et al. Surveillance or metastasis-directed therapy for oligometastatic prostate cancer recurrence: a prospective, randomized, multicenter phase II trial. J Clin Oncol. 2018;36(5):446–53.

33. Boeve LMS, Hulshof M, Vis AN, Zwinderman AH, Twisk JWR, Witjes WPJ, et al. Effect on survival of androgen deprivation therapy alone compared to androgen deprivation therapy combined with concurrent radiation therapy to the prostate in patients with primary bone metastatic prostate cancer in a prospective randomised clinical trial: data from the HORRAD trial. Eur Urol. 2019;75(3):410–8.

34. Parker CC, James ND, Brawley CD, Clarke NW, Hoyle AP, Ali A, et al. Radiotherapy to the primary tumour for newly diagnosed, metastatic prostate cancer (STAMPEDE): a randomised controlled phase 3 trial. Lancet. 2018;392(10162):2353–66.

35. You R, Liu YP, Huang PY, Zou X, Sun R, He YX, et al. Efficacy and safety of locoregional radiotherapy with chemotherapy vs chemotherapy alone in de novo metastatic nasopharyngeal carcinoma: a multicenter phase 3 randomized clinical trial. JAMA Oncol. 2020;6(9):1345–52.

36. Van Cutsem E, Cervantes A, Adam R, Sobrero A, Van Krieken JH, Aderka D, et al. ESMO consensus guidelines for the management of patients with metastatic colorectal cancer. Ann Oncol. 2016;27(8):1386–422.

37. Planchard D, Popat S, Kerr K, Novello S, Smit EF, Faivre-Finn C, et al. Metastatic non-small cell lung cancer: ESMO Clinical Practice Guidelines for diagnosis, treatment and follow-up. Ann Oncol. 2018;29(Suppl 4):iv192–237.

38. Cardoso F, Paluch-Shimon S, Senkus E, Curigliano G, Aapro MS, Andre F, et al. 5th ESO-ESMO international consensus guidelines for advanced breast cancer (ABC 5) (dagger). Ann Oncol. 2020;31(12):1623–49.

39. Parker C, Castro E, Fizazi K, Heidenreich A, Ost P, Procopio G, et al. Prostate cancer: ESMO Clinical Practice Guidelines for diagnosis, treatment and follow-up. Ann Oncol. 2020;31(9):1119–34.

Brachytherapy of Primary Liver Lesions

8

Konrad Mohnike and Matthias Lampe

Interstitial brachytherapy (iBT) of primary liver tumors—hepatocellular and chol-angiocellular carcinomas—has by now become established at specialized centers. There are a number of features that distinguish these procedures from iBT of, for example, colorectal liver metastases. This affects the choice of dose and also certain safety aspects, in consideration of the liver's pre-interventional function. Moreover, for hepatocellular carcinoma (HCC) there are other recognized local therapeutic procedures such as surgical resection, transarterial chemoembolization (TACE), and radio-frequency ablation (RFA); these are dealt with in the respective guidelines and there is thus a need for a well-founded indication for iBT (Fig. 8.1). Tumor size (above 3–5 cm) and location (hilum of the liver, gall-bladder bed, subcapsular loca-tion, or proximity to large blood-vessels) are relative or absolute contraindications for RFA, as are the absence of a tumor blush in angiography, a portal-arterial throm-bosis on the tumor side, and, for TACE, tumor size [1–3]. Furthermore, there are patients who can profit more from ^{90}Y radioembolization or from one of the sys-temic therapy options. Patients who meet the Milan criteria will also be considered for a potentially curative liver transplantation, and the choice of bridging therapy is of especial importance for such patients (Fig. 8.2, Milan criteria).

A prospective, explorative study of iBT was conducted with 83 HCC patients (Child–Pugh class A 64%, class B 36%; BCLC stage A 61%, stage B 14%, stage C

K. Mohnike (✉)
Department of Diagnostics, Department of Interventional Oncology & Radionuclide Therapy, Diagnostic Therapeutic Center Berlin, Berlin, Germany

Department of Radiology and Nuclear Medicine, University Hospital Magdeburg, Magdeburg, Germany
e-mail: konrad.mohnike@berlin-dtz.de

M. Lampe
Department of Radiation Oncology, Diagnostic Therapeutic Center Berlin, Berlin, Germany
e-mail: matthias.lampe@berlin-dtz.de

© The Author(s), under exclusive license to Springer Nature Switzerland AG 2021
K. Mohnike et al. (eds.), *Manual on Image-Guided Brachytherapy of Inner Organs*, https://doi.org/10.1007/978-3-030-78079-1_8

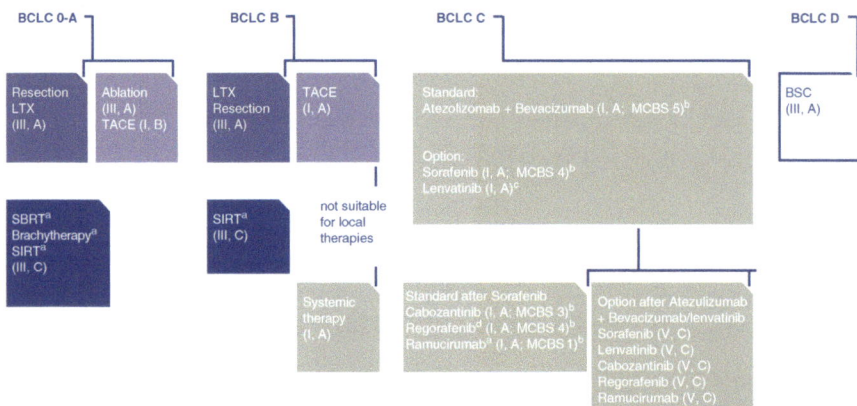

Fig. 8.1 Hepatocellular carcinoma: Treatment options according to the ESMO guidelines and depending on BCLC stage. [a]Non-standard, alternative treatment. [b]ESMO-MCBS v1.1 score for new therapy/indication approved by the EMA since 1 January 2016. The score has been calculated by the ESMO-MCBS Working Group and validated by the ESMO Guidelines Committee. [c]Non-inferiority to sorafenib established; no evaluable benefit. [d]Regorafenib is not recommended in TKI-naive patients. [e]Ramucirumab is only recommended in patients with an AFP level ≥ 400 ng/mL

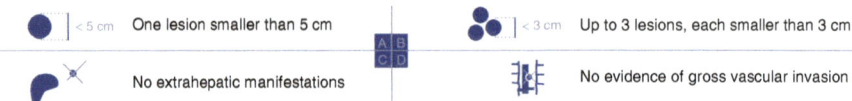

Fig. 8.2 Milan criteria, applied for liver transplantation as a curative treatment for patients with hepatocellular carcinoma and liver cirrhosis

24%) and a total of 140 liver lesions. The patients' planned doses were between 15 and 25 Gy. Of the 126 lesions followed up by imaging, 5 (4%) recurred locally. The median diameter of the largest lesion in each patient was 5.2 cm (range 1–15 cm). No dependence upon dose within the planned range of 15–25 Gy was observed; therefore, in clinical routine, HCC is treated according to the individual's tumor characteristics with a planned dose between 15 and 20 Gy. In the study, 114 lesions (median tumor diameter 3.1 cm, range 1–12 cm) were ablated unilaterally and 12 very large HCCs (median tumor diameter 11.3 cm, range 6–15 cm) were treated bi- or trilaterally. The local freedom from recurrence (LFR) rate after 12 months was 96% for the smaller, unilaterally treated HCCs and 91% for the larger, multilaterally treated HCCs. Thus, even with this relatively small patient collective, it proved possible to show that large or very large tumors also respond well to—if appropriate, multilateral—treatment.

The primary endpoint was time to any progression of disease (time to progression, TTP). Median TTP was 12 months for the smaller, unilaterally treated lesions; for the larger, multilaterally treated ones it was 8.4 months. The median follow-up time for overall survival (OS) was 33.8 months, and the median OS for all patients was 19.4 months.

A univariate analysis revealed that OS—after inclusion in the study or after the first diagnosis of HCC—depended upon the CLIP score (for CLIP = 0, 46.3 and 58.9 months, respectively; for CLIP ≥ 3, 8.3 and 13.5 months) and upon the BCLC stage and tumor diameter. Multivariate analysis detected only the CLIP score as a significant factor. A matched-pair analysis was performed with 57 pairs of patients who fulfilled all criteria for matching; each pair comprised one patient treated by iBT and one patient from a control group of patients who had been treated by a different regimen not including iBT. A significant difference in OS following initial diagnosis was found: 37.5 months in der brachytherapy group and 18 months in the control group ($p < 0.001$) [4].

An interesting study of the multimodal, systemic, and interventional treatment of intrahepatic cholangiocellular carcinoma (CCC) has been performed. Patients had been treated both by local therapies such as iBT, but also by RFA or locoregional procedures such as radioembolization (RE), or by intraarterial chemotherapy with 5-fluorouracil, or by systemic chemotherapy. iBT (the procedure predominantly used) at a planned dose of 20 Gy, alongside RFA, achieved the best result in terms of complete response. Median OS, from the time of first diagnosis or first intervention, was 33.1 and 16 months, respectively [5]. In a study by another group, 15 patients were treated; the mean tumor target volume was 131 mL (range 10–257 mL) and a median LFR of 10 months with a median OS of 14 months was achieved [6] (Fig. 8.3, patient example CCC).

Collettini et al. have reported on the efficacy of iBT in large (diameter 5–7 cm) and very large (7–12 cm) HCC tumors in patients with liver cirrhosis in Child–Pugh stage A or B. The mean planned dose was 15.8 Gy. After a median follow-up period of 12.8 months, two local recurrences were identified (2 of 30 patients with imaging follow-up, 7%), both were treated successfully by repeated brachytherapy. The mean OS was 15.4 months [7].

Tselis et al. treated 41 patients with 50 liver tumors of various kinds and a tumor size of more than 4 cm (median clinical target volume 84 cm³, range 38–1348 cm³) that were close to the liver hilum. Unlike other groups, they used a fractionation scheme with fractions between 4 and 14 Gy being administered once or twice a day, amounting to a median physical dose of 20 Gy (range 7–32 Gy). After a median follow-up period of 12.4 months, the 12-month LFR for liver metastases was 73%, and for primary liver tumor 81% [8].

The evidence adduced above demonstrates the efficacy of iBT even for large tumors and for those in difficult locations (Fig. 8.4, patient example HCC).

Interstitial Brachytherapy and Transarterial Chemoembolization in Patients with Hepatocellular Carcinomas: Comparison in a Randomized Study

Early studies demonstrated the high local efficacy of iBT, even in large hepatocellular carcinomas, but at the same time they revealed a higher complication rate compared with the treatment of metastases, especially in patients with advanced

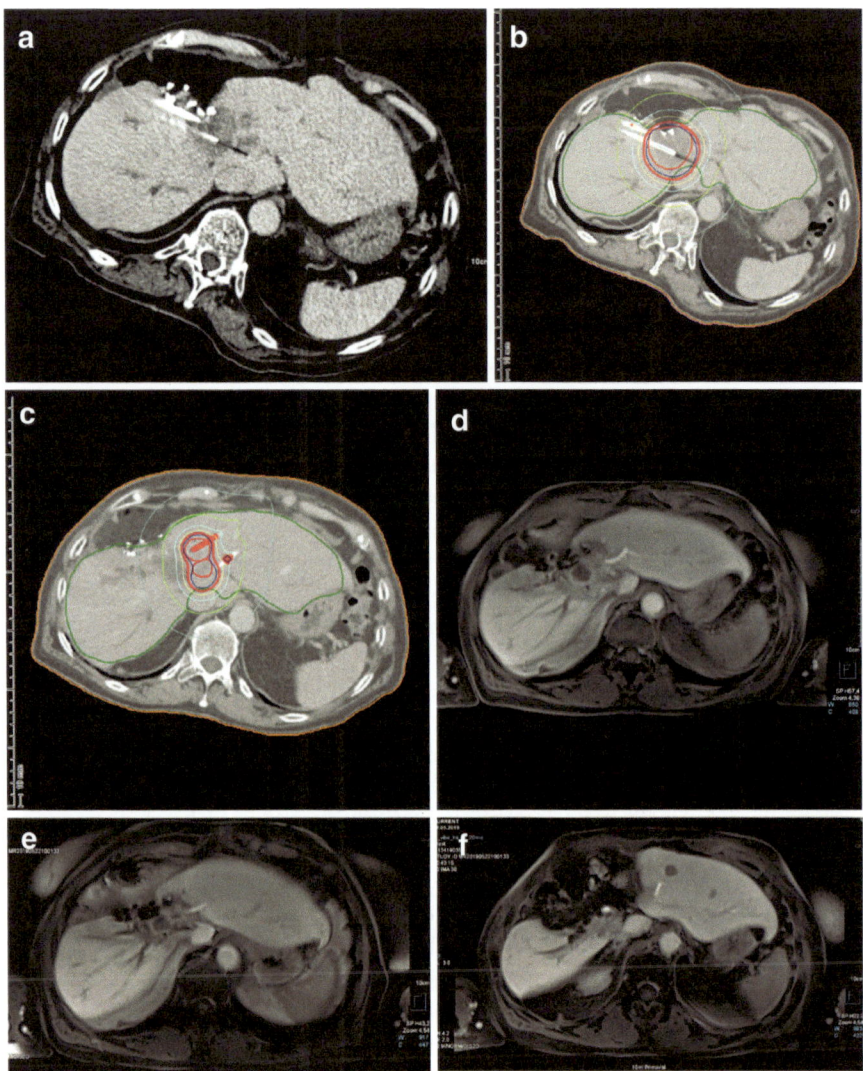

Fig. 8.3 Patient example: 80-year-old female patient with recurrent cholangiocellular carcinoma. Extended resection of segment 4 with cholecystectomy in June 2016. Local relapse (LR) in 2018 (**a**). CT-guided brachytherapy of the LR and satellite lesions in two treatment sessions in October and November 2018 (**b**, **c**). Remission in the MRI-scan 3 months (**d**) and 6 months (**e**) after treatment; 6 months after treatment new lesion in segment 3 (**f**), subsequent third iBT (**g**)

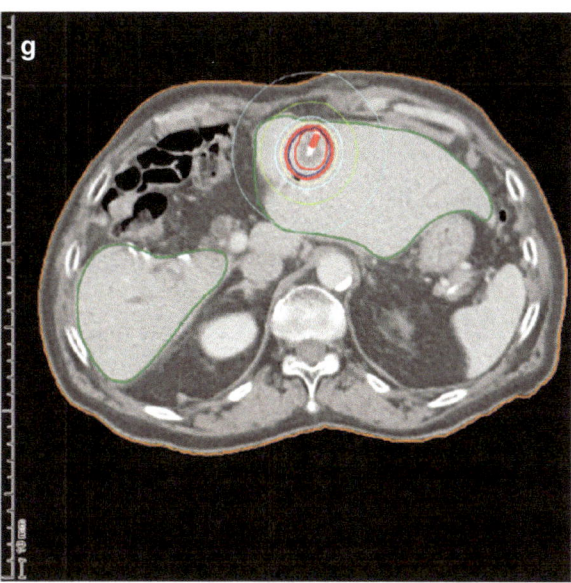

Fig. 8.3 (continued)

liver cirrhosis. These complications include above all intervention-related effects such as hemorrhage [4, 9].

TACE is the standard therapeutic procedure for patients in BCLC stage B [10]. In randomized studies performed in the early 2000s, patients treated by TACE showed a significant advantage in terms of survival compared with those receiving tamoxifen or only best supportive care [11].

In a prospective, randomized study, 77 patients with HCC were treated either by CT-guided iBT or by conventional transarterial chemoembolization (cTACE, with Lipiodol and doxorubicin). The primary endpoint was the time to untreatable progression (TTUP), in this case to local progression that was no longer treatable by the modality to which the patient had been randomized. Secondary endpoints included TTP and OS. Major inclusion criteria were a histologically confirmed HCC (44%) or, if liver cirrhosis was present, an image-confirmed HCC (66%), according to the criteria of the European Association for the Study of the Liver (EASL); non-resectability; and an estimated life expectancy of more than 16 weeks [12, 13]. Principal exclusion criteria were portal-vein thrombosis (PVT) on the tumor side, extrahepatic manifestations, liver cirrhosis at Child–Pugh stage C and any other carcinoma. The treatment arm and the control group did not differ in respect of numerous aspects such as BCLC stage, Child–Pugh stage, age, α-1-fetoprotein (AFP) level, tumor diameter, number of lesions or etiology; only the pre-therapeutic bilirubin level in the cTACE group (18.9 µmol/L; interquartile range (IQR) 11.4–28.9 µmol/L) was significantly higher than in the iBT group (12.2 µmol/L; IQR 9.9–15.7 µmol/L; $p = 0.007$). 84% of the patients in the iBT group and 88% of those in the cTACE group were therapy-naïve. After untreatable progression (cf. the

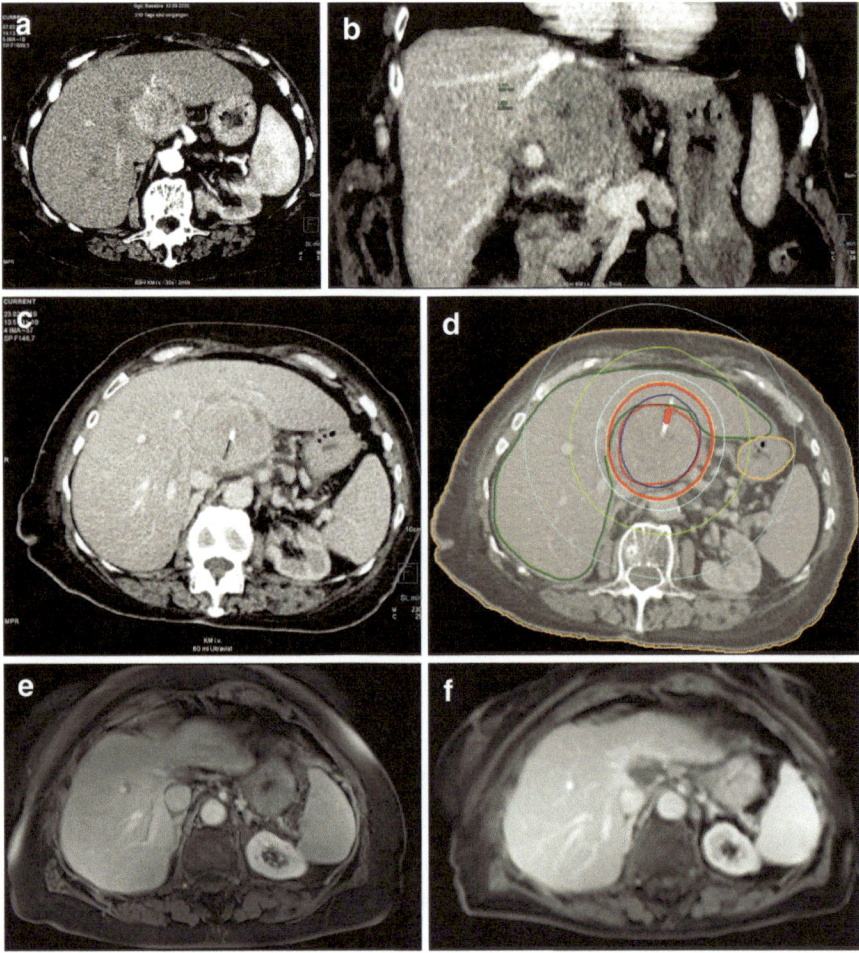

Fig. 8.4 Patient example: 79-year-old female patient (comorbidities: diabetes mellitus type 2, Parkinson's disease, COPD, permanent atrial fibrillation (Xarelto)) with hepatocellular carcinoma. History of breast cancer. 01/2018 First diagnosis of a hepatocellular carcinoma with central/left liver lobe; adjacent is a breast cancer liver metastasis (CT-guided biopsy proven). (**a, b**) Pre-interventional CE-CT scan. (**c**) CT scan after implantation of the iBT catheter. (**d**) Radiotherapy plan, isodose lines. (**e**) MRI, venous phase, 3 months after intervention. (**f**) MRI, venous phase, 30 months after intervention

primary endpoint, above) had been reached, there were no restrictions as regarded further therapies so that 14 patients in der cTACE group received iBT after the study had ended, while one patient in the iBT group received post-study cTACE (35% vs. 3%; $p < 0.001$). To avoid any bias that might have been introduced by the various (technically unavoidable and prospectively defined) withdrawal criteria, the patients concerned were censored on discovery at the time of occurrence (examples of such withdrawal criteria were for cTACE a PVT on the tumor side or the occurrence of arterioportal shunts; for iBT uncontrollable ascites or a severe coagulation disorder).

The study population analyzed comprised 39 per protocol (PP) patients in the iBT group and 38 in the cTACE group (intention to treat, 37 and 40, respectively). Longer TTUP and TTP were found for the patients in the iBT arm than for those in the cTACE arm, with a hazard ratio (PP) of 0.49 ($p = 0.019$ for TTUP and 0.011 for TTP). Especially patients at BCLC stage B profited more from iBT than from cTACE, which is significant, as BCLC stage B is the stage for which the guidelines recommend cTACE. The observation that this advantage was not reflected in OS may be associated with the limitations of this study, in which, in consequence of the study design, patients from the cTACE arm received iBT treatment once the primary endpoint had been reached.

Neither tumor diameter nor number of lesions had a statistically significant impact upon the variables for treatment outcome, in either the univariate or the multivariate analysis of the study results.

No significant differences in severe complications (Grade 3 or higher) were seen between the treatment arms in an intervention-based PP analysis (for iBT, 120 Interventions, for cTACE 163 interventions) [14].

The patient collective included patients at all BCLC stages and revealed relevant heterogeneity. In a pilot study, a matched-pair analysis of HCC patients with and without iBT had been performed, and this had revealed a significantly extended median OS for the patients in the iBT group (37.5 vs. 18 months, $p < 0.001$) [4].

For BCLC stage A, no advantage of iBT was detected in respect of the primary or secondary endpoints. On the one hand, iBT and cTACE were obviously similarly effective, for a limited number and size of lesions. On the other, it should be remarked that for small HCCs RFA offers an effective and guideline-compliant method that—especially for tumors up to 2 cm diameter—achieves good tumor control, with shorter hospital stays and lower procedural morbidity than those associated with surgical resection [15]. The frequently postulated oncological equivalence of RFA with surgical resection of HCC in early and very late stages, even with very early-detected HCCs of size below 2 cm, has been questioned in recent meta-analyses; these indicate a higher recurrence rate and lower 3- and 5-year survival rates among the RFA-treated patients. A selection bias appears possible [16, 17].

Interstitial Brachytherapy as a Bridging Therapy Before Liver Transplantation

Against the background of the dearth of donated organs in Germany and the consequently frequent need for bridging therapy for HCC patients on the transplantation list—including patients both within and, sometimes, outside the Milan criteria—a matched-pair analysis was conducted [18, 19].

To this end, 12 patients who had received iBT as a bridging therapy before liver transplantation were matched according to various criteria with 12 patients who had received TACE for the same purpose. In the histopathological assessment of outcomes after the liver transplantation, it was found that the lesions treated by iBT showed better tumor response than those treated by TACE; for complete tumor necrosis the respective response rates were 33 and 5%, for partial necrosis 58 and 36% ($p < 0.05$).

The overall tumor-volume necrosis rates (mean ± standard deviation) were 63% ± 10% for iBT and 22% ± 7% for TACE ($p = 0.002$). Among the assessable tumors with partial necrosis, the HCCs treated by iBT showed a lower degree of differentiation than those treated by TACE ($p = 0.041$). Puncture-tract metastases were not observed. In the histological assessment, 100% of the iBT-treated patients and 75% of the TACE-treated patients met all the Milan criteria. In a subgroup analysis of the patients who met the Milan criteria before bridging therapy, none experienced tumor recurrence after transplantation.

Despite the small number of patients, the result of this study is to be regarded as clinically relevant, on account of the correlation between the clinical and histopathological results. The value of iBT as a bridging therapy before liver transplantation should be tested more rigorously in larger-scale, prospective studies [20].

Prognostic Factors

Prognostically relevant factors were investigated in the multimodal therapy of 55 patients with CCC who had been treated with iBT, RFA, RE, and/or TACE, in some cases combined with intraarterial or intravenous chemotherapy. Median OS was 33.1 months from first diagnosis and 16 months from inclusion in the study. Multivariate regression analysis took account of—independently of one another—the number of tumor lesions, the level of the tumor markers CEA and CA-19 9, and the objective tumor response [5].

In univariate regression analysis of 83 prospectively assessed patients with HCC and a median OS of 19.4 months after first brachytherapy treatment, OS was correlated with CLIP score, BCLC stage, and the diameter of the respective patient's largest lesion, while in the multivariate analysis only the CLIP score's predictive power reached the significance level. In the meantime, BCLC stage has become established for the pre-therapeutic stratification of patients with HCC; this result was also obtained in a randomized study, as described above [4, 14]. The study in question revealed, in multivariate regression analysis, that significant factors influencing TTUP, independently of one another, were: female sex (HR 0.21, $p < 0.001$), belonging to the iBT arm (HR = 0.49, $p = 0.019$), AFP level (HR = 1.13, $p = 0.001$), and Child–Pugh stage B (HR = 3.81, $p = 0.036$). Significant factors independently influencing TTP were: belonging to the iBT arm (HR = 0.49, $p = 0.011$) and Child–Pugh stage B (HR = 3.12, $p = 0.045$). Significant factors independently influencing OS were: female sex (HR = 3.46, $p = 0.002$), AFP level (HR = 1.17, $p < 0.001$), and Child–Pugh stage B (HR = 5.76, $p = 0.006$).

Neither the univariate nor the multivariate analysis pointed to tumor diameter or number of lesions as having an influence, at the significance level, upon the outcome variables.

An intervention-based PP analysis (iBT, 120 interventions; cTACE, 163 interventions) revealed no significant difference between the two treatment arms in the numbers of serious complications (Grade 3 or above). A surprising result was the poorer outcome (overall and in both treatment groups) for the female patients, in respect both of TTUP (HR = 4.21) and of OS (HR = 3.6). This stands in contrast to current literature, at least for HBV-associated HCC, and should be investigated in further studies [21]. The influence of the stage of liver cirrhosis was considerable, as expected (HR = 3.81 for TTUP and 5.76 for OS) [14].

Safety

Safety aspects, against the background of liver cirrhosis, are discussed in detail in Chaps. 11 and 17. However, because of their importance, they are described briefly here as well.

To assess the influence of brachytherapy (and of ^{90}Y radioembolization) upon liver function in patients with an HCC and liver cirrhosis (Child–Pugh A or B), a study was performed in which liver-specific laboratory values were determined 3 days, 6 weeks, and 12 weeks after the intervention. For the 12 patients who received brachytherapy, the pre-therapeutic liver volume ranged from 708 to 2268 cm^3, CTV from 3.1 to 72.5 cm^3 (mean value 21 cm^3), and the 5 Gy volume of the liver from 2.6 to 20.3%. Low-grade elevations of aspartate aminotransferase and γ-glutamyl transferase were registered immediately after the intervention, while cholinesterase declined slightly. All relevant variables reverted after at most 12 weeks to their initial values. Thus, under the conditions of the study, it was shown that brachytherapy, even of large volumes within overall relatively small livers (for example, after partial resection of the liver) could safely be conducted in patients with cirrhosis and reduced liver function [22].

In pilot studies, a purely quantitatively higher 30-day mortality was observed in patients with HCC and liver cirrhosis (3/83, 4%) than in patients with colorectal liver metastases (0/73, 0%) [4, 23]. Moreover, in the abovementioned study with 83 HCC patients, among these patients two atypical, possible cases of RILD were observed.

In a study that is described in detail in Chap. 17, 192 patients were treated by liver iBT in 343 Interventions. The primary tumors included inter alia colorectal carcinomas, HCCs, CCCs, mammary carcinomas, and bronchial carcinomas. Of all tumors, 34.4% were between 5 and 10 cm in diameter, and 6.3% were above 10 cm. Of all patients, 26% had liver cirrhosis in Child–Pugh stage A or B. Two patients died within 30 days, one because of a fulminant hemorrhage of oesophageal varices and one because of neutropenic sepsis incurred through chemotherapy.

There was no instance of classical RILD. One patient with an HCC and hepatitis C, who received first iBT 22 months after partial liver resection, developed an atypical form of RILD with ascites and icteric elevation of hepatic enzymes. The patient received drug therapy, corresponding to prophylaxis of RILD, and after 7 months these values had completely returned to normal; the patient died slightly less than 2 years after receiving the last brachytherapy.

Severe bleeding occurred exclusively after intervention in patients with liver cirrhosis (5/89 vs. 0/254 patients, $p = 0.001$), and among these the group with moderately to severely impaired liver function predominated (Child–Pugh stage B, 3/13; stage A, 2/230; $p < 0.001$; Table 8.1). The pre-therapeutic thrombocyte count was a significant risk factor for this ($p = 0.043$), but the number of catheters inserted, prothrombin time, history of portal-vein thrombosis, and age were not (Table 8.1).

Table 8.1 Complications after iBT and subsequent treatments

Complication	No. of cases (%)[a]	Therapy[b]	Interval[c]
Major			
Bleeding CTCAE IV	1 (0.29)	Surgery, resolved	24 hours
Bleeding CTCAE III	4 (1.17)	DSA and/or PRBC, resolved	24 hours
Ascites CTCAE III	1 (0.29)[d]	Drainage and diuretics, resolved	48 hours
Ulcer, GI	3 (0.87)	Endoscopic intervention, resolved	5 weeks–8 months
Non-classic RILD	1 (0.5)[e]	Symptomatic, UDC[f], resolved	7 weeks
Liver abscess	4 (1.17)[g]	Drainage and antibiotics, resolved	4 days–8 months
Bile duct occlusion[h]	1 (0.29)	Endoscopic stenting, resolved	1 week
30-day mortality	2 (1.0)[e]		
Minor			
Bleeding CTCAE I	9 (3.21)	None, resolved	24 hours
Pleural effusion CTCAE I	31 (10.8)	None, resolved	24–72 hours
Pleural effusion CTCAE II	4 (1.40)[i]	Thoracentesis, resolved	24–72 hours
Pneumothorax CTCAE I	4 (1.40)	None, resolved	24 hours
Pneumothorax CTCAE II	1 (0.35)	Chest tube, resolved	24 hours
Ascites CTCAE I	2 (0.71)	None, resolved	24–72 hours

[a]Percentages for major complications: based on total of 343 iBT procedures; for minor complications: based on the number of imagings performed 3 days after intervention (abdomen: 280, chest: 286)

[b]Therapy to treat given event, *DSA* digital subtraction angiography with embolization, *PBRC* packed red blood cells

[c]Usual time after iBT that event was observed. Some cases of hematoma/hemorrhage, pneumothorax occurred during the procedure, *h* hour, *d* day, *w* week, *m* month

[d]Increased from pre-interventional Grade I

[e]Percentage: patient-based

[f]*UDC* ursodeoxycholic acid

[g]One abscess was related to percutaneous transhepatic cholangio drainage

[h]Oedema-related occlusion of a central bile tract

[i]Two increased from pre-interventional Grade I

Against this background, possible accompanying anticoagulatory treatment with low-molecular-weight heparin (LMWH) should be viewed especially critically. In a study, 446 cancer patients were treated for tumors located in the liver, lung, kidney, lymph nodes, and elsewhere; this included 781 tumor ablations (669 with iBT and 112 with RFA), with ($N = 260$) or without ($N = 521$) peri-interventional administration of LMWH, intended as prophylaxis. A total of 63 bleeding events (of any grade) were observed, and these were significantly more frequent in the group of patients who received prophylaxis than among those who did not (for all interventions, respectively 11.7% and 6.3%, $p = 0.0127$; for hepatic interventions 12.7% and 7.1%, $p = 0.0416$). In uni- and multivariate analyses of the results, the administration of LMWH was the only factor found to be constantly and significantly associated with frequency of bleeding events. The 30- and 90-day mortality rates were independent of the subsequent therapy (angiographic embolization or surgery) and were considerably higher (23.1% and 38.5%, respectively) among the patients with severe bleeding than among those with no bleeding events or only mild ones (0.5% and 2.3%; $p < 0.0001$). Post-interventional administration of LMWH did not raise the frequency of bleedings [24].

There are indications that the presence of a biliodigestive anastomosis increases the post-interventional rate of abscess occurrence, as is known to be the case for TACE and TAE [25–27]. Our own experience from an as yet unpublished study of iBT combined with drug-based tumor therapy in CCC supports this.

Key Points
- iBT is capable of achieving high to very high rates of tumor control in primary liver tumors, up to >90% after 12 months, even for large or very large tumors.
- A dose-dependence was demonstrated, and primary liver tumors could be brought excellently under control with a 15–20 Gy radiation dose.
- In a randomized study, superiority of iBT compared with transarterial chemoembolization was shown, with significantly longer time to progression and time to untreatable progression.
- For iBT in the treatment of patients with hepatocellular carcinoma and advanced liver cirrhosis, there are indications of a greater risk of hemorrhage compared with patients who have secondary neoplasms, although the total number of severe bleedings is still low to moderate.
- A biliodigestive anastomosis or history of papillotomy may increase the risk of post-interventional cholangitis or liver abscesses.
- Classical radiation-induced liver disorders have not been observed in our own studies or reported in the literature by other centers, although isolated, atypical cases of icteric increase in liver enzymes or ascites have been observed.

References

1. Marcacuzco Quinto A, Nutu OA, San Román Manso R, et al. Complications of transarterial chemoembolization (TACE) in the treatment of liver tumors. Cir Esp. 2018;96:560–7.
2. Nakazawa T, Kokubu S, Shibuya A, et al. Radiofrequency ablation of hepatocellular carcinoma: correlation between local tumor progression after ablation and ablative margin. AJR Am J Roentgenol. 2007;188:480–8.
3. Sacco R, Tapete G, Simonetti N, et al. Transarterial chemoembolization for the treatment of hepatocellular carcinoma: a review. J Hepatocell Carcinoma. 2017;4:105–10.
4. Mohnike K, Wieners G, Schwartz F, et al. Computed tomography-guided high-dose-rate brachytherapy in hepatocellular carcinoma: safety, efficacy, and effect on survival. Int J Radiat Oncol Biol Phys. 2010;78:172–9.
5. Seidensticker R, Seidensticker M, Doegen K, et al. Extensive use of interventional therapies improves survival in unresectable or recurrent intrahepatic cholangiocarcinoma. Gastroenterol Res Pract. 2016;2016:8732521.
6. Schnapauff D, Denecke T, Grieser C, et al. Computed tomography-guided interstitial HDR brachytherapy (CT-HDRBT) of the liver in patients with irresectable intrahepatic cholangiocarcinoma. Cardiovasc Intervent Radiol. 2012;35:581–7.
7. Collettini F, Schnapauff D, Poellinger A, et al. Hepatocellular carcinoma: computed-tomography-guided high-dose-rate brachytherapy (CT-HDRBT) ablation of large (5-7 cm) and very large (>7 cm) tumours. Eur Radiol. 2012;22:1101–9.
8. Tselis N, Chatzikonstantinou G, Kolotas C, Milickovic N, Baltas D, Zamboglou N. Computed tomography-guided interstitial high dose rate brachytherapy for centrally located liver tumours: a single institution study. Eur Radiol. 2013;23:2264–70.
9. Mohnike K, Wolf S, Damm R, et al. Radioablation of liver malignancies with interstitial high-dose-rate brachytherapy : complications and risk factors. Strahlenther Onkol. 2016;192:288–96.
10. Bruix J, Reig M, Sherman M. Evidence-based diagnosis, staging, and treatment of patients with hepatocellular carcinoma. Gastroenterology. 2016;150:835–53.
11. Llovet JM, Bruix J. Systematic review of randomized trials for unresectable hepatocellular carcinoma: chemoembolization improves survival. Hepatology. 2003;37:429–42.
12. Bruix J, Sherman M, Llovet JM, et al. Clinical management of hepatocellular carcinoma. Conclusions of the Barcelona-2000 EASL conference. European Association for the Study of the Liver. J Hepatol. 2001;35:421–30.
13. Bruix J, Sherman M, Practice Guidelines Committee, American Association for the Study of Liver Diseases. Management of hepatocellular carcinoma. Hepatology. 2005;42:1208–36.
14. Mohnike K, Steffen IG, Seidensticker M, et al. Radioablation by image-guided (HDR) brachytherapy and transarterial chemoembolization in hepatocellular carcinoma: a randomized phase II trial. Cardiovasc Intervent Radiol. 2019;42:239–49.
15. Livraghi T, Meloni F, Di Stasi M, et al. Sustained complete response and complications rates after radiofrequency ablation of very early hepatocellular carcinoma in cirrhosis: is resection still the treatment of choice? Hepatology. 2008;47:82–9.
16. Xu XL, Liu XD, Liang M, Luo BM. Radiofrequency ablation versus hepatic resection for small hepatocellular carcinoma: systematic review of randomized controlled trials with meta-analysis and trial sequential analysis. Radiology. 2018;287:461–72.
17. Yin Z, Jin H, Ma T, Zhou Y, Yu M, Jian Z. A meta-analysis of long-term survival outcomes between surgical resection and radiofrequency ablation in patients with single hepatocellular carcinoma </= 2cm (BCLC very early stage). Int J Surg. 2018;56:61–7.
18. Bismuth H, Chiche L, Adam R, Castaing D, Diamond T, Dennison A. Liver resection versus transplantation for hepatocellular carcinoma in cirrhotic patients. Ann Surg. 1993;218:145–51.
19. Mazzaferro V, Regalia E, Doci R, et al. Liver transplantation for the treatment of small hepatocellular carcinomas in patients with cirrhosis. N Engl J Med. 1996;334:693–9.

20. Denecke T, Stelter L, Schnapauff D, et al. CT-guided interstitial brachytherapy of hepatocellular carcinoma before liver transplantation: an equivalent alternative to transarterial chemoembolization? Eur Radiol. 2015;25:2608–16.
21. Li Y, Xu A, Jia S, Huang J. Recent advances in the molecular mechanism of sex disparity in hepatocellular carcinoma. Oncol Lett. 2019;17:4222–8.
22. Ruhl R, Seidensticker M, Peters N, et al. Hepatocellular carcinoma and liver cirrhosis: assessment of the liver function after Yttrium-90 radioembolization with resin microspheres or after CT-guided high-dose-rate brachytherapy. Dig Dis. 2009;27:189–99.
23. Ricke J, Mohnike K, Pech M, et al. Local response and impact on survival after local ablation of liver metastases from colorectal carcinoma by computed tomography-guided high-dose-rate brachytherapy. Int J Radiat Oncol Biol Phys. 2010;78:479–85.
24. Mohnike K, Sauerland H, Seidensticker M, et al. Haemorrhagic complications and symptomatic venous thromboembolism in interventional tumour ablations: the impact of peri-interventional thrombosis prophylaxis. Cardiovasc Intervent Radiol. 2016;39:1716–21.
25. Wieners G, Schippers AC, Collettini F, et al. CT-guided high-dose-rate brachytherapy in the interdisciplinary treatment of patients with liver metastases of pancreatic cancer. Hepatobiliary Pancreat Dis Int. 2015;14:530–8.
26. Huang SF, Ko CW, Chang CS, Chen GH. Liver abscess formation after transarterial chemoembolization for malignant hepatic tumor. Hepatogastroenterology. 2003;50:1115–8.
27. Kim W, Clark TW, Baum RA, Soulen MC. Risk factors for liver abscess formation after hepatic chemoembolization. J Vasc Interv Radiol. 2001;12:965–8.

Ablation of Liver Metastases by Brachytherapy

Max Seidensticker and Marc Mühlmann

Various local ablative and locoregional therapeutic techniques have been shown to be safe and effective in treating liver metastases of different cancer entities. It is critical to recognize that not only treatment modality, but also patient selection can have a profound impact both on the success of the treatment and on the safety and well-being of the patient. In general, local techniques such as brachytherapy allow complete tumor ablation with excellent local tumor control (LTC), thereby making possible a curatively intended therapeutic approach, as compared with locoregional techniques, which frequently only achieve partial remission and therefore are more commonly used in a palliative setting. Thus, local ablation is the preferred approach, where this is possible. The choice of technique (local ablation or locoregional treatment) is influenced mainly by the tumor(s) number, size, and location. Local thermoablative techniques are more suitable in the treatment of fewer (<3, possibly up to 5) and smaller (<3 cm, possibly up to 5 cm) tumors which are not located adjacent to the liver hilum or the surrounding organs (stomach, colon, duodenum, heart). Accordingly, not all tumors qualify for thermal ablation: (1) Proximity of the target to large intrahepatic vessels (veins and portal branches) leads to a heat-sink effect in the ablation zone and an increased risk of incomplete ablation (applies mainly for RFA, in part for MWA) [1]; (2) proximity of the target to the liver hilum entails the risk of damage to heat-vulnerable structures (mainly bile ducts) [2, 3]; (3) a peripheral location of the target, with proximity to heat-vulnerable organs (gall bladder, stomach, colon, duodenum, heart) entails the risk of organ damage or perforation [4]. Tumors with these characteristics can sometimes be treated by hepatic resection, especially when they are located at the periphery. In many cases where the

M. Seidensticker (✉) · M. Mühlmann
Department of Radiology, Ludwig Maximilian University (LMU) Hospital Munich, Munich, Germany
e-mail: Max.seidensticker@med.uni-muenchen.de; Marc.muehlmann@med.uni-muenchen.de

patient is considered unsuitable for surgery, locoregional techniques—including TACE, ^{90}Y radioembolization (TARE), or SBRT—are used as an alternative treatment, albeit with a potentially higher nontarget tissue exposure and a limited applicability in larger tumors. However, local radioablation by image-guided brachytherapy (iBT) expands the scope of application of true local ablation to lesion sizes above 5 cm and to tumor locations unfavorable for thermoablation.

In this chapter, we summarize the literature on local radioablation by iBT for various tumor entities, and we present data on local control rate and overall survival (OS).

It should be noted, as a general point, that local ablation in more common cancers (e.g., CRC) and in relatively rare ones (e.g., sarcoma or oesophageal carcinoma) was, in most of the literature reviewed here, performed in heavily pretreated patients and in the presence of oligometastatic disease. (The latter could possibly be defined as non-rapid progressive disease with metastasis in up to two or three organ sites and up to five manifestations, predominantly visceral or lymph-nodal) [5]. This could be a source of bias; therefore, the data summarized (especially OS data) should be interpreted with this in mind. Consequently, the focus should be on local control rate.

Local Radioablation by Catheter-Based Radiotherapy (Brachytherapy)

In contrast to thermally based ablative techniques, iBT employs radiation to induce tumor apoptosis. For this purpose, a radioactive source (Iridium-192, for high dose rate) is positioned temporarily within the lumen of a catheter that was placed fluoroscopically within the tumor under guidance by CT or MRI. Frequently, several catheters are used, to aid the organ-sparing 3D dosimetry. The aim is to cover the whole tumor in a single session, with a local tumor-enclosing dose D100 of 15–25 Gy (depending on the tumor entity). Since the radiation is applied from inside to outside, the complications and restrictions associated with stereotactic irradiation can be avoided or minimized. Nontarget radiation exposure is lower in iBT, as more precise dosimetry can be performed without accounting for movement of the liver during radiation application. From a technical point of view tumor size, heat-sink effect, and, in part, proximity to vulnerable adjacent structures constitute far less strict limitations upon iBT—in some cases no limitations at all (for case examples see Fig. 9.1). In addition, the exposure of adjacent organs can be decided during dosimetry planning, and known normal tissue tolerance doses can be included in the dosimetry planning in order to avoid toxicity in the normal tissue; further measures, such as temporarily inserted inflatable balloons, can decrease the exposure of adjacent tissue and allow full dose coverage of the target tumors [6].

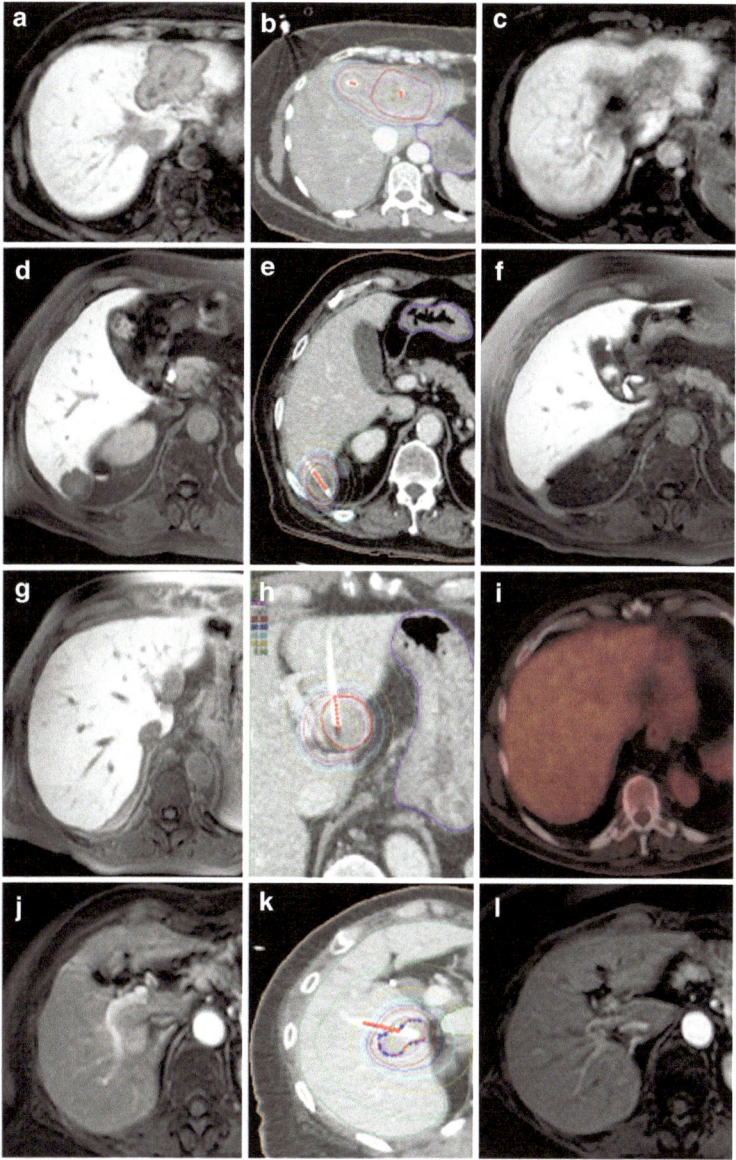

Fig. 9.1 Case examples. (**a–c**) Patient with metastatic breast cancer (**a**, pretreatment MRI, hepatobiliary phase, with a large metastasis in the left liver lobe; **b**, iBT with a D100 of 15 Gy; **c**, 12-month follow-up MRI with complete necrosis and residual hepatic scar). (**d–f**) Patient with metastatic colorectal cancer (**d**, pretreatment MRI, hepatobiliary phase, with a small metastasis in liver segment 6; **e**, iBT with a D100 of 25 Gy; **f**, 18-month follow-up MRI with complete necrosis). (**g–i**) Patient with metastatic colorectal cancer (**g**, pretreatment MRI, hepatobiliary phase, with a small metastasis in liver segment 3 with close proximity to the main left bile duct; **h**, iBT with a D100 of 25 Gy; **i**, 2.5-year follow-up PET CT with complete remission). (**j–l**) Patient with metastatic neuroendocrine cancer (**j**, pretreatment MRI, portal-venous phase, with a large metastasis in direct proximity to the main right portal stem; **k**, iBT with a D100 of 20 Gy; **l**, 24-month follow-up MRI (arterial phase) with complete response and patent adjacent vascular structures

Local Tumor Control

Colorectal Cancer Liver Metastases

The efficacy of iBT is high, as displayed by local control rate ranges from 76 to 88.3% (at 12 months) for 138 ablated lesions with sizes of 1–12 cm (median 4.6 cm) and 179 ablated lesions with sizes of 0.8–10.7 cm (median 2.85 cm) [7, 8]. Local tumor control after iBT of colorectal liver metastases demonstrated a strong dose dependence. Local tumor progression occurred in 1 of 33 (3%) lesions treated with a D100 of 18.8 Gy (46.3 months median time to local progression), compared with local tumor progression of 34.7% among 98 lesions treated with a D100 of only 12.8 Gy (27.1 months median time to local progression) [9]. If possible, 25 Gy should be administered as D100.

Breast Cancer Liver Metastases

The efficacy of iBT is very high, as exemplified by local control rates from 93.5% to 94.6% (at 12 months) for 115 tumors with sizes of 1.0–11 cm (median 4.4 cm) and 80 tumors 0.8–7.4 cm (median 2.6 cm), respectively [10, 11]. Breast cancer is radiosensitive, and a D100 of 15 Gy is sufficient to achieve ablation.

Neuroendocrine Tumors Liver Metastases

The efficacy of iBT is very high, as demonstrated by local control rates of 92% (at 12 months) and 83% (at 36 months) for 52 ablated tumors with sizes of 0.7–11.0 cm (median 2.1 cm) when treated with a D100 of 15–20 Gy [12].

Renal Cancer Liver Metastases

The efficacy of iBT is very high, as demonstrated by local control rates from 92.6% (at 10.2 months) to 93.8% (at 21.6 months) for 16 lesions with sizes of 1–8.2 cm (median 3.8 cm) and for 54 ablated tumors with the size of 0.5–13.9 cm (median 1.8 cm), the latter irradiated with a median D100 of 16 Gy [13, 14].

Liver Metastases of Other Cancer Entities

Regardless of entity, the efficacy of liver metastasis treated by iBT, as described by the local control rate, remains high.

For liver metastases of anal carcinoma, the local control rate has been reported as 97.4% (at 15.2 months) for 28 lesions with sizes of 0.4–6.2 cm (median 1.2 cm) when ablated with a mean D100 of 16.2 Gy [15].

For GIST metastases the local control rate has been reported as 97.5% (at 25 months) for 40 ablated tumors (30 liver, 10 peritoneal) with sizes of 0.6–11.2 cm (median 2.4 cm) when ablated with a mean D100 of 15 Gy [16].

For gastroesophageal carcinoma, the local control rate has been reported to range from 89 to 100% (at 8.3 months) in 36 tumors (location: 29 liver, 2 nodal, 5 others) with sizes of 1–10.2 cm (median 2 cm) when treated with (on average) a D100 of 19.9 Gy, and for 12 tumors with sizes of 1.4–6.8 cm (median 4.6 cm) when ablated with a target dose for D100 of 15–20 Gy [17, 18]. An overview of the studies reviewed is provided in Table 9.1.

Overall Survival/Survival Rate

As stated above, OS numbers are probably biased by lead time and selection. Furthermore, published results are for cohorts at single centers and patient numbers are small.

For example, we have only a few data about the context of treatment (treatment of progressive lesions under chemotherapy or treatment of stable or residual lesions after chemotherapy). However, overall, data are in line with published data on thermal ablation. Therefore, we can cautiously conclude that the results from thermal ablation can be extended to iBT treatment of tumors that are not eligible for thermal ablation but may be eligible for iBT.

Colorectal Cancer Liver Metastases

Median OS after iBT of colorectal liver metastases has been reported to range from 18 to 23.4 months and peaks around 26.3 months when iBT is combined with chemotherapy. Patients were usually pretreated by chemotherapy or had been chemorefractory [8, 9].

Breast Cancer Liver Metastases

The median OS after iBT of breast cancer liver metastases has been reported to range from 18 to 21.9 months. Patients were mostly pretreated by chemotherapy (83.8–95% of the patients) or had been chemorefractory [11, 19].

Neuroendocrine Tumors Liver Metastases

The median OS after iBT of neuroendocrine cancer liver metastases has been reported as 36 months. Patients were mostly pretreated by chemotherapy and/or had been chemorefractory [12].

Table 9.1 Brachytherapy of liver metastases. *CRC* colorectal carcinoma, *NET* neuroendocrine tumor, *GIST* gastrointestinal stroma tumor, *GE-CA* gastroesophageal carcinoma, *CTX* chemotherapy, *LTC* local tumor control, *HAIC* hepatic arterial infusion chemotherapy, *STRT* stereotactic radiotherapy, *n/a* no information available, *FU* follow-up, *m* month(s), *avg* average

Entity	Study (year)	Patients (% male)	Lesion count	Lesion size	D100	LTCR at FU (month)	OS median (range)	Additional information
CRC	Collettini (2014)	80 (75%)	179	2.85 cm (0.8–10.7 cm)	19.1 Gy (15–20 Gy)	88.3% at 12 m 81.2% at 24 m 68% at 36 m	18 m	Heavily pretreated patients (Ctx, surgical), LTC depended on size
	Ricke (2009)	73 (67.1%)	200	3.6 cm (1–13.5 cm)	3 dose groups 12.8–18.8 Gy	74.9% at 34 m	23.4 m (26 m with CTX)	LTC depended on shape not size, dose level estimation
	Wieners (2009)	33 (56.3%)	138	4.6 cm (1–12 cm)	3 dose groups 14.2–21.2 Gy	87% at 6 m 76% at 12 m 69% at 24 m	n/a	Brachytherapy, and HAI
Breast CA	Collettini (2012)	37 (0%)	80	2.6 cm (0.8–7.4 cm)	18.6 Gy (±2.27 Gy)	94.6% at 12 m	18 m (3–39 m)	Multimodal pretreatment (surgical, Ctx, STRT)
	Wieners (2011)	41 (0%)	115	4.4 cm (1.0–11 cm)	18.5 Gy (12–25 Gy)	97% at 6 m 93.5% at 18 m	n/a	Survival rates: 97%, 79% 60% at 6 m, 12 m, and 18 m
NET	Schippers (2016)	27 (48.1%)	52	2.1 cm (0.7–11.0 cm)	15–20 Gy (target)	92% at 1 y 83% at 3 y	36 m (4.2–106.1 m)	Survival rates: 96% at 1 y, 96% at 3 y, 63% at 5 y
Renal CA	Geisel (2012)	10 (70%)	16	3.8 cm (1–8.2 cm)	n/a	93.8% at avg. FU 21.6 m ± 13.7 m	n/a	Extrahepatic progression limited OS
	Omari (2019)	14 (64.3%)	54	1.8 cm (0.5–13.9 cm)	16.1 Gy	92.6% avg. FU 10.2 (range 2.4–73.6 m)	51.2 m (1.0–27.8 m)	

GIST	Omari (2018)	10 (90%)	40[a]	2.4 cm (0.6–11.2 cm)	15 Gy (6.7–21.96 Gy)	97.5% at 25 m median FU	37.3 m (11.4–89.7 m)
Anal CA	Heinze (2018)	7 (28.5%)	38[b]	1.2 (0.4–6.2 cm)	16.2 (12.0–32.6 Gy)	97.4% at 15 m	25.2 m (6.5–51 m)
Pancreas CA	Wieners (2015)	41 (55%)	49	2.9 cm (1.0–7.3 cm)	18.1 Gy	91% at 12 m	8.6 m (1.5–55.3 m)
GE-CA	Geisel (2012b)	8 (50%)	12	4.6 cm (1.4–6.8 cm)	21 Gy (5–29 Gy)	100% at 8.4 m (±6.8 m FU)	n/a
	Omari (2019)	12 (83.3%)	36[c]	2 cm (1–10.2 cm)	19.9 Gy (5.4–22.5 Gy)	89% at 8.3 m median FU	11.4 m (4.3–47 m)

[a]30 liver- and 10 peritoneal-metastasis were treated
[b]28 liver, 9 lung, 1 nodal metastasis were treated
[c]29 liver, 5 pancreatic, and 2 nodal lesions were treated

Renal Cancer Liver Metastases

The median OS after iBT of renal cancer liver metastases has been reported as 51.2 months. Patients were mostly pretreated with chemotherapy and/or had been chemorefractory [13].

Liver Metastases of Other Cancer Entities

As mentioned above, OS data can be of limited validity, and this is especially true for rare cancer entities. However, in the light of the low complication rate and the limited alternative treatment options available, reported OS data may be considered adequate to support individual, rather aggressive treatment decisions. This applies especially for tumor dynamics and for distributions that meet the criteria for oligo-metastatic disease.

Median OS of more than 2 years was observed after iBT of liver metastases from (1) GIST (at 37.3 months) and (2) anal CA (at 25.2 months) [15, 16].

Median OS less than 1 year was observed in (1) pancreatic carcinoma (8.6–8.9 months) and (2) gastroesophageal CA (11.4 months) [17, 20, 21].

Special Considerations

Damage to Adjacent Organs

In tumors located peripherally, there is an inherent risk of radiation damage to adjacent organs (e.g., stomach, duodenum, colon, gall bladder, heart). However, in contrast to thermal energy, exposure to radiation can be predicted in dosimetry planning and, if needed, adjusted if relevant overexposure of an organ at risk is identified. Thus, tumors in locations not eligible for thermal ablation can be ablated by iBT. Planned dose exposure of hollow organs should not exceed 11 Gy/mL [22]. In order to achieve an effective dose administration to the target while sparing the organ at risk, spacing by temporarily placed inflatable balloons has been stated to be safe and effective [6]. For a case example see Fig. 9.2.

Abscess

Post-iBT abscess formation has been reported, with a frequency of up to 2% [23, 24]. As with thermal ablation, the risk of abscess development is deemed higher in presence of hepaticojejunostomy or compromised ampulla of Vater [23].

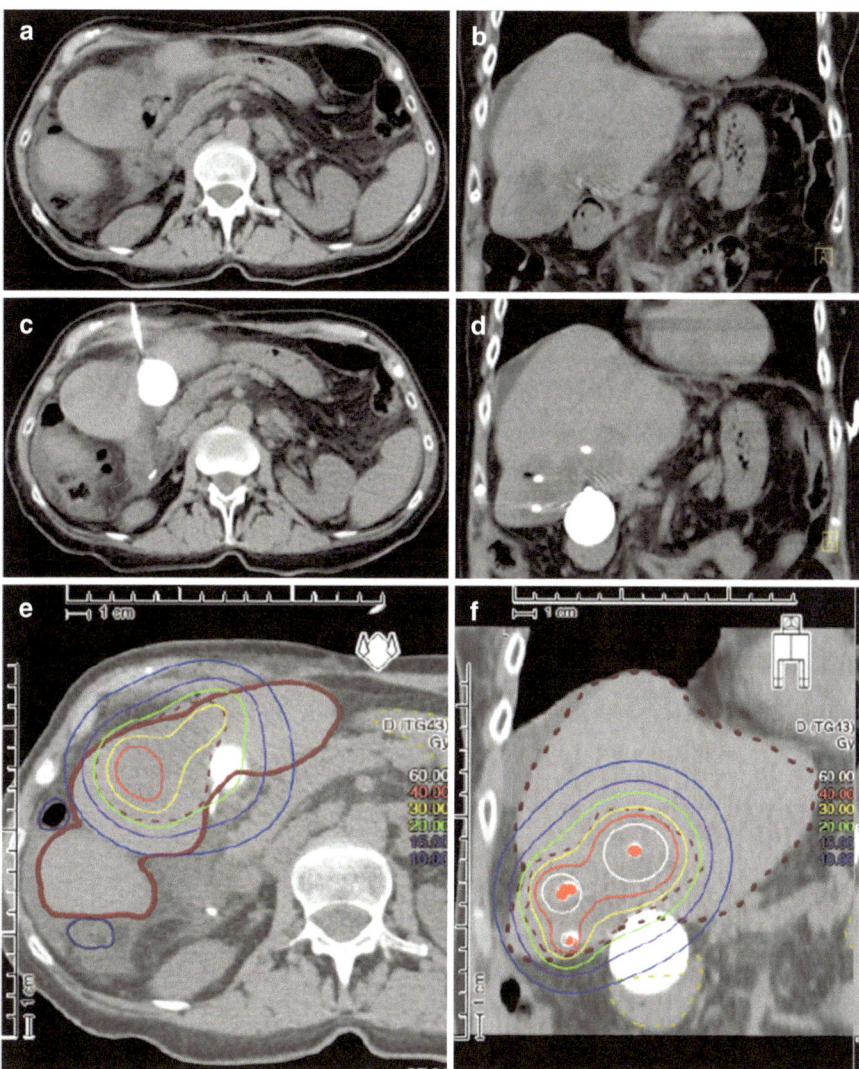

Fig. 9.2 Case example: A 75-year-old female with hepatic metastases from colorectal cancer, after hepatic resection and chemotherapy, had become chemorefractory and developed liver metastases. According to the multidisciplinary tumor board, the patient was scheduled for iBT. Planning CT (**a** axial, **b** coronal) without contrast showed confluent metastases in liver segment 4b/5. Note the proximity to the stomach (distal) and duodenum (proximal). After CT-guided placement of three catheters, a balloon was inserted and inflated to 4 cm, in order to increase the distance between the liver and stomach/duodenum(**c, d**). (**e, f**) Show the dosimetry in axial (**e**) and coronal (**f**) orientation. D100 was 20 Gy, but most parts of the tumor were encircled by the 25 Gy isodose. Note the 20 Gy isodose (green) crossing the balloon, i.e., the former position of the stomach/duodenum

Bile Duct Damage

High peak doses at main bile ducts can lead to bile duct necrosis and bile duct stenosis. Unlike thermoablation, dosimetric planning for iBT allows exact prediction of potential exposure and adjustment of the dosimetry if exposure is considered too high. In the literature, a threshold of approximately 20 Gy is reported for the development of bile duct complications [25]; thus, restrictions upon treatment for local ablation of central tumors with iBT are smaller than for thermal ablation.

> **Key Points**
> - Local radioablation by brachytherapy expands the scope of application of true local ablation to liver lesion sizes above 5 cm and to tumor locations unfavorable for thermoablation.
> - High local tumor control for liver metastases of different tumor entities was shown.
> - Overall survival depends highly on patient selection. The target population for brachytherapy comprises patients with controlled oligometastatic disease.
> - Rates of side effects of brachytherapy of liver metastases are within an acceptable range and can be reduced by cautious dosimetry planning and by paying attention to potential risk factors.

References

1. Berber E, Siperstein A. Local recurrence after laparoscopic radiofrequency ablation of liver tumors: an analysis of 1032 tumors. Ann Surg Oncol. 2008;15(10):2757–64.
2. Ohnishi T, et al. Intraductal chilled saline perfusion to prevent bile duct injury during percutaneous radiofrequency ablation for hepatocellular carcinoma. J Gastroenterol Hepatol. 2008;23(8 Pt 2):e410–5.
3. Kim YS, et al. Intrahepatic recurrence after percutaneous radiofrequency ablation of hepatocellular carcinoma: analysis of the pattern and risk factors. Eur J Radiol. 2006;59(3):432–41.
4. Livraghi T, et al. Treatment of focal liver tumors with percutaneous radio-frequency ablation: complications encountered in a multicenter study. Radiology. 2003;226(2):441–51.
5. Van Cutsem E, et al. ESMO consensus guidelines for the management of patients with metastatic colorectal cancer. Ann Oncol. 2016;27(8):1386–422.
6. Hass P, et al. First report on extended distance between tumor lesion and adjacent organs at risk using interventionally applied balloon catheters: a simple procedure to optimize clinical target volume covering effective isodose in interstitial high-dose-rate brachytherapy of liver malignomas. J Contemp Brachytherapy. 2019;11(2):152–61.
7. Wieners G, et al. Phase II feasibility study on the combination of two different regional treatment approaches in patients with colorectal "liver-only" metastases: hepatic interstitial brachytherapy plus regional chemotherapy. Cardiovasc Intervent Radiol. 2009;32(5):937–45.
8. Collettini F, et al. Unresectable colorectal liver metastases: percutaneous ablation using CT-guided high-dose-rate brachytherapy (CT-HDBRT). Rofo. 2014;186(6):606–12.

9. Ricke J, et al. Local response and impact on survival after local ablation of liver metastases from colorectal carcinoma by computed tomography-guided high-dose-rate brachytherapy. Int J Radiat Oncol Biol Phys. 2010;78(2):479–85.
10. Wieners G, et al. Treatment of hepatic metastases of breast cancer with CT-guided interstitial brachytherapy—a phase II-study. Radiother Oncol. 2011;100(2):314–9.
11. Collettini F, et al. Percutaneous computed tomography-guided high-dose-rate brachytherapy ablation of breast cancer liver metastases: initial experience with 80 lesions. J Vasc Interv Radiol. 2012;23(5):618–26.
12. Schippers AC, et al. Initial experience with CT-guided high-dose-rate brachytherapy in the multimodality treatment of neuroendocrine tumor liver metastases. J Vasc Interv Radiol. 2017;28(5):672–82.
13. Omari J, et al. Radioablation of hepatic metastases from renal cell carcinoma with image-guided interstitial brachytherapy. Anticancer Res. 2019;39(5):2501–8.
14. Geisel D, et al. Treatment for liver metastasis from renal cell carcinoma with computed-tomography-guided high-dose-rate brachytherapy (CT-HDRBT): a case series. World J Urol. 2013;31(6):1525–30.
15. Heinze C, et al. Image-guided interstitial brachytherapy in the management of metastasized anal squamous cell carcinoma. Anticancer Res. 2018;38(9):5401–7.
16. Omari J, et al. Treatment of metastatic, imatinib refractory, gastrointestinal stroma tumor with image-guided high-dose-rate interstitial brachytherapy. Brachytherapy. 2019;18(1):63–70.
17. Omari J, et al. Treatment of metastatic gastric adenocarcinoma with image-guided high-dose rate, interstitial brachytherapy as second-line or salvage therapy. Diagn Interv Radiol. 2019;25(5):360–7.
18. Geisel D, et al. Treatment of hepatic metastases from gastric or gastroesophageal adeno-carcinoma with computed tomography-guided high-dose-rate brachytherapy (CT-HDRBT). Anticancer Res. 2012;32(12):5453–8.
19. Seidensticker M, et al. Locally ablative treatment of breast cancer liver metastases: identification of factors influencing survival (the Mammary Cancer Microtherapy and Interventional Approaches (MAMMA MIA) study). BMC Cancer. 2015;15:517.
20. Wieners G, et al. CT-guided high-dose-rate brachytherapy in the interdisciplinary treatment of patients with liver metastases of pancreatic cancer. Hepatobiliary Pancreat Dis Int. 2015;14(5):530–8.
21. Drewes R, et al. Treatment of hepatic pancreatic ductal adenocarcinoma metastases with high-dose-rate image-guided interstitial brachytherapy: a single center experience. J Contemp Brachytherapy. 2019;11(4):329–36.
22. Streitparth F, et al. In vivo assessment of the gastric mucosal tolerance dose after single fraction, small volume irradiation of liver malignancies by computed tomography-guided, high-dose-rate brachytherapy. Int J Radiat Oncol Biol Phys. 2006;65(5):1479–86.
23. Boning G, et al. Complications of computed tomography-guided high-dose-rate brachytherapy (CT-HDRBT) and risk factors: results from more than 10 years of experience. Cardiovasc Intervent Radiol. 2020;43(2):284–94.
24. Mohnike K, et al. Radioablation of liver malignancies with interstitial high-dose-rate brachy-therapy: complications and risk factors. Strahlenther Onkol. 2016;192(5):288–96.
25. Powerski M, et al. Biliary duct stenosis after image-guided high-dose-rate interstitial brachy-therapy of central and hilar liver tumors: a systematic analysis of 102 cases. Strahlenther Onkol. 2019;195(3):265–73.

Daya Nand Sharma and Gokula Kumar Appalanaido

Magnitude of the Problem: Epidemiology of Liver Malignancies

The liver as an organ is often inflicted by various types of malignancies—both primary and secondary in nature. The most common primary malignancy affecting the liver is hepatocellular carcinoma (HCC) [1]. Cholangiocarcinoma, angiosarcoma, and hepatoblastoma are rarer malignancies of the liver. HCC is a major problem in parts of Asia, with the highest rate of HCC in the world among men occurring in Eastern Asia and South-East Asia (SEA), with age-standardized rates (ASR) of 31.9 and 22.2 per 100,000, respectively [1]. On the basis of the Globocan 2018 estimate, nearly three-quarters of the newly diagnosed primary liver malignancies are from the Asian region, with China alone contributing 50% of the cases [2]. Various causes have been ascribed to this high incidence including, but not limited to, endemicity of hepatitis B, the presence of aflatoxins in stored maize and groundnut, and the prevalence of hepatitis C infection [3]. Public health interventions such as universal hepatitis B immunization and improved awareness of modes of transmission of hepatitis B and C viruses, as well as changing agricultural practices to reduce food contamination with aflatoxins, have led to a decreased incidence of HCC in Asia in recent years [4–8]. In India, the available data indicate that the age-adjusted incidence rate of HCC is low, ranging from 0.7 to 7.5 per 100,000 in men and 0.2 to 2.2 per 100,000 in women per year [9]. The incidence of HCC in patients suffering from cirrhotic liver in India is 1.6% per year [9]. Liver is also a common site for metastases of malignancies from other sites in the body. Among the 2.4 million cancer patients registered in the SEER database from 2010 to 2015, 5.14% were diagnosed

D. N. Sharma (✉)
Department of Radiation Oncology, All India Institute of Medical Sciences, New Delhi, India

G. K. Appalanaido
Universiti Sains Malaysia, Penang, Malaysia

© The Author(s), under exclusive license to Springer Nature
Switzerland AG 2021
K. Mohnike et al. (eds.), *Manual on Image-Guided Brachytherapy of Inner Organs*, https://doi.org/10.1007/978-3-030-78079-1_10

117

with liver metastasis at the time of primary cancer diagnosis. For women between 20 and 50 years old, breast cancer is the most common metastatic disease of the liver, whereas for men aged between 20 and 50 years colon cancer was the most common cause, followed by rectal, lung, and pancreatic cancers [10]. With the likely reduction in the incidence of HCC due to active hepatitis B vaccination, metastatic tumors in the liver, especially colorectal liver metastasis (CRLM), will become a significant burden for healthcare facilities in Asia. The incidence of colorectal cancer in Asia—especially in China, Japan, South Korea, and Singapore—has increased significantly compared with historical data, and the estimated cumulative incidence of CRLM is 15.1% and 16.9% at 5 years and 10 years, respectively [11, 12].

The Barcelona clinic liver cancer (BCLC) staging system is the most widely used staging system in HCC for treatment allocation and prognostication. It divides HCC patients into five groups: 0 (very early), A (early), B (intermediate), C (advanced), and D (end-stage). 30–40% of HCC patients present in stage 0 or A [13]. The role of local ablative therapy (LAT) using high-dose-rate interstitial brachytherapy (iBT) in HCC is defined primarily for early stages and is particularly preferred in situations where radiofrequency or microwave ablation is contraindicated or deemed inadequate to achieve good local control. Its role in more advanced disease is still evolving. Table 10.1 summarizes the BCLC staging and the commonly prescribed iBT dose in HCC. The role of iBT in liver metastases is discussed later.

Local Ablative Therapy (LAT) of Primary Liver Malignancies in Asia

The management of primary HCC in Asia generally conforms to the ESMO guidelines, with most recommendations being accepted as guidelines for practice in the respective countries. The *Pan-Asian adapted ESMO Clinical Practice Guidelines for the management of patients with intermediate and advanced/relapsed hepatocellular carcinoma* (a TOS–ESMO initiative endorsed by CSCO, ISMPO, JSMO, KSMO, MOS, and SSO) have been published in the annals of oncology [14]. Unfortunately, unlike the main ESMO guidelines, iBT is not stated in these Pan-Asian adapted guidelines to be an alternative treatment for tumors less than 5 cm in size and when there are fewer than three lesions.

Local Ablative Therapy (LAT) in Liver Metastases

There are several treatment options (surgical resection and LAT) for liver metastases. Among the LAT options, iBT is generally indicated for relatively large lesions (even up to 10 cm) in patients presenting with oligometastatic disease. Extensive local ablations with iBT can be part of multimodal therapeutic management, e.g., conducted intermittently during systemic chemotherapy, or to control the local

Table 10.1 BCLC staging and the role of brachytherapy

BCLC stage	Stage definition	Standard treatment(s)	Additional comments	Role of brachytherapy	Dose of HDR brachytherapy	Level of evidence for brachytherapy
0	Single lesion <2 cm Preserved liver function PS 0	Liver resection Liver transplantation Radiofrequency (RFA) or microwave (MWA) ablation Trans-arterial chemo-embolization (TACE)	RFA or MWA is indicated in <3 cm lesions For RFA, the lesion should be away from any vessel >5 mm in size (to prevent cooling effect and loss of efficacy) RFA or MWA also not preferred if lesion near gall bladder, exophytic growth, or near bowel	**As an alternative to RFA and MWA** Preferred to RFA in lesions 3–7 cm in size Preferred if lesion is close to vessel Preferred in exophytic growth and lesion close to gall bladder	15–25 Gy Single session	IIIC
A	Single or up to 3 lesions <3 cm Preserved liver function PS 0	Liver resection Liver transplantation Radiofrequency (RFA) or microwave (MWA) ablation Trans-arterial chemo-embolisation (TACE)		Preferred to RFA in lesions 3–7 cm in size Preferred if lesion is close to vessel Preferred in exophytic growth and lesion close to gall bladder	15–25 Gy Single session	IIIC

(continued)

Table 10.1 (continued)

BCLC stage	Stage definition	Standard treatment(s)	Additional comments	Role of brachytherapy	Dose of HDR brachytherapy	Level of evidence for brachytherapy
B	Multi-nodular Unresectable Preserved liver function PS 0	TACE		Can be considered if needle placement possible to cover all nodules (up to four nodules) Size <7 cm	15–25 Gy Single session if dose constraints met. Otherwise multiple sessions Dose constraints: To preserve the liver parenchyma, dosing adjusted such that not more than two-thirds of the normal liver tissue received >5 Gy. The maximum exposure limited to 15 Gy per 1 mL for the stomach and intestine and 8 Gy per 1 mL for the spinal cord	IIIC [14, 15]
C	Portal invasion Extra-hepatic spread Preserved liver function PS 1–2	Sorafenib Regorafenib		No role Trials running in combining radiotherapy with HDAc inhibitors and immunotherapy		
D	Not transplantable PS 3–4 End-stage liver function	Best supportive care		No role		

tumor while the patient is on chemotherapy holiday in view of side effects that decrease the patient's quality of life. Most of the treatment centers in Asia follow the ESMO consensus guidelines on the indications for local ablative therapy in CRLM, which is adapted by the pan-Asian group [11–13, 15]. The adopted consensus guideline for LAT in CRLM is shown in Table 10.2.

The use of LAT for other primary liver tumors such as cholangiocarcinoma or metastatic tumors to the liver from other malignancies excluding the CRLM is not a well-established practice backed by strong evidence as in the rest of the world, though is practiced at some centers in Asia [16, 17]. LATs for liver metastasis commonly used in Asia are radiofrequency ablation (RFA), percutaneous ethanol injection, percutaneous acetic acid injection, cryoablation, microwave coagulation therapy, and high-intensity focused ultrasound (HIFU) [18].

Status of Liver Brachytherapy in Asia

Interstitial brachytherapy for liver lesions is practiced at a limited number of centers in Asia. To the best of the authors' knowledge, only three centers in India and one center in Malaysia practice liver iBT. It was first introduced in New Delhi, India, in the year 2009 by Sharma et al. [19, 20]. Subsequently, Appalanaido did the same in Malaysia, in 2018 [21]. Encouraged by the initial results from these reports [19–21], some other centers in India also started iBT for liver tumors [22, 23]. With growing awareness about liver brachytherapy and an increase in the number of HDR brachytherapy machine installations, its use in India is likely to increase in the future.

Table 10.2 Pan-Asian adapted ESMO consensus guidelines for the management of patients with metastatic colorectal cancer: a JSMO-ESMO initiative endorsed by CSCO, KACO, MOS, SSO, and TOS

Recommendation 15: local ablation techniques
15a. In patients with unresectable liver metastases only, or OMD, local ablation techniques such as thermal ablation or high conformal radiation techniques (e.g., SBRT. HDR brachytherapy) can be considered. The decision should be taken by a MDT based on local experience, tumor characteristics, and patient preference [IV, B]
15b. In patients with lung only or OMD of the lung, ablative high conformal radiation or thermal ablation may be considered if resection is limited by comorbidity, the extent of lung parenchyma resection, or, other factors [IV, B]
15c. SBRT is a safe and feasible alternative treatment of oligometastatic colorectal liver and lung metastases in patients not amenable to surgery or other ablative treatments [IV, B]
15d. RFA can be used in addition to surgery with the goal of eradicating all visible metastatic sites [II, B]

OMD Oligometastatic disease, *SBRT* Stereotactic Body Radiotherapy, *HDR* High Dose Rate
Voting process: [A = accept completely, B = accept with some reservation, C = accept with major reservations, D = reject with some reservation, and E = reject completely]
[I–IV]; level of evidence based on the adapted version of the "Infectious Diseases Society of America—United States Public Health Service Grading System"
Reproduced with permission

Clinical Experience with Liver iBT in Asia

Sharma et al. reported their experience of using CT-guided iBT in liver metastases [19]. A total of 10 patients with 12 metastatic lesions in the liver were enrolled in this prospective trial. Patients with any bleeding diathesis, low platelets, abnormal liver function tests, and Karnofsky performance status below 70 were excluded. Also, patients with more than three lesions, pediatric patients, patients with metastases from Wilms' tumor, choriocarcinoma, seminomas, or other chemo-sensitive tumors, patients with metastases to more than one visceral organ and those with previous irradiation to the liver (including SBRT) were also excluded. Lesions up to 7 cm in size (median size 3.8 cm) were included in this study. The procedure was carried out in the CT scan room under local anesthesia (2% xylocaine). In the breath-hold position, a 16-gauge blind-end stainless steel or rigid plastic brachytherapy needle was inserted into the center of the lesion by the percutaneous route. The needle tip was preferably advanced 3–5 mm beyond the lesion since the needle tip is blind and the radioactive source cannot reach the edge of the needle. Caution was taken not to introduce the needle during breathing movement, in order to avoid tissue tearing. Numbers of iBT needles were decided by the size and shape of the tumor: a single iBT needle is sufficient for lesions up to 3 cm and more needles are needed for lesions above 3 cm in diameter. The distance between two adjacent needles was kept at approximately 2–3 cm. The needles were then secured with screws (Fig. 10.1). If required, needles were sutured to the skin for additional securing. CT scan images were acquired with a slice thickness of 3 mm and transferred to the treatment-planning system. A single dose of 20 Gy was prescribed for the CTV. No margin was added to the CTV for defining PTV; thus PTV was equivalent to CTV. The volume of normal liver (excluding the PTV) receiving 5 Gy was kept below 30%. The needle was removed in the breath-hold position immediately after the completion of treatment, and the puncture site was sealed. Pain was the most frequent complication, witnessed in 25% of patients. No patient developed bleeding

Fig. 10.1 Clinical photograph showing percutaneously inserted needles secured with screws. Adapted from: Sharma DN et al. High-dose-rate interstitial brachytherapy for liver metastases: first study from India. J Contemp Brachy 2013; 5(2): 70–75

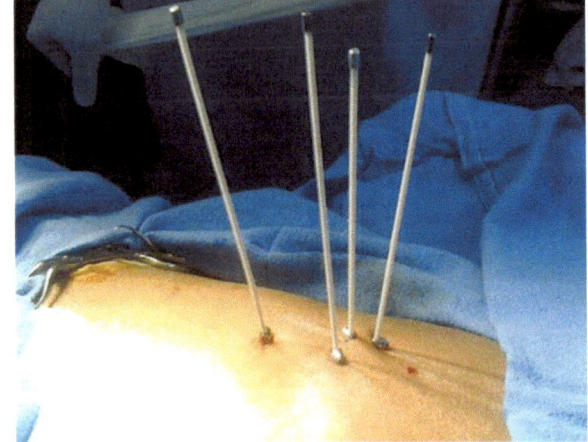

or needle-tract progression. Local control rate at 12 months was 75%. The 1-year local-progression-free survival rate (LPFS) was 33%.

Appalanaido et al. presented their series at the 2019 annual ASCOMOS meeting in Malaysia. The updated series comprised a total of 51 patients, with 84 lesions, treated from December 2018 to December 2020 at Universiti Sains Malaysia. The largest dimension of a metastatic lesion treated was 14.5 cm (Fig. 10.2). In this patient, with CRLM, the lesion was treated in a planned two-stage manner, with the second fraction of brachytherapy administered after 4 months to the residual lesion inducing complete metabolic response. The largest number of lesions treated in single patient was 16. Though experience with HCC was limited, one patient with a 16.2 cm primary HCC showed a complete radiological response after a low peripheral dose of 11.8 Gy covering the tumor (Fig. 10.3). Patient selection criteria are adopted from Mohnike et al. with no limit to the lesion size and a maximum of five lesions treated in a session [23]. The prescription dose covering the GTV range from 10 to 15 Gy for HCC and 20 Gy for other metastatic lesions such as those from breast, nasopharynx, and pancreas. A higher dose of 25 Gy is used for colorectal liver metastasis. The technique of implantation is similar to that of Sharma et al., who use CT guidance and stainless steel needles rather than plastic brachytherapy

Fig. 10.2 iBT plan of a patient with colorectal cancer liver metastasis. The yellow line shows a prescription isodose line of 15 Gy

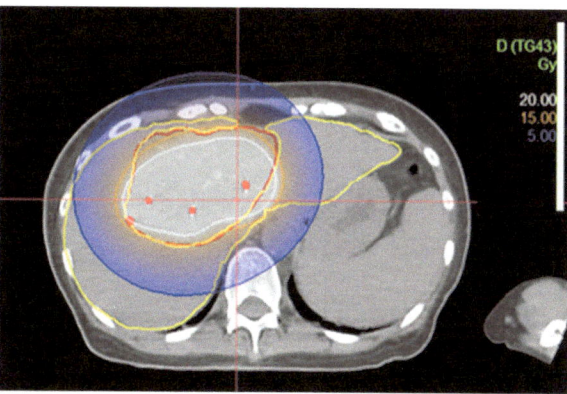

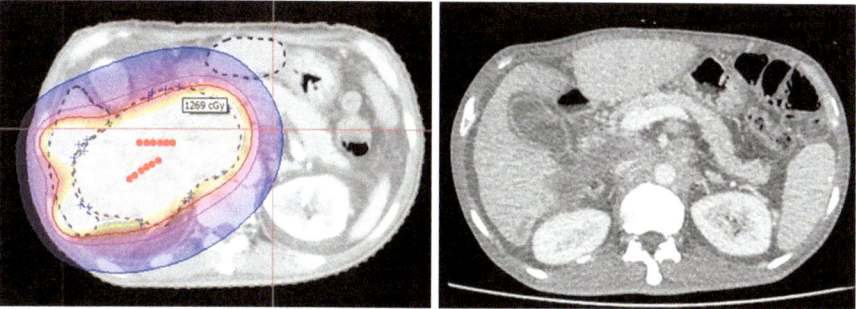

Fig. 10.3 iBT plan and posttreatment CT Scan showing complete response in a patient with large hepatocellular carcinoma. The yellow line shows a prescription isodose line of 12 Gy

catheters. As in the experience of Sharma et al., pain is the most common toxicity, and most patients with lesions larger than 5 cm treated have a spike of temperature within few hours of completing the treatment. Three patients had significant subcapsular bleeding that needed transfusion. Otherwise, no significant long-term toxicity was noted in follow-up. Analysis of the first 32 patients, with 43 lesions, within the first year of the liver brachytherapy program (presented at ASCOMOS, not published to date), no patient had progressive disease of the treated lesion in the liver. However, most patients were treated within the 6 months immediately before the presentation of the data so that the follow-up interval was too short to allow a final conclusion. Full data on the control rates will be published after completion of the ongoing final statistical analysis with a longer follow-up period.

Vishwanathan et al. from Bangalore, India reported the use of image-guided robotic iBT to treat a large (12.5 cm) pediatric unresectable HCC; this was not suitable for any other treatment modality, such as liver transplantation, liver resection or RFA, and it was refractory to medical treatment. The procedure was done under local anesthesia. The interstitial needle with an angiographic sheath attached to a robotic arm was introduced and was replaced with a 5–6F flexible single leader brachytherapy catheter (Fig. 10.4). Inter-catheter distance was kept to 3–4 cm. A dose of 30 Gy in 2 fractions was prescribed for the CTV, using the iBT afterloader

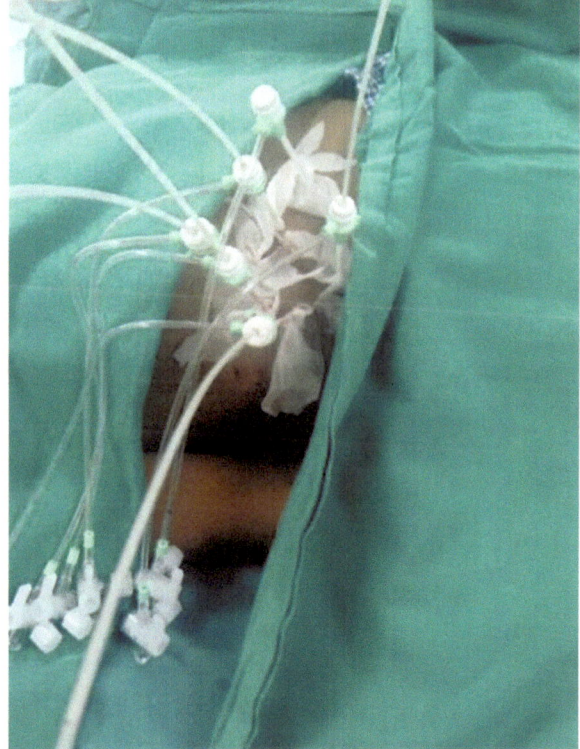

Fig. 10.4 Clinical image depicting placement of HDR brachytherapy catheters. Adapted from: Vishwanathan et al. Image-guided robotic interstitial brachytherapy, a new innovative treatment for malignancies. Hematology and Medical Oncology 2018; 3 (1): 1–4

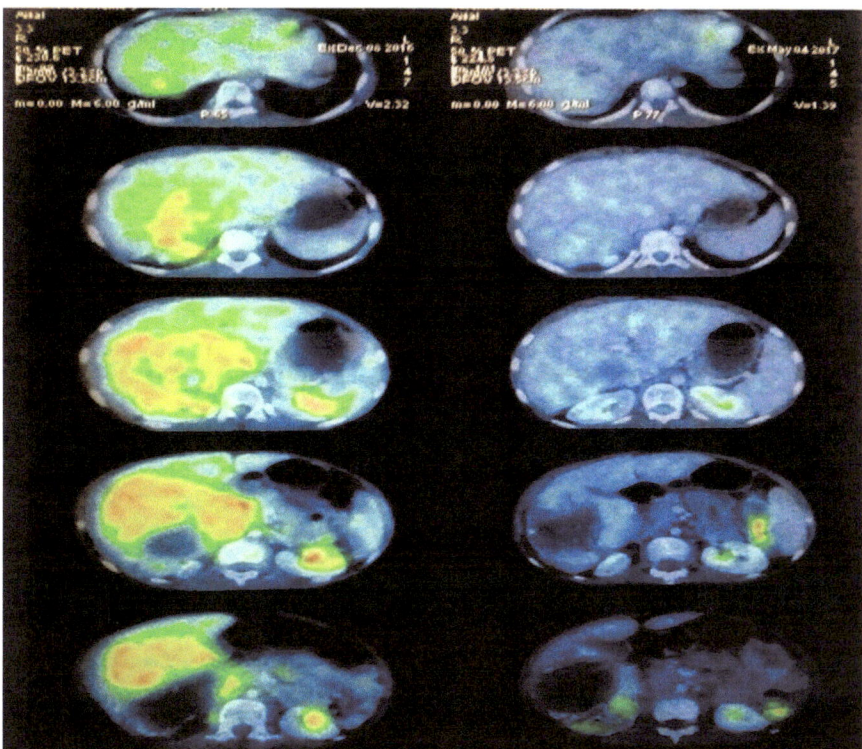

Fig. 10.5 PET scan images showing response to HDR brachytherapy. Adapted from: Vishwanathan et al. Image-guided robotic interstitial brachytherapy, a new innovative treatment for malignancies. Hematology and Medical Oncology 2018; 3 (1): 1–4

system. There were no intraoperative or immediate postoperative complications. After 6 months of follow-up, the patient achieved partial response and near-complete metabolic response [22] (Fig. 10.5).

Agrawal and Singh from Lucknow, India treated a patient with liver metastases (size 4 cm) from colorectal cancer with iBT. The procedure was conducted under the guidance of ultrasound and fluoroscopy. A dose of 15 Gy in a single fraction was prescribed for the CTV. There were no intraoperative or perioperative complications. The patient had an overall survival of 13 months [23].

Future of Liver Brachytherapy

Although the *Pan-Asian adapted ESMO Clinical Practice Guidelines for the management of patients with metastatic colorectal cancer* did endorse liver iBT as an option in CRLM with some reservations, it is a different story for primary HCC in Asia [11]. *The Pan-Asian adapted ESMO Clinical Practice Guidelines for the management of patients with intermediate and advanced/relapsed HCC* [14] do not mention brachytherapy as a form of local ablative therapy for primary HCC. This is despite the fact that primary HCC is known to be a very radiosensitive tumor compared with CRLM.

This is not surprising, given the fact that iBT of the liver is not widely known or offered in the Asiatic region. A more concerted effort, that includes a comprehensive brachytherapy module in the radiation oncologist residency training programs, post-qualification training of radiation oncologists and active promotion, is needed in increasing the recognition and in promoting the very effective technique of iBT in the local treatment of liver metastasis and primary HCC.

An image-guided brachytherapy facility is readily available in many radiotherapy centers in Asia; however, its services are usually limited to gynecological brachytherapy, and, rarely, prostate brachytherapy. With the active human papillomavirus (HPV) vaccination program in most parts of Asia, it is very likely that the rates of cervical cancers will decline over time and this will translate into underuse of the available brachytherapy facilities. Therefore, it is time for radiation oncologists to explore other anatomical sites—such as esophagus, tongue, breast, and liver—for iBT treatment. Furthermore, iBT of the liver does have certain advantages over other LAT modalities, such as RFA, which is known to have many limitations based on the anatomical location of the tumor [18].

A serious review and incorporation of non-gynecological brachytherapy applications into the radiation oncology training curriculum should be emphasized, to ensure that this important skill is not lost to future generations of radiation oncologists. With the renewed interest in liver brachytherapy, the future can be expected to witness interesting developments in this field.

Key Points
- Hepatocellular carcinoma is a major problem in certain parts of Asia. The liver is also very commonly afflicted by metastases from various primary malignancies.
- The majority of patients (>80%) with primary/metastatic hepatic tumors are not suitable for surgical resection.
- There are several local ablative therapies (radiofrequency ablation, cryoablation, high-intensity focused ultrasound, interstitial brachytherapy, etc.) available as nonsurgical options.
- High-dose-rate iBT is a relatively new therapy but has excellent therapeutic potential owing to its highly conformal dosimetry.
- HDR iBT practice in Asia is limited to a few centers in India and Malaysia. Clinical experience at these centers has so far been very promising.

References

1. Liver E, Cancer E. EASL–EORTC Clinical Practice Guidelines: management of hepatocellular carcinoma. J Hepatol. 2012;56:908–43.
2. Liver-fact-sheet [Internet]. 2018. https://gco.iarc.fr/today/data/factsheets/cancers/11-Liver-fact-sheet.pdf.
3. Goh GB-B, Chang P-E, Tan C-K. Changing epidemiology of hepatocellular carcinoma in Asia. Best Pract Res Clin Gastroenterol. 2015;29:919–28.
4. Jemal A, Bray F, Center M, Ferlay J, Ward E, Forman D. Global cancer statistics. CA Cancer J Clin. 2011;61:69–90.
5. Liang X, Bi S, Yang W, Wang L, Cui G, Cui F, et al. Epidemiological serosurvey of hepatitis B in China—declining HBV prevalence due to hepatitis B vaccination. Vaccine. 2009;27(47):6550–7.
6. Ni YH, Chang MH, Huang LM, Chen HL, Hsu HY, Chiu TY, et al. Hepatitis B virus infection in children and adolescents in a hyperendemic area: 15 years after mass hepatitis B vaccination. Ann Intern Med. 2001;135(9):796–800.
7. Liu Y, Chang CC, Marsh GM, Wu F. Population attributable risk of aflatoxin-related liver cancer: systematic review and meta-analysis. Eur J Cancer. 2012;48(14):2125–36.
8. Chen JG, Egner PA, Ng D, Jacobson LP, Muñoz A, Zhu YR, et al. Reduced aflatoxin exposure presages decline in liver cancer mortality in an endemic region of China. Cancer Prev Res (Phila). 2013;6(10):1038–45.
9. Acharya S. Epidemiology of hepatocellular carcinoma in India. J Clin Exp Hepatol. 2014;4:S27–33.
10. Horn S, Stoltzfus K, Lehrer E, Dawson L, Tchelebi L, Gusani N, et al. Epidemiology of liver metastases. Cancer Epidemiol. 2020;67:101760.
11. Yoshino T, Arnold D, Taniguchi H, Pentheroudakis G, Yamazaki K, Xu RH, et al. Pan-Asian adapted ESMO consensus guidelines for the management of patients with metastatic colorectal cancer: a JSMO-ESMO initiative endorsed by CSCO, KACO, MOS, SSO and TOS. Ann Oncol. 2018;29(1):44–70.
12. Landreau P, Drouillard A, Launoy G, Ortega-Deballon P, Jooste V, Lepage C, et al. Incidence and survival in late liver metastases of colorectal cancer. J Gastroenterol Hepatol. 2015;30(1):82–5.
13. Richani M, Kolly P, Knoepfli M, Herrmann E, Zweifel M, Von Tengg-Kobligk H, et al. Treatment allocation in hepatocellular carcinoma: assessment of the BCLC algorithm. Ann Hepatol. 2015;15:82–90.
14. Chen LT, Martinelli E, Cheng AL, Pentheroudakis G, Qin S, Bhattacharyya GS, et al. Pan-Asian adapted ESMO Clinical Practice Guidelines for the management of patients with intermediate and advanced/relapsed hepatocellular carcinoma: a TOS-ESMO initiative endorsed by CSCO, ISMPO, JSMO, KSMO, MOS and SSO. Ann Oncol. 2020;31(3):334–51.
15. Van Cutsem E, Cervantes A, Adam R, Sobrero A, Van Krieken JH, Aderka D, et al. ESMO consensus guidelines for the management of patients with metastatic colorectal cancer. Ann Oncol. 2016;27(8):1386–422.
16. Yun BL, Lee JM, Baek JH, Kim SH, Lee JY, Han JK, et al. Radiofrequency ablation for treating liver metastases from a non-colorectal origin. Korean J Radiol. 2011;12(5):579–87.
17. Hao W, Binbin J, Wei Y, Kun Y. Can radiofrequency ablation replace liver resection for solitary colorectal liver metastasis? A systemic review and meta-analysis. Front Oncol. 2020;10(1912):561669.
18. Wu M-C, Tang Z-Y, Ye S-L, Fan J, Qin S-K, Yang J-M, et al. Expert consensus on local ablation therapies for primary liver cancer. Chin Clin Oncol. 2012;1(1):14.

19. Sharma DN, Thulkar S, Sharma S, Gandhi AK, Haresh KP, Gupta S, et al. High-dose-rate inter-stitial brachytherapy for liver metastases: first study from India. J Contemp Brachytherapy. 2013;5(2):70–5.
20. Sharma D, Thulkar S, Kumar R, Rath G. Interstitial brachytherapy for liver metastases and assessment of response by positron emission tomography: a. J Contemp Brachytherapy. 2010;3:114–6.
21. Appalanaido GK, editor. HDR Liver brachytherapy. In: 31st Annual Scientific Congress of Malaysian Oncological Society (ASCOMOS). 2019.
22. Vishwanathan B, Mandal S, Kumar R, Ramprakash HV. Image guided robotic intersti-tial brachytherapy, a new innovative treatment for malignancies. Hematol Med Oncol. 2018;3(1):1–4.
23. Sushma Agrawal ASS, Lucknow, India. HDR Brachytherapy for liver metastases. Personal communication. 2018.

Matthias P. Fabritius and Ricarda Seidensticker

A key limiting factor in the radiotherapy of liver malignancies is the relatively low tolerance of the liver parenchyma to radiation. This can lead to subclinical focal or generalized injury of the liver parenchyma. Any catheter-based radiotherapy (image-guided brachytherapy, iBT) leads to unavoidable radiation-induced damage to the adjacent liver parenchyma, a so-called focal radiation-induced liver injury (fRILI). Liver tolerance dose levels extracted by looking at liver function after percutaneous radiotherapy cannot necessarily be adopted for iBT. This is because available clinical data from percutaneous radiotherapy of parts of the liver do not reflect the intrinsic tolerance of the liver parenchyma and are highly biased by the variable extent of volume exposure. Only data from percutaneous whole-liver radiotherapy provide information on intrinsic liver tolerance dose, indicating a tolerance dose of 30 Gy, fractionated [1]. For iBT, there are data showing that magnetic-resonance imaging with hepatocyte-specific contrast media can specifically display the fRILI after iBT [2]. By correlation of the extent of the fRILI in follow-up MRI (with hepatocyte-specific contrast media) with the former dose exposure during iBT, it was shown that the minimum hepatic tolerance dose is around 10 Gy in median (with fRILI peaking at about 6 weeks after iBT) [2, 3]. If this single-fractioned 10 Gy dose is converted to a fractionated regimen, data correlate well with the abovementioned 30 Gy liver tolerance dose from fractioned whole-liver radiotherapy [1]. However, when the extent of RILI exceeds the functional reserve of the liver, clinical complications appear, with deterioration of liver function and hepatic failure, typically 2 weeks to 4 months after the intervention [3, 4]. This syndrome is described as radiation-induced liver disease (RILD) and is characterized by jaundice,

M. P. Fabritius · R. Seidensticker (✉)
Department of Radiology, Ludwig Maximilian University (LMU) Hospital Munich, Munich, Germany
e-mail: Matthias.fabritius@med.uni-muenchen.de; Ricarda.seidensticker@med.uni-muenchen.de

129

development of ascites, hyperbilirubinemia, and hypoalbuminemia in the absence of tumor progression or biliary obstruction. The pathological correlate of fRILI/RILD is veno-occlusive disease (VOD). VOD in the context of liver damage was first described for patients undergoing external-beam radiation therapy and is thought primarily to comprise injury to endothelial cells of small branches of the hepatic veins, which leads to focal deposition of fibrin, resulting in a fibrin network which is finally replaced by collagen, causing fibrous occlusion and atrophy of the hepatocytes [4–6].

The rate of RILD occurrence after iBT is generally low (0.5%), most probably owing to conservative restrictions upon dose exposure of the liver parenchyma (see below) [7]. However, in clinical practice, patients with a low functional liver remnant due to their medical history (prior hepatotoxic chemotherapies, large tumor volumes, prior liver resection, or multiple and recurrent lesions requiring repeated irradiation) are at risk of developing liver dysfunction even in this setting. To preserve liver function after irradiation, one attempts to keep the dose below 5 Gy per one-third of the normal liver parenchyma in clinical routine. (5 Gy represents the lowest liver tolerance level, as detected in analyses of hepatobiliary MRI studies (see above) and derived from data on normal tissue tolerance doses in percutaneous radiotherapy [8].)

To monitor potential post-therapeutic liver damage, regular clinical and laboratory follow-up, including assessment of liver-specific parameters as well as imaging follow-up employing MRI with hepatocyte-specific contrast media, is necessary. The following laboratory values should be assessed 1 day before the intervention, at discharge, and 6 weeks and 3 months after the intervention: total bilirubin and γ-glutamyl transpeptidase as indicators of detoxification function, albumin and cholinesterase as reflectors of the synthetic function of the liver, and alanine aminotransferase, aspartate aminotransferase, and alkaline phosphatase as indicators of damage to liver tissue. Mild changes in liver function parameters are common shortly after radiation therapy. Deviant laboratory values normally return to baseline levels within 6 weeks. RILD is suggested by ascites, by hepatomegaly, and by elevation of alkaline phosphatase level to 3–10 times normal or elevation of transaminases to twice the upper limit of the normal or pretreatment level [4, 9]. In addition, functional hepatobiliary MRI can allow visualization of the extent of fRILI and can—in cases of liver decompensation—rule out massive disease progression as an alternative cause of liver decompensation [2, 3] (Fig. 11.1). As stated above, the histopathological evidence for fRILI correlates well with the absence of uptake of hepatobiliary MRI contrast media by hepatocytes. The development of areas of fRILI is greatest 6–8 weeks after iBT, which correlates with the peak incidence of RILD [10].

Medication designed to reduce RILI can improve the safety of radiotherapy as well as making possible more aggressive radiotherapy. As mentioned above, prior exposure and concomitant chemotherapy are thought to increase the risk of RILD, and RILD is therefore a relatively common complication, for example, after conditioning therapy (chemotherapy plus whole-body irradiation) performed before bone-marrow transplantation (BMT), where it occurs in 5–60% of patients [4,

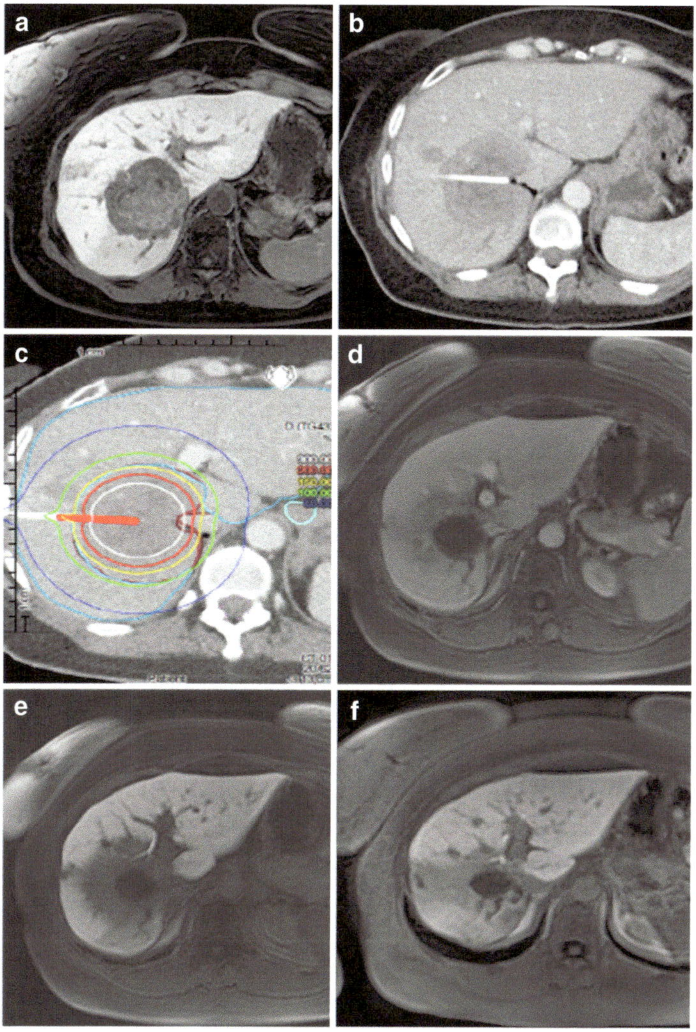

Fig. 11.1 Case example. A 51-year-old patient with breast cancer liver metastases. Stable disease under chemotherapy/anti-hormonal therapy. The multidisciplinary tumor board recommended local ablation by catheter-based brachytherapy. (**a**) MRI with hepatocyte-specific contrast medium with a large metastasis in the central right liver lobe. (**b**) Contrast-enhanced planning CT after catheter insertion (further catheters at other levels, not shown). Small satellite metastasis in liver segment 5 (not in-plane in A). (**c**) Dosimetry of radiotherapy. D100: 15 Gy. Green isodose resemble 15 Gy. (**d**) MRI venous phase 12 weeks after treatment shows a partial remission. Residual tumor is non-vascularised thus avital. Residual tumor is surrounded by a hypointense zone, which is demarcated in (**e**) (hepatobiliary phase) as parenchymal zone with lost capacity to take up the hepatocyte-specific contrast medium. Parenchymal defect extends to the former 10 Gy isodose. Thus, liver parenchyma with a dose exposure of >10 Gy showed no uptake of hepatocyte-specific contrast medium and suffered a local veno-occlusive disease (VOD). (**f**) MRI with hepatocyte-specific contrast medium 24 weeks after treatment. Avital residual of the tumor shows further shrinkage. Partial recovery of the liver parenchyma from local VOD, accompanied by liver volume decrease of the exposed liver parenchyma and compensatory growth of the left liver

11–14]. Clinical studies have shown with varying strength of evidence that VOD/RILD after pre-BMT conditioning therapy can be ameliorated by pentoxifylline (PTX), ursodeoxycholic acid (UDCA), and low-molecular-weight heparin (LMWH) [15–22]. These drugs, alone or in combination, probably influence the pathomechanism of VOD/RILD to protect the liver through their anti-inflammatory and anticoagulant features. UDCA reduces the concentration of potentially hepatotoxic bile acids and presumably downregulates proinflammatory cytokines such as tumor necrosis factor α (TNF-α) and interleukin-1 [23, 24]. PTX downregulates TNF-α and stimulates noninflammatory prostaglandin synthesis [15]. LMWHs are believed to prevent thrombosis of hepatic venules after endothelial damage [22]. Further studies could also confirm the efficacy of the drug combination in local ablative procedures including iBT: Post-therapeutic application of PTX (oral, 400 mg t.i.d.), UDCA (oral, 250 mg t.i.d.), and LMWH (s.c. injection, 40 mg q.d.) for 8 weeks reduced significantly the extent and incidence of fRILI as assessed 6 weeks after brachytherapy [25]. On the basis of the low toxicity profile of these medications and the promising study results, this drug combination should be prescribed preventively for at least 8 weeks to patients with increased risk of RILD if there are no contraindications. Note however that there is evidence for an increased risk of bleeding events after iBT when LMWH is used pre-interventional [26].

Defibrotide, a mixture of single-stranded oligonucleotides with a poorly understood effect mechanism, is approved for the treatment of severe hepatic VOD in patients after BMT [27]. However, this therapy has not been tested in patients with RILD after radiotherapy. Therefore, treatment of RILD is directed mainly at controlling symptoms. Drugs that can be used for supportive care include diuretics for fluid retention, paracentesis for ascites, correction of coagulopathy, steroids to reduce hepatic congestion, and the use of anticoagulants for relieving hepatic vein thrombosis [28].

Key Points
- iBT leads to predictable local radiation-induced damage to the adjacent liver parenchyma.
- The minimum intrinsic hepatic tolerance dose is around 10 Gy in median.
- Clinical complications (liver decompensation) appear when the extent of radiation-induced liver injury exceeds the functional reserve of the liver. Generally, the rate of RILD occurrence after iBT is low (0.5%).
- To preserve liver function after irradiation, the dose should be kept below 5 Gy per one-third of the normal liver parenchyma.
- Prophylactic medication can reduce radiation-induced liver damage.

References

1. Jacobs P, Miller JL, Uys CJ, Dietrich BE. Fatal veno-occlusive disease of the liver after chemotherapy, whole-body irradiation and bone marrow transplantation for refractory acute leukaemia. S Afr Med J. 1979;55(1):5–10.
2. Seidensticker M, Seidensticker R, Mohnike K, Wybranski C, Kalinski T, Luess S, et al. Quantitative in vivo assessment of radiation injury of the liver using Gd-EOB-DTPA enhanced MRI: tolerance dose of small liver volumes. Radiat Oncol (London, England). 2011;6:40.
3. Ricke J, Seidensticker M, Ludemann L, Pech M, Wieners G, Hengst S, et al. In vivo assessment of the tolerance dose of small liver volumes after single-fraction HDR irradiation. Int J Radiat Oncol Biol Phys. 2005;62(3):776–84.
4. Lawrence TS, Robertson JM, Anscher MS, Jirtle RL, Ensminger WD, Fajardo LF. Hepatic toxicity resulting from cancer treatment. Int J Radiat Oncol Biol Phys. 1995;31(5):1237–48.
5. Fajardo LF, Colby TV. Pathogenesis of veno-occlusive liver disease after radiation. Arch Pathol Lab Med. 1980;104(11):584–8.
6. Reed GB Jr, Cox AJ Jr. The human liver after radiation injury. A form of veno-occlusive disease. Am J Pathol. 1966;48(4):597–611.
7. Mohnike K, Wolf S, Damm R, Seidensticker M, Seidensticker R, Fischbach F, et al. Radioablation of liver malignancies with interstitial high-dose-rate brachytherapy: complications and risk factors. Strahlenther Onkol. 2016;192(5):288–96.
8. Emami B, Lyman J, Brown A, Coia L, Goitein M, Munzenrider JE, et al. Tolerance of normal tissue to therapeutic irradiation. Int J Radiat Oncol Biol Phys. 1991;21(1):109–22.
9. Ruhl R, Seidensticker M, Peters N, Mohnike K, Bornschein J, Schutte K, et al. Hepatocellular carcinoma and liver cirrhosis: assessment of the liver function after Yttrium-90 radioembolization with resin microspheres or after CT-guided high-dose-rate brachytherapy. Dig Dis. 2009;27(2):189–99.
10. Seidensticker M, Burak M, Kalinski T, Garlipp B, Koelble K, Wust P, et al. Radiation-induced liver damage: correlation of histopathology with hepatobiliary magnetic resonance imaging, a feasibility study. Cardiovasc Intervent Radiol. 2015;38(1):213–21.
11. Farthing MJ, Clark ML, Sloane JP, Powles RL, McElwain TJ. Liver disease after bone marrow transplantation. Gut. 1982;23(6):465–74.
12. McDonald GB, Sharma P, Matthews DE, Shulman HM, Thomas ED. Venocclusive disease of the liver after bone marrow transplantation: diagnosis, incidence, and predisposing factors. Hepatology (Baltimore, MD). 1984;4(1):116–22.
13. McDonald GB, Sharma P, Matthews DE, Shulman HM, Thomas ED. The clinical course of 53 patients with venocclusive disease of the liver after marrow transplantation. Transplantation. 1985;39(6):603–8.
14. Shulman HM, Hinterberger W. Hepatic veno-occlusive disease—liver toxicity syndrome after bone marrow transplantation. Bone Marrow Transplant. 1992;10(3):197–214.
15. Bianco JA, Appelbaum FR, Nemunaitis J, Almgren J, Andrews F, Kettner P, et al. Phase I-II trial of pentoxifylline for the prevention of transplant-related toxicities following bone marrow transplantation. Blood. 1991;78(5):1205–11.
16. Attal M, Huguet F, Rubie H, Huynh A, Charlet JP, Payen JL, et al. Prevention of hepatic veno-occlusive disease after bone marrow transplantation by continuous infusion of low-dose heparin: a prospective, randomized trial. Blood. 1992;79(11):2834–40.
17. Attal M, Huguet F, Rubie H, Charlet JP, Schlaifer D, Huynh A, et al. Prevention of regimen-related toxicities after bone marrow transplantation by pentoxifylline: a prospective, randomized trial. Blood. 1993;82(3):732–6.
18. Clift RA, Bianco JA, Appelbaum FR, Buckner CD, Singer JW, Bakke L, et al. A randomized controlled trial of pentoxifylline for the prevention of regimen-related toxicities in patients undergoing allogeneic marrow transplantation. Blood. 1993;82(7):2025–30.

19. Essell JH, Schroeder MT, Harman GS, Halvorson R, Lew V, Callander N, et al. Ursodiol prophylaxis against hepatic complications of allogeneic bone marrow transplantation. A randomized, double-blind, placebo-controlled trial. Ann Intern Med. 1998;128(12 Pt 1):975–81.
20. Ohashi K, Tanabe J, Watanabe R, Tanaka T, Sakamaki H, Maruta A, et al. The Japanese multicenter open randomized trial of ursodeoxycholic acid prophylaxis for hepatic veno-occlusive disease after stem cell transplantation. Am J Hematol. 2000;64(1):32–8.
21. Ruutu T, Eriksson B, Remes K, Juvonen E, Volin L, Remberger M, et al. Ursodeoxycholic acid for the prevention of hepatic complications in allogeneic stem cell transplantation. Blood. 2002;100(6):1977–83.
22. Forrest DL, Thompson K, Dorcas VG, Couban SH, Pierce R. Low molecular weight heparin for the prevention of hepatic veno-occlusive disease (VOD) after hematopoietic stem cell transplantation: a prospective phase II study. Bone Marrow Transplant. 2003;31(12):1143–9.
23. Kowdley KV. Ursodeoxycholic acid therapy in hepatobiliary disease. Am J Med. 2000;108(6):481–6.
24. Neuman MG, Shear NH, Bellentani S, Tiribelli C. Role of cytokines in ethanol-induced cytotoxicity in vitro in Hep G2 cells. Gastroenterology. 1998;115(1):157–66.
25. Seidensticker M, Seidensticker R, Damm R, Mohnike K, Pech M, Sangro B, et al. Prospective randomized trial of enoxaparin, pentoxifylline and ursodeoxycholic acid for prevention of radiation-induced liver toxicity. PLoS One. 2014;9(11):e112731.
26. Mohnike K, Sauerland H, Seidensticker M, Hass P, Kropf S, Seidensticker R, et al. Haemorrhagic complications and symptomatic venous thromboembolism in interventional tumour ablations: the impact of peri-interventional thrombosis prophylaxis. Cardiovasc Intervent Radiol. 2016;39(12):1716–21.
27. Richardson P, Aggarwal S, Topaloglu O, Villa KF, Corbacioglu S. Systematic review of defibrotide studies in the treatment of veno-occlusive disease/sinusoidal obstruction syndrome (VOD/SOS). Bone Marrow Transplant. 2019;54(12):1951–62.
28. Guha C, Kavanagh BD. Hepatic radiation toxicity: avoidance and amelioration. Semin Radiat Oncol. 2011;21(4):256–63.

Lung Brachytherapy: Experience from Germany

12

Nils Peters

Introduction

Cancer was the second leading cause of death globally in 2018. Among all cancers, lung cancer is the most common type in men and the third most common among women. It represents the leading cause of cancer death globally. Worldwide, more than two million new cases of lung cancer were estimated in 2018, with an estimated 1.8 million deaths [1]. About one-third of the patients are >75 years old and many of them present with comorbidities due to age and tobacco use.

Non-small-cell lung cancer (NSCLC) is the most common of all lung cancers, with approximately 87% of lung cancer diagnoses; of these, about 21% are at stage I of disease on first presentation [2]. For patients with early-stage (stage IA–IIA) NSCLC, lobectomy has been the gold standard for surgery and provides the best chance of cure [3]. However, about 25% of patients are not candidates for lobectomy [4].

At the same time, the lung is the second most frequent site of metastatic focus. About 25–30% of all patients with malignant tumors will eventually develop pulmonary metastases. Tumors that often metastasize to the lungs include colorectal cancer, breast cancer, renal cancer, and melanoma. Conventional therapies are similar to localized lung cancer, with the addition of systemic approaches for diffuse metastatic disease. Often, surgical options are not feasible, or are not desirable, because of critical risk/benefit considerations. Here, minimally invasive ablative procedures such as brachytherapy can play an important part in oncological therapy concepts. The last two decades have seen a rise of such techniques, as alternatives to surgery for patients either with high medical risk and localized disease or with metastatic disease. These techniques include radiation (SBRT, brachytherapy) and

N. Peters (✉)
Department of Radiation Oncology, Diagnostic Therapeutic Center Berlin, Berlin, Germany
e-mail: nils.peters@berlin-dtz.de

135
K. Mohnike et al. (eds.), *Manual on Image-Guided Brachytherapy of Inner Organs*, https://doi.org/10.1007/978-3-030-78079-1_12

thermal ablative procedures such as laser-induced thermo-therapy (LITT), irreversible electroporation (IRE), radio-frequency ablation (RFA), or microwave ablation (MWA) [5–12].

The general acceptance of local therapy in oligometastasized patients and in the context of multimodal, interdisciplinary therapy settings has continued to increase in the past decade, but it had to fight hard for its status at the beginning. Hellmannn and Weichselbaum had created a theoretical foundation for this in 1995, in their postulation of oligometastasis as an intermediate disease state, and they thus set a starting point for its transfer into practice [13, 14]. In recent years, extensive experience has been gained with various methods of local therapy independent of, or in combination with, systemic therapies in the treatment of early-stage lung cancer and lung metastasis.

After the implementation of interventional, CT-guided interstitial brachytherapy in the early 2000s by Ricke, Wust et al. at the Charité in Berlin, a wide range of applications of the technique have emerged [15–26]. Beside liver metastasis, early-stage lung cancers and lung metastases were early targets [27–29]. In various hospitals, mostly in Germany, comprehensive experience has been gained in CT-guided interstitial brachytherapy of the lung, with encouraging results in respect of both safety and effectivity [7, 30–34].

The method has been developed from a combination of conventional brachytherapy, mostly used for gynecological cancers and CT-guided interventional procedures such as frequently used for tissue sampling. It differs from endobronchial brachytherapy, where the applicator is placed inside the airways by bronchoscopy to perform image-guided high-dose-rate (HDR) brachytherapy (iBT), and also from interstitial low-dose-rate (LDR) brachytherapy, where radioactive ^{125}I seeds are placed permanently inside the tumor. Differences also exist with respect to other interventional, mostly hyperthermic, ablative procedures such as radio-frequency ablation (RFA) and microwave ablation (MWA). These thermal procedures are often limited by tumor size and localization, and blood vessels can disperse the thermal energy by a "heat sink" effect.

In brachytherapy the energy deposition is physically defined and is therefore highly predictable; additionally, it is not strongly influenced by neighboring structures. These circumstances allow treatment even in difficult locations, where thermal procedures can only be performed with difficulty. Also, the size limit inherent in other procedures does not pose a problem in brachytherapy because more applicators can be used to cover the volume to be irradiated. Owing to the steep dose gradient in brachytherapy, structures at risk outside of the target volume can be spared high doses. After brachytherapy, delayed tissue degradation with slow fibrotic alteration is common; as a consequence, organ integrity will not be disrupted suddenly, and this may reduce the risk of side effects.

Another radiotherapeutic modality is stereotactic body radiation therapy (SBRT), which emerged from stereotactic radiosurgery (SRS) for the treatment of extracranial targets. Here, high single doses of radiation are directed toward pulmonary nodules. Accounting for breathing motion, techniques such as tracking or gating are commonly applied. With the advancing technology in linear accelerators, SBRT has become a standard treatment with widespread availability in recent years [6, 35].

One major goal for the future is the development of standardized treatment protocols for different manifestations of metastasis and oligometastasis, such as oligoprogression and oligorecurrence, employing the full variety of different treatment approaches.

General Indications and Contraindications

Patients with early-stage NSCLC (TNM T1–2), with no involvement of lymph nodes or patients with pulmonary metastases from various tumors can be evaluated for lung brachytherapy if surgical options are not feasible or desired. Predominantly, patients with singular lesions or oligometastatic disease will benefit from local treatment. In the context of metastatic disease, the lesions treated should be of prognostic significance, with the remaining burden of disease either in treatment or under stable control.

Local difficulties such as recurrent or persistent disease, rapid progression, compression of pulmonary structures, pain, or impending problems could be further indications for brachytherapy on an individual basis.

Contraindications include:

- Poor performance status (e.g., ASA physical status > ASAIII) [36]
- Insufficient coagulation
- Uncontrolled systemic disease

Generally, metastatic disease should be treated according to a comprehensive oncological therapy concept and decisions should be made on an individual basis with consensus by a supporting multidisciplinary tumor board.

Assessment and Preparation

At our institution, during the first personal appointment we obtain written informed consent from the patient. The information given to the patient includes risks, benefits, and treatment alternatives regarding:

- Sedation and analgesia
- Image-guided intervention for insertion of therapy probes including administration of contrast agents
- Interstitial brachytherapy

The assessment includes:

- Current imaging of the treatment area
- Medical and oncological history
- Clinical signs for high-risk interventions
- Pulmonary, renal, and hepatic function
- ASA physical status [36]
- Allergies, hypersensitivities
- Current medications
- History of opioid treatment
- Surgical and anesthetic history
- Indications for a specific assessment by an anesthesiologist [37]

All drugs that may interfere with normal blood coagulation must be discontinued appropriately according to standard perioperative surgical procedures [38]. Metformin should be paused 3 days ahead of therapy to avoid interaction with iodine-containing contrast agents. Preliminary laboratory checks include blood-cell count, albumin, creatinine, total bilirubin, CRP, ASAT, ALAT, GGT, and coagulation values. For patients with impaired pulmonary function, initial spirometry is recommended and this should be repeated after the procedure at follow-up.

Histological confirmation of the malignancy should always be provided. However, in patients where the malignant nature of the evaluated lesion is beyond doubt, for instance through the patient's medical history, it can be omitted on an individual basis. In newly diagnosed lung malignancies, PET/CT and cMRI are required diagnostic approaches for staging.

Interventional Technique

Generally, the procedure can be seen as a four-step process starting with CT-guided catheter application under procedural sedation, then computer-aided 3D-irradiation treatment planning, then the actual administration of single-fraction high-dose-rate brachytherapy employing the afterloading technique, and finally retraction of the interventional material with simultaneous sealing of the access canal with fibrin adhesive.

Interventional Team

The interventional team comprises at least five persons:

- Physician (interventional radiologist, catheter application)
- Physician (radiation oncologist, treatment planning)
- Medical physicist (provisioning of the treatment unit and treatment planning)
- OP nurse or interventional assistant

- Radiographer
- One person administering the analgosedation (in practice, this can be done intermittently by the radiation oncologist)

Patient Positioning

Whenever possible, the patient should be lying in the supine position with both arms resting comfortably above the head (see Fig. 12.1). For difficult dorsal or dorsolateral target locations, a lateral or prone position can be chosen if a stable and comfortable position can be achieved. In any case, the patient must be able to remain in the chosen position until the end of the entire procedure, which normally takes at least 2–3 h. For patients in a lateral or prone position, a urinary catheter is required.

Then, a first native CT scan is performed to determine the access area to be prepared for the intervention (see Fig. 12.2).

Fig. 12.1 OP nurse delineating the skin area to be disinfected before the procedure

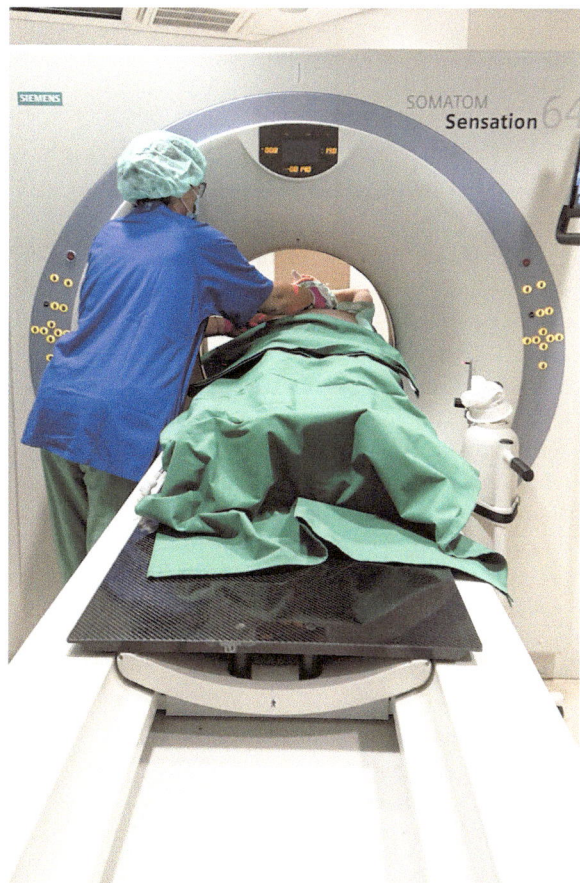

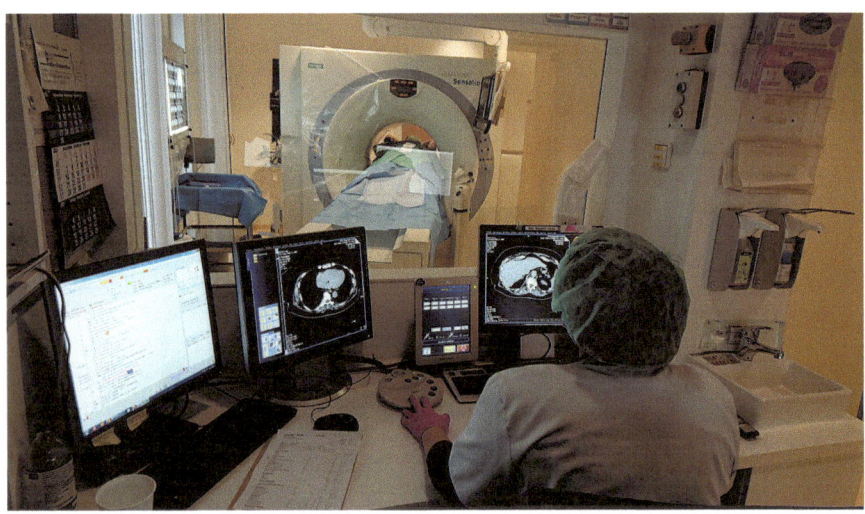

Fig. 12.2 CT-control room set-up at the Diagnostisch Therapeutisches Zentrum (DTZ) in Berlin. The patient is placed in a supine position with the arms rested comfortably over the head. An initial native CT scan is performed for a diagnostic survey and to identify the access area for skin disinfection

Anesthesiological Management

Usually, the procedure is performed employing procedural sedation (also known as analgosedation). Monitoring of vital parameters including pulse, blood pressure, and oxygenation is mandatory until the end of strict bed rest, for a total time of about 8–10 h (see Fig. 12.3). Oxygen supplementation should be 1–2 L/min starting at patient positioning. Sedative and analgesic effects must be achieved by titration. One should aim for minimum to moderate sedative effects according to level 1–2 as defined by the American Society of Anaesthesiologists [36, 39], where patients are relaxed but can fully cooperate and hold their breath on request. Sedation procedures should start well ahead of the intervention to allow for slow titration to adequate sedation. The anesthesiologist should be prepared for significant dose differences between individual patients based, for example, on the patient's weight, hydration, general constitution, and medication history. Because of these differences, constant communication with the patient during the procedure has been proven beneficial. Patients should be asked to report a possible onset of pain and should be kept informed during maneuvers that entail a higher chance of discomfort.

Application of midazolam should start 10–15 min and fentanyl 5–10 min ahead of catheter placement, with starting doses of 0.5–1 mg of midazolam and 50 μg of fentanyl, both given by slow i.v. drip. Additional single doses should not exceed 0.5 mg of midazolam or 50 mcg of fentanyl and must not be given before the

Fig. 12.3 Rearview of the interventional CT gantry. This is the connection area to the patient for the administration of the procedural sedation. Patient monitor and medications are easily accessible from here

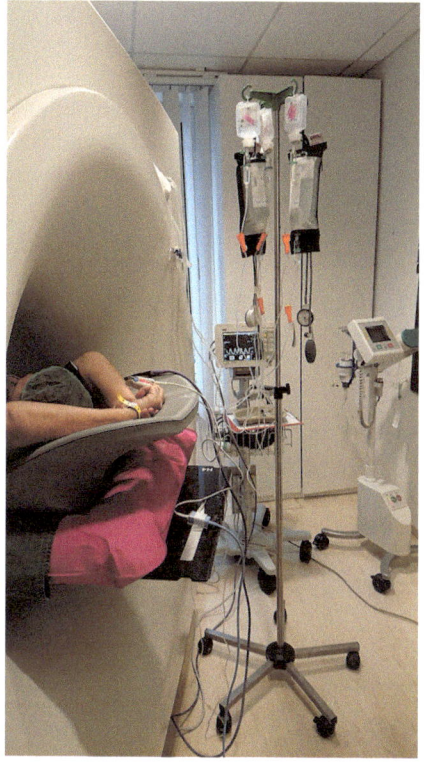

previous dose has fully taken effect. During prolonged interventions, the anesthesiologist must be prepared to repeat doses of fentanyl every 10–15 min for persistent analgesia. Antidotes for midazolam (flumazenil) and fentanyl (naloxone) should be quickly accessible in case of unwanted side effects such as can definitely occur within the regular dose range [39]. Additionally, local anesthesia with xylocaine is applied at the point of entry for the needle. At the end of catheter positioning, additional analgosedation might be necessary, but usually at larger intervals of 30 min or more.

When analgosedation is properly applied, the most common adverse effect seems to be mild bradycardia. In cases of heart rate <50 beats per minute, atropine can be given intravenously at a dose of 0.5 mg.

If adequate analgesia cannot be achieved, drugs from another class of analgesics can be considered for a different mode of action. Following that principle, an i.v. drip of 2 g metamizole has generally proven successful.

According to differences in local laws, guidelines or standards of care, analgosedation can be performed either by anesthetists or by non-anesthesia sedation teams; appropriate account should be taken of this [40]. Additional and more detailed information is provided in the "CIRSE Standards of Practice on Analgesia and Sedation" and the guidelines of the European Society of Anaesthesiology [37, 39].

Additional Medications

Pre-interventional dexamethasone (8 mg) and ondansetron (8 mg) are administered as an intravenous drip. O_2 is supplied routinely through a nasal cannula at an initial flow rate of 1–2 L/min and should be maintained until the sedative effects wear off. Additionally, prophylactic i.v. antibiotics should be considered if an elevated risk of local inflammation is suspected.

Catheter Positioning

Catheter positioning is performed employing image guidance by computed tomography (CT) fluoroscopy (see Figs. 12.4 and 12.5). After local anesthesia of the access site, the target lesion is punctured with a 17-gauge coaxial needle (KLS Martin GmbH, Freiburg, Germany). During the protraction of the needle, a breath-hold technique is performed by the patient. This is repeated several times until the target is reached. After optimum positioning of the needle centrally in the target area (see Figs. 12.6a and 12.7a) the spacer of the needle is retracted and replaced by a stiff angiography guide wire (Amplatz, Boston Scientific, USA) by using the

Fig. 12.4 Side view of the CT gantry with sterile covering of the patient and the gantry in place

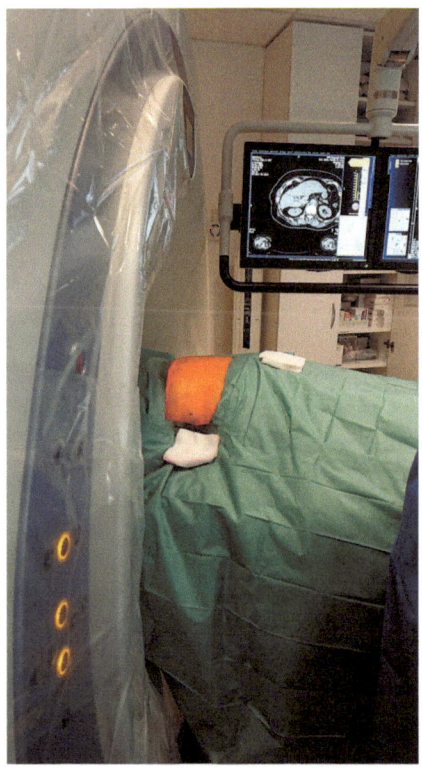

Fig. 12.5 Readily
prepared instrument table
with angiography sheath,
guidewire, and
brachytherapy catheter
(blue) among standard
equipment

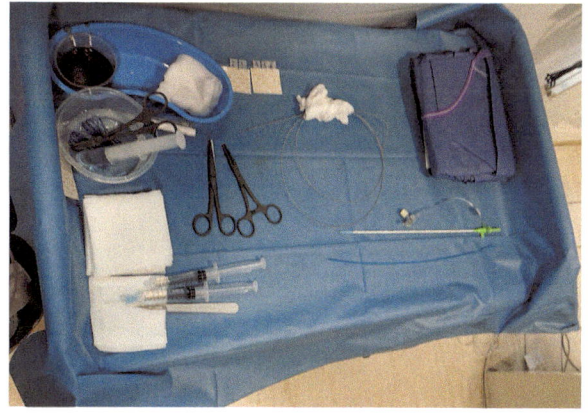

Seldinger technique. Then the outer hollow needle itself is retracted and replaced by a 6F angiography sheath with a hydrophilic coating (Radifocus Introducer II, Terumo, Japan) over the guidewire. After retraction of the guidewire, the 6F brachytherapy applicator (Primed, Halberstadt Medizintechnik GmbH, Halberstadt, Germany) is positioned inside the sheath so that the tip of the catheter is in line with the sheath or beyond, to ensure that the tip is visible in the planning CT scan. The number of applicators used depends on the size and configuration of the lesion to be treated. Single lesions up to 4 cm in diameter can usually be treated with a single applicator, a central location inside the target provided. For larger tumors, catheters should be placed at intervals, 1–2 cm apart. Physically, irradiation time and volume are defined by the largest distance between the target and the applicator, and can of course be decreased by using more applicators. If a central position cannot be achieved and the catheter only touches the lesion tangentially, full coverage of the target can only be accomplished with a significantly higher treated volume and also longer treatment time. It should be noted that by increasing treatment complexity through higher numbers of applicators one may also increase interventional risks so that a thoughtful balance between precision and simplicity is desirable.

Irradiation Treatment Planning

After positioning of the applicators, a spiral CT scan is performed, usually without contrast agents. These images are transferred to the dedicated irradiation treatment planning workstation (Brachyvision, Varian Medical Systems, Charlottesville, VA, USA; or Oncentra, Nucletron, Elekta AB, Stockholm, Sweden).

Treatment planning is performed employing target doses and constraints for risk structures [41] by a physicist, an interventional radiologist, and a radio-oncologist. First, catheter positions are entered into the program by digitizing the length of the applicators. For each pulmonary lesion, an individual target volume is defined. The planning target volume (PTV) represents the gross tumor volume (GTV) in the CT

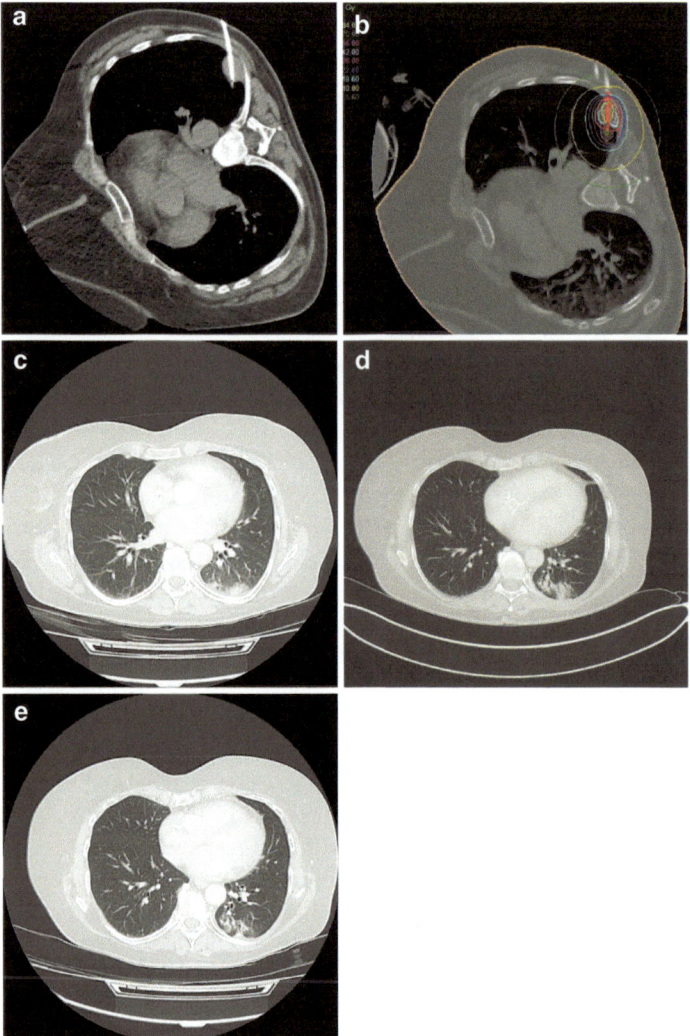

Fig. 12.6 (**a**) Case presentation 1: 64-year-old female patient with three pulmonary metastases from rectal cancer (only one shown); ID 2016 cT3 N2 M0; neoadjuvant radiochemotherapy, rectum amputation, pT3 pN0 (0/13), no regression of primary tumor, 11/2017 RFA of the right lung, 12/2017 brachytherapy of the left lung. Shown here interventional imaging with the brachytherapy sheath in place central in the dorsal metastasis. The patient is positioned on the right side for ease of access. (**b**) After irradiation treatment planning the target volume is completely confined by the 28 Gy isodose. Note the isodose distribution and the steep dose gradient to the periphery. The average dose to the spinal cord is 5.6 Gy. (**c**) First follow-up imaging 3 months after treatment shows mild post-therapeutic consolidation of the treatment area. A second paravertebral consolidation represents a second target volume (not demonstrated here). Patient is now examined in supine position. (**d**) Second follow-up after 6 months shows wider and more diffuse changes of the lung parenchyma. No solid tumor tissue determinable. (**e**) Third follow-up 9 months after irradiation. Further contraction of the consolidation with a dense pleural nodule discernible, corresponding to necrosis

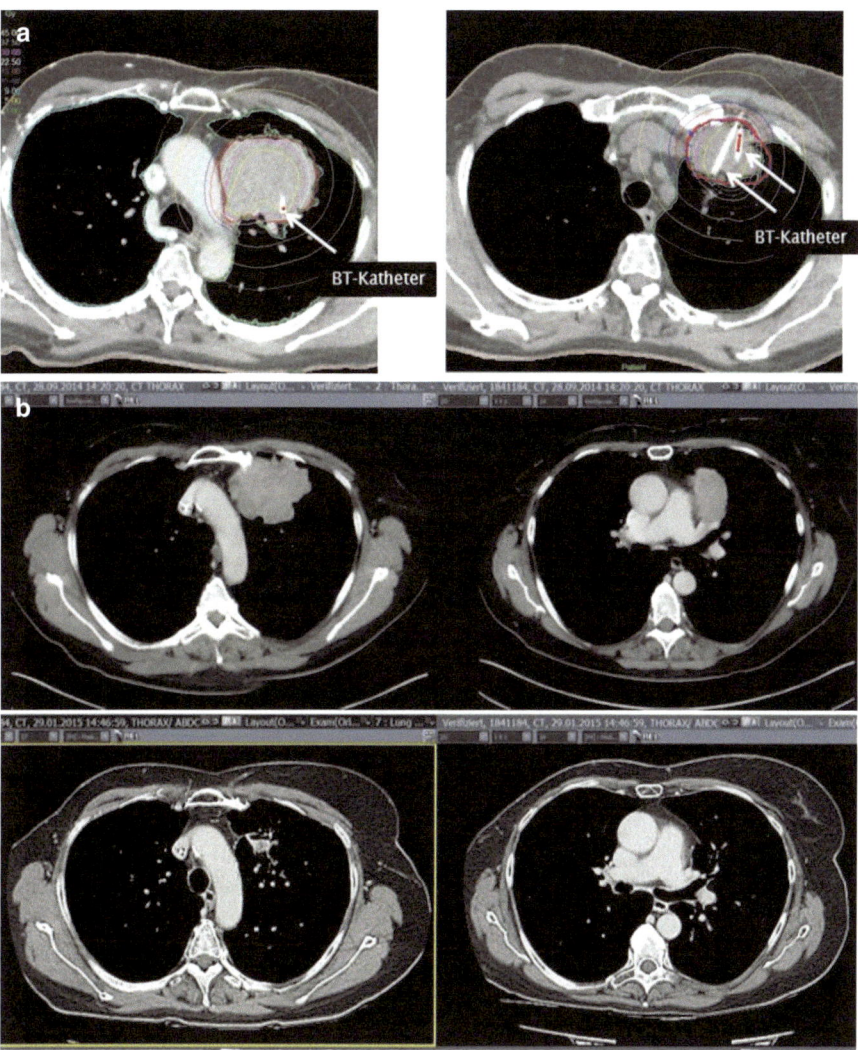

Fig. 12.7 (**a**) Case presentation 2: 63-year-old female patient with a progredient pulmonary lesion from breast cancer; ID 2008 pT4 pN1b M0; ablatio mammae, palliative radiotherapy of a sternal metastasis, treatment with bisphosphonate and 05/2013 pulmonary + mediastinal lesions; 06–10/2013 6× EC-Chemotherapy, Tamoxifen; 01/2014 PD: 12× Taxol, result = PR; 05/2014 start Exemestane; 08/2014 PD of a pulmonary oligo-recurrent metastasis left; 09–10/14 2× interstitial brachytherapy 15G (first upper, then lower part of the lesion); Isodoses: red line = 15 Gy isodose; left: first brachytherapy 09/2014; right: second brachytherapy 10/2014. (**b**) The same patient, comparison of pretherapeutic CT (above) and restaging 3 months after second brachytherapy (below); the contrast-enhanced CT shows rapid remission with only minimal residual tumor. (By kind permission, adopted from Hass et al.) [32]

lung window, with an additional margin of suspected subclinical spread to generate the clinical target volume (CTV), which is equivalent to the PTV in this instance, since no relative movement between the target and the applicator is expected.

Organs and structures close to the target volume should be specified as organs at risk (OAR). During treatment planning, dose distributions in these structures can be quantified and assessed.

Source dwell points and times are initially computed by the planning system, in complex situations using the HIPO (hybrid inverse planning and optimization) algorithm, and then optimized manually to achieve full coverage of the target volume with the prescribed dose of (usually) 20–25 Gy. Dose maxima of >50 Gy in central tumor areas are acceptable and can be admitted without restriction. Close to structures at risk or areas that have previously been treated, doses must be reduced to safe levels. For practical reasons, a total of three treated lesions per intervention should not be exceeded. It is to be explicitly noted that only unilateral treatment can be performed, to avoid the risk of bilateral pneumothorax.

During planning, the patient is prepared for transferral to the treatment room by covering the treatment area to preserve sterile conditions. In the treatment room, the transfer tubes are attached to the brachytherapy applicators (see Fig. 12.8), again with sterile conditions being maintained.

Irradiation

Treatment is performed as a single-fraction HDR irradiation using an afterloading system (Gammamed™, Varian Medical Systems, Charlottesville, VA, USA; or microSelectron HDR, Nucletron, Elekta AB, Stockholm, Sweden) employing an iridium-192 (^{192}Ir) source with a nominal activity of 10 Ci and a diameter of <1 mm.

During irradiation, the patient is locked into the treatment area while being continuously monitored with cameras and microphones from the outside. The average treatment time may be expected to be some 10–40 min, depending on the number and size of the lesions and the activity of the ^{192}Ir source.

Fig. 12.8 Directly before the irradiation: Connection of transfer tube and afterloading unit with the brachytherapy catheter (blue) mostly inside the angiography sheath (white and green). Precise positioning without displacement of the catheter is necessary

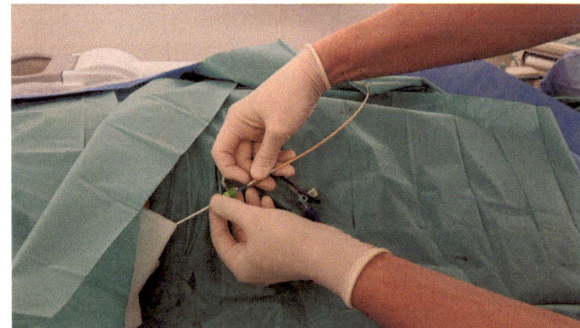

Fig. 12.9 After irradiation: The brachytherapy catheter is removed from the sheath before retraction of the sheath itself. Fibrin adhesive will be applied through the sheath to seal the intervention canal

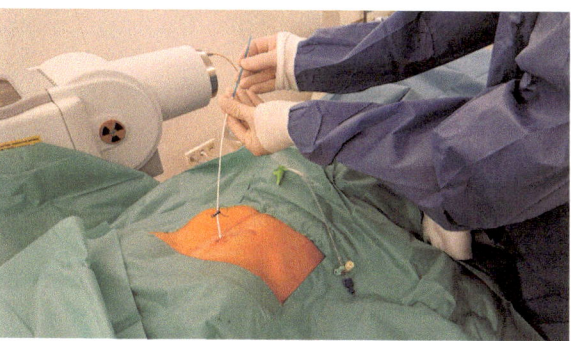

Material Retraction

When the end of irradiation is reached, each brachytherapy catheter is removed (see Fig. 12.9) and the angiographic introducer sheath is slowly retracted while less than 1 mL of fibrin tissue adhesive (Tissucol™, Baxter, Unterschleißheim, Germany) is injected. This seals the access canal, to reduce the risk of hemorrhage.

Post-procedural and Inpatient Management

After termination of the intervention, we perform a native CT scan of the thorax to check for side effects such as hemorrhage or pneumothorax. If these have been ruled out, we allow another hour of recovery for the patient before transportation back to the ward.

At the ward, patients should be monitored and should keep strict bed rest for another 6 h. We recommend blood tests for inflammation and hemoglobin for the two subsequent days, after which the patient can be discharged if no anomalies have developed.

In cases of pain, breathing difficulties, signs of hemorrhage, or inflammation during the stay, further diagnostic procedures such as ultrasound imaging or CT scans may be advisable.

Dose Prescription and Reporting

Although all dose prescription and reporting is managed according to ICRU standards, internally we employ a simplified system which is based on prescribing the dose to 100% of the PTV. For reporting, we specify the realized minimum dose in that volume (D100). Since the dose–volume relationship cannot be represented adequately by a single number, we also routinely state the dose in 95 and 90% of the PTV, giving a basic idea about conformality and dose distribution. Typically, the prescribed doses are in the range of 20–25 Gy.

Follow-Up Care of Patients, Quality Control

Patients should receive follow-up checks at intervals of 3, 6, 9, and 12 months (see Figs. 12.6a–e and 12.7a, b), including routine blood tests and CT scans of the thorax with additional contrast-enhanced imaging when necessary. Treatment success should be assessed following the modified WHO cancer treatment response criteria [42]. Any adverse events should be recorded by following the CTCAE criteria where applicable [43].

On detection of local progression, recurrent or persistent disease of the treated lesion, patients should be reevaluated by the tumor board with a view to possible further treatment.

Oncological Outcomes

In a retrospective study of 174 patients, we analyzed 156 patients with lung metastases and 18 patients with primary NSCLC [32]. Patients were treated in a period between 2006 and 2015 with a total of 359 lesions in 276 mostly single-fraction CT-guided brachytherapies. A median of 1 lesion was treated per intervention, with a range of 1–7. A median of 2 (1–11) brachytherapy catheters was used per treatment. Among metastasized patients a wide range of primary tumors was treated; of these, colorectal carcinoma (CRC) was the most frequent at 56%, malignant melanomas (17%), followed by renal cell carcinomas and mammary carcinomas. The malignomas were irradiated with median single doses of 20.5 Gy, enclosing 100% of the PTV.

We were able to achieve local control rates of 77% after 12 months with overall 12-month survival of 78%. Interestingly, in a subgroup analysis of different tumor entities, we could demonstrate significant differences between the histological types examined and the local control rates with renal cell carcinomas (100%), malignant melanomas (88%), adenocarcinomas (77%), squamous cell carcinomas (44%), and others (96%). For tumor entities that respond especially poorly, higher single doses should be considered, as experienced in other organs [20, 32].

Safety, Complications, and Management

Generally, treatment was well tolerated, with minimal patient discomfort and low complications. Local bleeding occurred in six cases (2.2%) which were quickly resolved by angiographic coiling. In 60 treatments (21.8%) a mild pneumothorax (<1 cm) could be observed; among them, 7 patients (2.5%) needed a temporary suction drainage to address the complication.

In five patients (2%) pneumonitis was associated with typical radiological findings; among them, two patients were given anti-inflammatory medication.

Although severe complications are rare, and could in our cases be resolved quickly, all necessary precautions should be taken to handle these comprehensively and rapidly. Especially hemorrhage and pneumothorax can lead to life-threatening situations, particularly in the elderly or in patients with relevant preexisting conditions; therefore, facilities for angiographic interventions and tube thoracostomy must be available.

Topical Challenges and Future Opportunities

After more than 15 years in clinical use, interventional interstitial brachytherapy continues to be a success story. It has even, in the case of hepatocellular carcinoma and liver metastases from colorectal carcinomas, been included in the European ESMO treatment guidelines [44, 45]. For the treatment of pulmonary lesions, the results are similarly promising, but the greatest challenge to this method is that it be generally accepted and broadly applied. Traditionally, tumor therapy has always been a challenge for interdisciplinary cooperation. In this respect, one of the great strengths of the method obviously also remains one of its major difficulties. To improve this situation, a clear-cut structural approach is required. This poses organizational and, not least, political difficulties for many institutions. The approach of interventional oncology, having emerged from a liaison between different disciplines, has developed into a novel field and is still just beginning its institutionalization. Interdisciplinary facilities must be established between departments which are able to accompany patients from initial presentation through therapy to periodic follow-up. The further creation of these structures must be encouraged.

Accurate selection of patients will also be decisive for the method's future long-term success. Further important issues will be the question of whether local therapy should be used alternatively or in addition to systemic approaches, the sequence of these procedures, and the question of how different types of local therapy are to be related to one another. We expect new insights from tumor and molecular biology to help us better differentiate between the various disease stages so that patients can be directed in a timely way to the appropriate treatment modalities [46, 47].

Fortunately, a number of local, ablative tumor therapies are now widely available—be they procedures from the field of radiation such as SBRT or brachytherapy, or thermal procedures such as RFA. Until now, the comparative value of these methods has not been conclusively established. Further clinical studies will be necessary to answer these questions.

Key Points

- CT-guided, interventional interstitial brachytherapy of the lung is a safe and effective procedure which can be performed with little patient discomfort.
- It is a multidisciplinary approach involving radiation oncology and interventional radiology.
- The method can be performed without general anesthesia by employing analgosedation.
- Early-stage lung cancers, as well as lung metastases from various cancer entities, can be targeted.
- Therapy decisions should be approved by a multidisciplinary tumor board.
- The diverse nature of local therapies should be utilized, to offer individual treatment options.

References

1. Bray F, Ferlay J, Soerjomataram I, Siegel RL, Torre LA, Jemal A. Global cancer statistics 2018: GLOBOCAN estimates of incidence and mortality worldwide for 36 cancers in 185 countries. CA Cancer J Clin. 2018;68(6):394–424.
2. Cronin KA, Lake AJ, Scott S, Sherman RL, Noone A-M, Howlader N, et al. Annual report to the nation on the status of cancer, part I: national cancer statistics. Cancer. 2018;124(13):2785–800.
3. Network NCC. NCCN clinical practice guidelines in oncology: non-small cell. Lung Cancer. 2017;2017. https://www.nccn.org/professionals/physician_gls/pdf/nscl.pdf.
4. Donington J, Ferguson M, Mazzone P, Handy J Jr, Schuchert M, Fernando H, et al. American College of Chest Physicians and Society of Thoracic Surgeons consensus statement for evaluation and management for high-risk patients with stage I non-small cell lung cancer. Chest. 2012;142(6):1620–35.
5. Ricke J, Jürgens JH, Deschamps F, Tselikas L, Uhde K, Kosiek O, et al. Irreversible electroporation (IRE) fails to demonstrate efficacy in a prospective multicenter phase II trial on lung malignancies: the ALICE trial. Cardiovasc Intervent Radiol. 2015;38(2):401–8.
6. Guckenberger M, Andratschke N, Dieckmann K, Hoogeman MS, Hoyer M, Hurkmans C, et al. ESTRO ACROP consensus guideline on implementation and practice of stereotactic body radiotherapy for peripherally located early stage non-small cell lung cancer. Radiother Oncol. 2017;124(1):11–7.
7. Peters N, Wieners G, Pech M, Hengst S, Ruhl R, Streitparth F, et al. CT-guided interstitial brachytherapy of primary and secondary lung malignancies: results of a prospective phase II trial. Strahlenther Onkol. 2008;184(6):296–301.
8. Nour-Eldin NA, Exner S, Al-Subhi M, Naguib NNN, Kaltenbach B, Roman A, et al. Ablation therapy of non-colorectal cancer lung metastases: retrospective analysis of tumour response post-laser-induced interstitial thermotherapy (LITT), radiofrequency ablation (RFA) and microwave ablation (MWA). Int J Hyperth. 2017;33(7):820–9.
9. Vogl TJ, Eckert R, Naguib NN, Beeres M, Gruber-Rouh T, Nour-Eldin NA. Thermal ablation of colorectal lung metastases: retrospective comparison among laser-induced thermotherapy, radiofrequency ablation, and microwave ablation. AJR Am J Roentgenol. 2016;207(6):1340–9.
10. Vogl TJ, Straub R, Lehnert T, Eichler K, Lüder-Lühr T, Peters J, et al. [Percutaneous thermoablation of pulmonary metastases. Experience with the application of laser-induced

thermotherapy (LITT) and radiofrequency ablation (RFA), and a literature review]. Rofo. 2004;176(11):1658–66.
11. Streitparth T, Schumacher D, Damm R, Friebe B, Mohnike K, Kosiek O, et al. Percutaneous radiofrequency ablation in the treatment of pulmonary malignancies: efficacy, safety and predictive factors. Oncotarget. 2018;9(14):11722–33.
12. Vogl T, Nour-Eldin N-E, Albrecht M, Kaltenbach B, Hohenforst-Schmidt W, Lin H, et al. Thermal ablation of lung tumors: focus on microwave ablation. RöFo. 2017;189(09):828–43.
13. Hellman S, Weichselbaum RR. Oligometastases. J Clin Oncol. 1995;13(1):8–10.
14. Weichselbaum RR, Hellman S. Oligometastases revisited. Nat Rev Clin Oncol. 2011;8(6):378–82.
15. Bretschneider T, Peters N, Hass P, Ricke J. [Update on interstitial brachytherapy]. Radiologe. 2012;52(1):70–3.
16. Mohnike K, Wieners G, Schwartz F, Seidensticker M, Pech M, Ruehl R, et al. Computed tomography-guided high-dose-rate brachytherapy in hepatocellular carcinoma: safety, efficacy, and effect on survival. Int J Radiat Oncol Biol Phys. 2010;78(1):172–9.
17. Streitparth F, Pech M, Bohmig M, Ruehl R, Peters N, Wieners G, et al. In vivo assessment of the gastric mucosal tolerance dose after single fraction, small volume irradiation of liver malignancies by computed tomography-guided, high-dose-rate brachytherapy. Int J Radiat Oncol Biol Phys. 2006;65(5):1479–86.
18. Wieners G, Mohnike K, Peters N, Bischoff J, Kleine-Tebbe A, Seidensticker R, et al. Treatment of hepatic metastases of breast cancer with CT-guided interstitial brachytherapy—a phase II-study. Radiother Oncol. 2011;100(2):314–9.
19. Wieners G, Pech M, Hildebrandt B, Peters N, Nicolaou A, Mohnike K, et al. Phase II feasibility study on the combination of two different regional treatment approaches in patients with colorectal "liver-only" metastases: hepatic interstitial brachytherapy plus regional chemotherapy. Cardiovasc Intervent Radiol. 2009;32(5):937–45.
20. Ricke J, Mohnike K, Pech M, Seidensticker M, Ruhl R, Wieners G, et al. Local response and impact on survival after local ablation of liver metastases from colorectal carcinoma by computed tomography-guided high-dose-rate brachytherapy. Int J Radiat Oncol Biol Phys. 2010;78(2):479–85.
21. Ricke J, Wust P. Computed tomography-guided brachytherapy for liver cancer. Semin Radiat Oncol. 2011;21(4):287–93.
22. Bretschneider T, Mohnike K, Hass P, Seidensticker R, Göppner D, Dudeck O, et al. Efficacy and safety of image-guided interstitial single fraction high-dose-rate brachytherapy in the management of metastatic malignant melanoma. J Contemp Brachytherapy. 2015;7(2):154–60.
23. Heinze C, Omari J, Othmer M, Hass P, Seidensticker M, Damm R, et al. Image-guided interstitial brachytherapy in the management of metastasized anal squamous cell carcinoma. Anticancer Res. 2018;38(9):5401–7.
24. Omari J, Heinze C, Wilck A, Hass P, Seidensticker M, Damm R, et al. Image-guided interstitial high-dose-rate brachytherapy in the treatment of metastatic esophageal squamous cell carcinoma. J Contemp Brachytherapy. 2018;10(5):439–45.
25. Bretschneider T, Ricke J, Gebauer B, Streitparth F. Image-guided high-dose-rate brachytherapy of malignancies in various inner organs—technique, indications, and perspectives. J Contemp Brachytherapy. 2016;3:251–61.
26. Wieners G, Pech M, Rudzinska M, Lehmkuhl L, Wlodarczyk W, Miersch A, et al. CT-guided interstitial brachytherapy in the local treatment of extrahepatic, extrapulmonary secondary malignancies. Eur Radiol. 2006;16(11):2586–93.
27. Ricke J, Wust P, Hengst S, Wieners G, Pech M, Herzog H, et al. [CT-guided interstitial brachytherapy of lung malignancies. Technique and first results]. Radiologe. 2004;44(7):684–6.
28. Ricke J, Wust P, Stohlmann A, Beck A, Cho CH, Pech M, et al. [CT-Guided brachytherapy. A novel percutaneous technique for interstitial ablation of liver metastases]. Strahlenther Onkol. 2004;180(5):274–80.

29. Ricke J, Wust P, Wieners G, Hengst S, Pech M, Lopez Hänninen E, et al. CT-guided interstitial single-fraction brachytherapy of lung tumors: phase I results of a novel technique. Chest. 2005;127(6):2237–42.
30. Collettini F, Schnapauff D, Poellinger A, Denecke T, Banzer J, Golenia MJ, et al. [Percutaneous CT-guided high-dose brachytherapy (CT-HDRBT) ablation of primary and metastatic lung tumors in nonsurgical candidates]. Rofo. 2012;184(4):316–23.
31. Chatzikonstantinou G, Zamboglou N, Baltas D, Ferentinos K, Bon D, Tselis N. Image-guided interstitial high-dose-rate brachytherapy for dose escalation in the radiotherapy treatment of locally advanced lung cancer: a single-institute experience. Brachytherapy. 2019;18(6):829–34.
32. Hass P, Sieber F, Willich C, Seidensticker M, Brunner T, Ricke J, et al., editors. CT-guided interstitial BT of pulmonary malignomas. Retrospecticve analysis of 174 patients. ESTRO37. Barcelona; 2018.
33. Tselis N, Ferentinos K, Kolotas C, Schirren J, Baltas D, Antonakakis A, et al. Computed tomography-guided interstitial high-dose-rate brachytherapy in the local treatment of primary and secondary intrathoracic malignancies. J Thorac Oncol. 2011;6(3):545–52.
34. Jonczyk M, Collettini F, Schnapauff D, Geisel D, Böning G, Feldhaus F, et al. Primary and metastatic malignancies of the lung: retrospective analysis of the CT-guided high-dose rate brachytherapy (CT-HDRBT) ablation in tumours <4 cm and ≥4 cm. Eur J Radiol. 2018;108:230–5.
35. Brada M, Pope A, Baumann M. SABR in NSCLC—the beginning of the end or the end of the beginning? Radiother Oncol. 2015;114(2):135–7.
36. Practice Guidelines for Moderate Procedural Sedation and Analgesia 2018: A Report by the American Society of Anesthesiologists Task Force on Moderate Procedural Sedation and Analgesia, the American Association of Oral and Maxillofacial Surgeons, American College of Radiology, American Dental Association, American Society of Dentist Anesthesiologists, and Society of Interventional Radiology. Anesthesiology. 2018;128(3):437–79.
37. Hinkelbein J, Lamperti M, Akeson J, Santos J, Costa J, De Robertis E, et al. European Society of Anaesthesiology and European Board of Anaesthesiology guidelines for procedural sedation and analgesia in adults. Eur J Anaesthesiol. 2018;35(1):6–24.
38. Mohnike K, Sauerland H, Seidensticker M, Hass P, Kropf S, Seidensticker R, et al. Haemorrhagic complications and symptomatic venous thromboembolism in interventional tumour ablations: the impact of peri-interventional thrombosis prophylaxis. Cardiovasc Intervent Radiol. 2016;39(12):1716–21.
39. Romagnoli S, Fanelli F, Barbani F, Uberoi R, Esteban E, Lee MJ, et al. CIRSE standards of practice on analgesia and sedation for interventional radiology in adults. Cardiovasc Intervent Radiol. 2020;43(9):1251–60.
40. Fernandez-Robles C, Oprea AD. Nonoperating room anesthesia in different parts of the world. Curr Opin Anaesthesiol. 2020;33(4):520–6.
41. Grimm J, LaCouture T, Croce R, Yeo I, Zhu Y, Xue J. Dose tolerance limits and dose volume histogram evaluation for stereotactic body radiotherapy. J Appl Clin Med Phys. 2011;12(2):3368.
42. WHO handbook for reporting results of cancer treatment. Geneva; 1979.
43. Institute NC. Common terminology criteria for adverse events: (CTCAE). 2010.
44. Schmoll HJ, Van Cutsem E, Stein A, Valentini V, Glimelius B, Haustermans K, et al. ESMO Consensus Guidelines for management of patients with colon and rectal cancer. a personalized approach to clinical decision making. Ann Oncol. 2012;23(10):2479–516.
45. Vogel A, Cervantes A, Chau I, Daniele B, Llovet JM, Meyer T, et al. Hepatocellular carcinoma: ESMO Clinical Practice Guidelines for diagnosis, treatment and follow-up. Ann Oncol. 2018;29(Suppl 4):iv238–iv55.
46. Pitroda SP, Weichselbaum RR. Integrated molecular and clinical staging defines the spectrum of metastatic cancer. Nat Rev Clin Oncol. 2019;16(9):581–8.
47. Gutiontov SI, Pitroda SP, Weichselbaum RR. Oligometastasis: past, present, future. Int J Radiat Oncol Biol Phys. 2020;108(3):530–8.

CT-Guided Interstitial HDR
Brachytherapy for Malignant Lung
Lesions: Experience from University
of California Los Angeles

13

Stephanie M. Yoon, Jie Deng, Kirsten Wong, Alan Lee,
Puja Venkat, and Albert J. Chang

Introduction

The lungs are a common site for primary and metastatic malignancies. Primary lung cancer is the second most common malignancy diagnosed in the United States and is the leading cause of cancer-related mortality with 5-year survival rates of less than 25% [1]. Lung cancer comprises two distinct subtypes, with 85% of lung cancers being non-small-cell lung cancer (NSCLC) and 15% being small-cell lung cancer (SCLC) [2]. NSCLC is further divided into three main histological subtypes—adenocarcinoma, squamous cell carcinoma, and large-cell (undifferentiated) carcinoma—each associated with its unique clinical presentation. SCLC is a high-grade neuroendocrine tumor and differs from NSCLC in its rapid growth and early development of disseminated metastasis. The majority of lung cancers are diagnosed in locally advanced or metastatic stages. Additionally, approximately 20–54% of extra-thoracic malignancies metastasize to the lungs thus making management of malignant lung lesions a common scenario faced by patients and oncologists [3].

The indications for treating primary or metastatic lung malignancies are evolving. First, malignant lung lesions can cause debilitating symptoms (such as cough, dyspnoea, hemoptysis, and airway obstruction) that greatly impact the quality of life. Palliation for obstructive tumors is of great value in this setting [4]. Secondly,

S. M. Yoon · J. Deng · A. Lee · P. Venkat · A. J. Chang (✉)
Department of Radiation Oncology, University of California Los Angeles,
Los Angeles, CA, USA
e-mail: SMYoon@mednet.ucla.edu; JieDeng@mednet.ucla.edu; AlaLee@mednet.ucla.edu;
PSVenkat@mednet.ucla.edu; AJChang@mednet.ucla.edu

K. Wong
David Geffen School of Medicine, University of California Los Angeles,
Los Angeles, CA, USA
e-mail: KCWong@mednet.ucla.edu

© The Author(s), under exclusive license to Springer Nature
Switzerland AG 2021
K. Mohnike et al. (eds.), *Manual on Image-Guided Brachytherapy of Inner Organs*, https://doi.org/10.1007/978-3-030-78079-1_13

153

the concept of treating all known sites of disease in patients with low metastatic disease burden (an "oligometastatic state") has been shown to prolong survival [5–7]. Combining local therapies with more effective systemic treatments, such as targeted therapies and immunotherapy, is increasingly being adopted into clinical practice for patients with oligometastatic disease. Therefore, locoregional therapy such as external-beam radiation or brachytherapy can remain of great value in the future, for both clinical and research purposes.

Lung Brachytherapy

Many patients with malignant lung lesions present with poor performance status or limited cardiopulmonary reserve, which precludes them from surgery. Alternative therapeutic options for medically inoperable patients are heterogeneous, and the choice of therapy is made on a case-by-case basis in a multidisciplinary setting. Brachytherapy is a minimally invasive therapy that can be used for malignant lung lesions. This therapy delivers high doses of radiation directly to the target tumor in a highly conformal manner. Depositing such tumoricidal radiation doses ensures high local control, while the steep dose drop-off minimizes exposure of nearby critical organs to radiation. Most reported experiences of brachytherapy in the United States have been in one of two settings.

One such setting is the treatment of endoluminal lesions by introducing a radioisotope through a catheter carrying a flexible bronchoscope. While endobronchial brachytherapy has been used in conjunction with external-beam radiotherapy (EBRT) to provide more curative treatments, it has primarily been used for palliation. Several collaborative groups, including the American Brachytherapy Society and the American College of Radiology, have recommended that endobronchial brachytherapy be used for palliation in patients with symptoms secondary to obstructive endobronchial tumors, especially if the patients were previously treated by EBRT [8–10]. Objective tumor response rates have ranged from 78 to 87%, while subjective relief from obstructive symptoms has been reported in 66–92% of patients [11, 12]. While combining EBRT with endobronchial brachytherapy may improve local tumor control, a recent Cochrane meta-analysis showed no advantage in disease-free or overall survival [8]. High-dose-rate (HDR) or pulse-dose-rate (PDR) is recommended over low-dose-rate (LDR) brachytherapy for endobronchial treatments [10].

The second common setting for lung brachytherapy is intraoperative or adjuvant treatment after surgery to address areas of potential local recurrence (from sublobar lung resections, incomplete resection, or close surgical margins) by implanting several LDR radioactive seeds. These radioactive seeds can be implanted at various locations throughout the thoracic cavity, either directly into residual tumor or near high-risk areas including the suture line in a grid or mesh pattern [10]. Various radioisotopes are available for LDR interstitial brachytherapy, including iodine-125 (^{125}I), palladium-103 (^{103}Pd), and caesium-131 (^{131}Cs). All sources are gamma emitters, with ^{103}Pd and ^{131}Cs having half-lives slightly shorter than that of

^{125}I. Radioisotopes with shorter half-lives deposit dose more rapidly, which can make the treatment of late radiation-responding tissues (such as the lung) more efficacious [13]. However, the decision to use a particular radioisotope must be balanced against the risk of depositing dose quickly in surrounding critical normal structures. Smaller institutional retrospective series demonstrated lower than expected local recurrence rates with the addition of intraoperative or adjuvant LDR brachytherapy [14–16]. However, the American College of Surgeons Oncology Group (ACOSOG) Z4032 phase 3 prospective randomized trial of sub-lobar resection with or without LDR interstitial brachytherapy showed no benefit in local control or overall survival with the addition of brachytherapy [17]. Two- and 3-year local control rates were respectively 12.3% and 12.3% with sub-lobar resection alone, and 9.3% and 12.0% with the addition of brachytherapy ($p = 0.47$ and $p = 0.96$) with a hazard ratio for local recurrence of 1.01 ($p = 0.98$). The local recurrence rate overall was lower than expected (7.7%) from the sub-lobar "resection only" group, and it was postulated that the study was underpowered for finding a difference in its primary endpoint of local recurrence. Therefore, interstitial LDR brachytherapy used either intraoperatively or adjuvantly is not routinely recommended in the United States except within the context of a clinical trial.

Outside the United States, there is growing experience with percutaneous interstitial brachytherapy for the management of malignant pulmonary lesions, with relatively more data on interstitial LDR brachytherapy than on HDR. In a recent meta-analysis that analyzed the safety and efficacy of ^{125}I brachytherapy combined with chemotherapy in 296 patients with advanced lung cancer from five randomized clinical trials, the addition of ^{125}I was found to be safe and did not significantly increase the incidences of adverse effects, with the exception of pneumothorax (RR = 4.93, 95% CI 1.94–12.55, $p < 0.001$) [18]. It was also associated with improved overall response rates (RR = 1.85, 95% CI 1.54–2.22, $p < 0.001$) and disease control rate (RR = 1.19, 95% CI 1.10–1.29, $p < 0.001$). There was no significant difference in 2-year overall survival (RR = 1.30, 95% CI 0.72–2.37, $p = 0.39$). Recent retrospective series have also shown that permanent ^{125}I interstitial brachytherapy led to disease-free and overall survival similar to those obtained by microwave ablation or second-line chemotherapy for patients who had pulmonary disease progression from first-line chemotherapy treatments; additional prospective studies in its utility for interstitial LDR brachytherapy are warranted [19, 20].

CT-guided interstitial HDR brachytherapy is, compared with LDR brachytherapy, a relatively new technique for treating pulmonary lesions, and it is practiced at UCLA. Few institutions have expertise with this technique, so reported experiences are few. It was initially introduced as a novel method for treating hepatic malignancies, and over recent years interest in applying this technique for treating malignant lung lesions has grown [21]. This method involves implanting an applicator percutaneously under CT guidance directly into a tumor of interest, and treating the tumor with an iridium-192 (^{192}Ir) source. This will be described in more detail in subsequent sections. Data on early outcomes suggest that interstitial HDR brachytherapy can achieve high local control with a favorable safety profile in treating pulmonary lesions [22–25]. A summary of contemporary studies of LDR and HDR interstitial brachytherapy is provided in Table 13.1.

One of the earliest experience with CT-guided interstitial HDR brachytherapy was published by Ricke et al. on the basis of a Phase I trial with 15 patients [22]. Thirty malignant lung lesions with mean tumor diameter of 2 cm (range 0.6–11 cm) were treated with at least 20 Gy in a single fraction administered to the tumor surface. After median follow-up of >5 months, local tumor control was 97%. With the exception of one patient who experienced nausea post-procedurally, no patients developed acute adverse events such as pneumothorax, hemoptysis, or abscesses. Another report from Peters et al. reported a 1-year local control rate of 91% after treating 30 patients with 83 primary and secondary lung malignancies to at least 20 Gy in a single fraction administered to the clinical target volume on a prospective, non-randomized trial [23]. One (2%) patient experienced a major pneumothorax requiring a chest tube placement for 24 hours. Moreover, six (12%) patients experienced minor pneumothorax (managed conservatively) and three (6%) patients had nausea after a median follow-up interval of 9 months. Tselis et al. also reported high 2- and 3-year local control rates in a retrospective review of 55 patients treated for 60 malignant lung lesions [24]. Unlike in the two trials described above, patients in this cohort received a multi-fractionated regimen to a median total dose of 20 Gy (range 7–32 Gy). Approximately half of the patients received twice daily treatment fractions of (median) 6 Gy per fraction, while the rest of the patients received several once daily fractions of (median) 8 Gy per fraction. After 14 months of follow-up, estimated 2- and 3-year local rates were both 82% for metastatic tumors. Estimated 2- and 3-year local control for primary/locally recurrent intrathoracic lesions was 79% and 73%, respectively. Relative tumor volume reduction was related to local control according to univariate analysis. Furthermore, pneumothorax occurred in 11.7% of procedures, but only one (1.8%) patient required post-procedural drainage.

Interventional Percutaneous Ablative Therapies

CT-guided interstitial HDR brachytherapy has the potential to overcome some limitations of other therapies for medically inoperable patients. One class of therapies comprises of image guided thermal ablations. These include radiofrequency ablation (RFA), microwave ablation (MWA), and cryoablation. RFA employs electromagnetic energy to create oscillating electric field lines which ultimately induce frictional heating in tissue. It is best utilized to ablate small, peripheral tumors, and can be performed in an outpatient setting. However, 2-year local control rates have been variable, ranging from ~15- 76%, and relapse rates tend to increase for tumors larger than 3 cm because of the inability to ablate to the tumor edge [26–30]. Tumors close to central lung, mediastinum, diaphragm, and vascular structures are also not ideal for thermal ablation. Moreover, vasculature reduces the efficacy of thermal ablation by the "heat-sink effect" or the loss of thermal energy through convection in the circulation [31].

Table 13.1 Contemporary studies summarizing low-dose-rate (LDR) and high-dose-rate (HDR) interstitial brachytherapy for malignant lung lesions

Study	Description	Year	Inclusion	Patient number	Dose fractionation	Tumor size	Response rate	Local control	Overall survival	Acute toxicity	Late toxicity
Wang et al. [19]	LDR (^{125}I)	2011	Inoperable NSCLC	21	Median matched peripheral dose 130 Gy (range, 100–160)	Median diameter, 4.6 cm (range 2.8–6.5)	30 months, 71.4% (CR, PR)	30 months, 85.7%	1-year, 42.4%, 2-year, 6.5%	19% patients with minor complications: pneumothorax, hemosputum, pleural effusion, or skin erythema	NA
Yue et al. [61]	LDR (^{125}I) + docetaxel or gemcitabine	2020	Age > 60, <3 localized NSCLC	50	Matched peripheral dose 110–140 Gy	≤2 cm diameter (30%) 2–3 cm (50%) ≥3 cm (20%)	6 months, CR 28%, PR 50%, SD 16%	Median PFS, 15.08 months	1-year, 88% 2-year, 54%	Pneumothorax (14%), cough/ hemoptysis (10%), pneumonitis (6%)	NA
Liu et al. [20]	LDR (^{125}I)	2020	Recurrent, unilateral NSCLC after first-line chemotherapy	32	Matched peripheral dose 120–160 Gy	<4 cm diameter	6 months, CR 40.63% 8 months, CR 100%	6 months, 100% 12 months, 96.9%	1-year, 96.9% 2-year, 90.6%	Pleural effusion (3.1%)	NA
Wang et al. [62]	LDR (^{125}I) + docetaxel or pemetrexed	2020	Oligo-recurrent NSCLC after first-line chemotherapy	25	Matched peripheral dose 100–140 Gy	≤3 cm diameter (48%) >3 cm (52%)	6 months, CR 4% PR 25% SD 42%	6 months, 70.8%	1-year, 59.5% 2-year, 23.9%	Pneumothorax (8%), hemoptysis (8%), fatigue (8%), nausea/ vomiting (4%)	NA

(continued)

Table 13.1 (continued)

Study	Description	Year	Inclusion	Patient number	Dose fractionation	Tumor size	Response rate	Local control	Overall survival	Acute toxicity	Late toxicity
Ricke et al. [22]	HDR (^{192}Ir)	2005	Primary NSCLC, lung metastasis	15	20 Gy/1 fx	Mean diameter, 2 cm (range 0.6–11.0)	NA	5+ months, 97%	NA	Nausea (7%), focal hemorrhage (7%)	Abscess (7%)
Peters et al. [23]	HDR (^{192}Ir)	2008	Primary NSCLC, lung metastasis	30	15–20 Gy/1 fx	Mean diameter 2.5 cm (0.6–11.0)	3 months, CR 0% PR 36% SD 64%	1 year, 91%	NA	Minor pneumothorax (12%), major pneumothorax (2%), nausea (6%)	Abscess (3%)
Tselis et al. [24]	HDR (^{192}Ir)	2011	Primary NSCLC, lung metastasis	55	Median total dose 25 Gy (range 10–32 Gy) in 4–15 Gy/fx BID *or* median total dose 10 Gy (range 7–32 Gy) in 4–20 Gy/fx QD	Median tumor volume, 160 cc (range 24–583)	Median 11 months, CR 18.1% PR 49.0% SD 27.2%	1-year, 86–93% 2-year, 79–82% 3-year, 73–82%	1-year, 63% 2-year 26% 3-year 7%	Minor pneumothorax (11.7%), major pneumothorax (1.8%)	NA
Sharma et al. [25]	HDR (^{192}Ir)	2011	Primary NSCLC, lung metastasis	8	20 Gy/1 fx	Median diameter 4 cm (range 3.0–5.5)	6 months, 75% (CR, PR, SD)	6 months, 75%	8 months, 100%	Hemoptysis (12%), pleural effusion (12%)	NA

NSCLC non-small-cell lung cancer, *CR* complete response, *PR* partial response, *SD* stable disease, *PFS* progression-free survival, *fx* fraction, *BID* twice daily, *QD* once daily

MWA also uses an electromagnetic source, but at higher wave frequencies to excite and oscillate water molecules within the tissue around a probe in order to ablate tumors [32]. Unlike RFA, it is less susceptible to the heat-sink effect and is thus potentially able to treat lesions near vasculature more effectively than RFA. Similar to RFA, MWA is limited to treating smaller lesions and is associated with risk of pneumothorax, hemoptysis, and post-procedural pain. There are fewer reported data on the use of MWA for pulmonary lesions than on RFA, but 2- and 3-year local control rates were respectively 64% and 56% in one large retrospective series [33]. Recurrence rates would also increase with tumors larger than 3 cm in diameter.

Alternatively, cryoablation utilizes freeze-and-thaw cycles to ablate small lesions by inducing intra and extracellular ice crystals that disrupt cellular membrane and processes. This therapy is well suited for smaller (<3 cm) tumors. It can also be safely applied for centrally located tumors because cellular architecture and collagenous tissue are preserved, and compared with thermal ablative techniques, it entails a lower risk of toxicity to major airways or mediastinal organs. The 2-year local progression-free survival rate in one large retrospective series of 210 tumors was 69% [34]. Additional interventional techniques are available to treat malignant endoluminal tumors, though these will not be the focus of this chapter. While quite effective under certain circumstances in controlling local growth, interventional percutaneous therapies have been associated with complication rates of pneumothorax, pleural effusion, and hemoptysis, as compared with percutaneous interstitial brachytherapy [31, 35]. Pneumothorax rates have reported to range from 11 to 67%, and chest tube insertions for drainage were required for 6–29% of patients after interventional therapies [36, 37].

Available data on CT-guided HDR interstitial brachytherapy have shown consistently high local control rates irrespective of tumor volume, which is not often possible with image guided thermal ablation. One-year local control rates have been >90%, and 2-year control rates have been 79–82% [22–24]. Achieving high control rates for larger tumors is possible as several catheters can be implanted, and/or treatment time can be adjusted, to achieve optimal dosing. HDR brachytherapy also delivers the necessary tumoricidal doses in a non-homogenous manner, which is advantageous for boosting dose to intratumoral areas that may exhibit radioresistance from a hypoxic tumor microenvironment [38]. Furthermore, 3D computer-generated planning systems for radiation treatment allow radiation oncologists to optimize dose distribution before treatment delivery. Precise dose measurements cannot be performed during image guided thermal ablation as several factors cannot be accounted for at the time of delivery, including thermal conductivity, capacity, impedance, perfusion, and tissue inhomogeneity. The sharp dose fall-off in brachytherapy also makes it possible to manage pulmonary lesions, adjacent to major blood vessels and central/ultra-central regions. Finally, interstitial HDR brachytherapy has so far been associated with similar or lower rates of complications, especially of pneumothorax. While the exact mechanism of this trend is not entirely understood, it is hypothesized that it may be attributed to differences in biological effects between the two treatment methods. Cytotoxic effects from radiation often occur over weeks to months, which may cause less immediate structural changes, whereas interventional ablative techniques lead to instantaneous cell death and necrosis. With less immediate structural changes from radiation, there may be slower tissue reorganization, and this may mitigate the formation of air cavities and pneumothorax compared with interventional ablation methods [25, 39]. A summary of the use of image guided thermal ablative techniques is provided in Table 13.2.

Stereotactic Body Radiotherapy

Another class of therapies considered for malignant lung lesions is external-beam radiation. Stereotactic body radiotherapy (SBRT) is a specialized technique in which high doses of radiation are delivered to a target over five or fewer treatments. It is commonly employed for medically inoperable early-stage NSCLC and increasingly for oligometastatic pulmonary metastases. Much as in brachytherapy, the entirety of the tumor can be treated to tumoricidal doses in a highly conformal manner. Image guidance ensures reproducibility and accuracy during each treatment delivery. Unlike brachytherapy, SBRT treatment planning includes a safety margin of normal lung tissue around the target lesion to account for uncertainties in tumor localization from respiratory motion as well as systematic and random errors. Therefore, a relatively larger volume of lung tissue will be irradiated with external-beam radiation compared with brachytherapy.

Early studies evaluating SBRT in early-stage NSCLC and metastatic lung lesions demonstrated high local tumor control of >90% [40–42]. Long-term results of the RTOG 0236 study demonstrated that 5-year primary tumor failure was 7% [42]. However, disease progression outside the radiation field remained common and 5-year overall survival was 40%. Delivering higher dose per treatment confers an increased risk for long-term toxicities, including radiation pneumonitis, bronchial stenosis, hemorrhage, and respiratory failure, especially if radiation is directed toward central or ultra-central lesions that are close to critical structures including major airways, great vessels, and mediastinal structures (i.e., the heart, esophagus) [43–46]. In a phase 2 trial evaluating SBRT doses of 60–66 Gy in 3 fractions for early-stage NSCLC in medically inoperable patients, 2-year freedom from severe toxicity was 54% for patients with centrally located tumors compared with 83% for those with peripherally located tumors [44]. Since then, more acceptable toxicity rates have been found to be achievable by delivering the total radiation dose over a greater number (~7–12) of treatment fractions [47–49]. For example, NRG/RTOG 0813 was a dose-escalation trial for a 5-fraction SBRT regimen in central tumors to determine the maximum tolerated dose (MTD) that would yield a dose-limiting toxicity of <20%. The study concluded that the MTD was 12.0 Gy per fraction, and the associated probability of dose-limiting toxicity was 7.2% [50]. Treating central and especially ultra-central tumors remain challenging in the modern era. Several studies have reported severe and even fatal toxicities when SBRT was used to treat

Table 13.2 Summary of minimally invasive therapeutic options for the management of malignant lung lesions

	Technique	Tumor size	Tumor location	Local control	Benefits	Pitfalls
Interventional ablation	Radiofrequency ablation (RFA) [26–30]	≤3 cm diameter	– Peripheral – Not ideal near vasculature or central location	2-year, 15–76%	– Immediate ablation – Predictable post-ablation radiographic changes	– Local control diminishes with larger tumors – "Heat-sink effect" near vasculature – Relatively high complication rate[a]
	Microwave ablation (MWA) [33]	≤3 cm diameter	– Peripheral and some central – Some lesions near vasculature	2-year, 64% 3-year, 56%	– Immediate ablation – Able to treat some lesions near central locations or vasculature better than RFA	– Relatively high complication rate
	Cryoablation [34]	≤3 cm diameter	– Peripheral and central – Lesions near vasculature	2-year, 69%	– Immediate ablation – Able to treat lesions near central locations or vasculature	– Relatively high complication rate
Radiation	Stereotactic body radiotherapy (SBRT) [40–50]	≤5 cm diameter	– Peripheral and central – Lesions near vasculature	5-year, 93%	– Noninvasive – Tumoricidal dose delivery – Conformal radiation delivery	– Multiple fractions – Account for respiratory motion on tumor location – Risk of severe (even fatal) toxicities without careful treatment planning, especially for central/ultra-central lesions
	Interstitial brachytherapy (HDR) [22–24]	No size constraint	– Peripheral, central, ultra-central – Lesions near vasculature or other critical structures	1-year, 86–93% 2-year, 79–82%	– Tumoricidal dose delivery – Conformal radiation delivery	– Risk of severe toxicities without careful treatment planning, especially for ultra-central lesions

[a]Common complications include pneumothorax, hemoptysis, and post-procedural pain. Major pneumothorax requires temporary chest tube insertion. Minor pneumothorax is often managed conservatively

ultra-central pulmonary lesions, and special considerations for neighboring organs need to be taken into account during treatment planning [45, 46]. Interstitial HDR brachytherapy can be advantageous over SBRT in treating central and ultra-central tumors safely and effectively. Future dosimetric comparisons between SBRT and interstitial HDR brachytherapy would be of high interest.

Procedure

Interstitial Catheter Implantation

Interstitial catheter insertions are performed in collaboration with the Department of Interventional Radiology. Patients undergo a diagnostic chest CT. The tumor is located under CT guidance, and a mark is placed on the overlying skin by the interventional radiologist. The skin is sterilely prepared and local anesthetic (lidocaine 2% and bupivacaine 0.5%) is administered subcutaneously. A single 17-gauge coaxial introducer needle is inserted percutaneously through the marked location up to the pleura, where additional bupivacaine is injected. Serial CT scans are taken to confirm accurate needle trajectory as the needle tip is advanced to the distal edge of the lesion (Fig. 13.1). A single 4 Fr brachytherapy catheter is subsequently introduced through the needle sheath until its tip is coincident with the tip of the needle sheath (Fig. 13.2). Additional needles and catheters are introduced as needed to ensure adequate coverage and dosing of the tumor. Several catheter insertions are often considered when the tumor diameter is greater than 3 cm or near previously irradiated areas. The point at which the inner catheter leaves the outer coaxial introducer needle when their tips are coincident is marked on the catheter. The distances between the inner and outer Luer locks from the catheter and coaxial needle, respectively, are measured as well. These marks are used to confirm accurate placement of the brachytherapy catheter with respect to the coaxial needle during the treatment planning process. The brachytherapy catheters and coaxial needles are affixed to each other and to the patient's skin with Mastisol liquid adhesive and Covidien or Transpore tape (Fig. 13.3).

Brachytherapy Planning and Treatment Delivery

Upon completion of catheter insertion, the patient undergoes a planning CT simulation scan using slice thickness of 2 mm. Acquired images are transferred to the treatment planning system (TPS). The radiation oncologist delineates the clinical target volume (CTV) on the CT planning simulation scan. The CTV includes the gross tumor volume (GTV) and suspicious areas shown on simulation or prior diagnostic chest scans. Critical nearby organs at risk (OAR) are contoured on each slice. The treatment catheter is reconstructed on the TPS. Inverse planning is utilized for a prescription dose to the CTV surface. Previous studies have shown significantly higher local tumor control when biologically effective doses (BED_3) of greater than 100 Gy were delivered to the tumor [40]. A systematic review in 2013 also found that

Fig. 13.1 Advancement of coaxial needle under CT guidance during brachytherapy catheter implantation. In this example, a coaxial needle was advanced percutaneously and placed directly into an ultra-central lesion in the right middle lobe abutting the heart

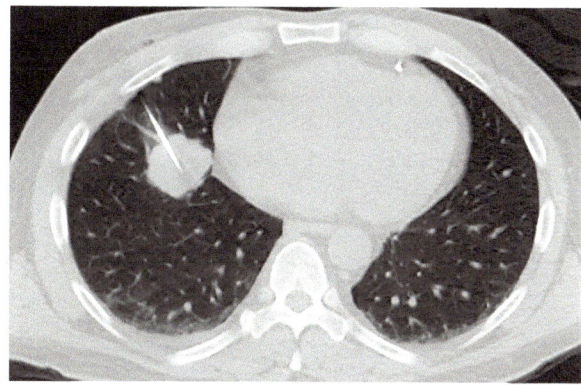

Fig. 13.2 The final position of a single 4 Fr brachytherapy catheter within percutaneous coaxial needle with both tips coincident with each other shown on the patient's skin surface. A black mark is made on the brachytherapy catheter to ensure accurate placement during the treatment planning and delivery processes

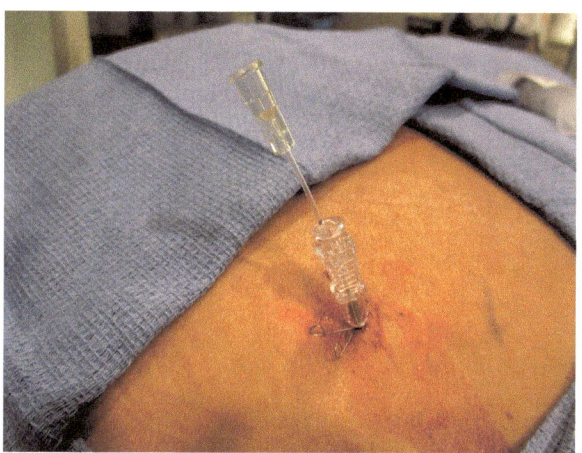

maintaining BED$_3$ below 210 Gy, especially for centrally located tumors, would keep the risk of treatment-related death to 1.0% [48]. From our institutional experience, the median prescription dose was 21.5 Gy (range 15–27.5 Gy) in a single fraction, corresponding to median BED$_3$ of 175.58 Gy. For a multi-fractionated regimen, the median dose prescribed was 24.75 Gy (range 24–25.5 Gy) in 2–3 fractions.

High target coverage was one of the primary goals during treatment planning and defined as 95% of the CTV to receive the full prescription dose (V100% ≥ 95%). Another dosimetric endpoint that was maximized when possible was the minimum dose that 90% of the tumor volume received (D90%). OAR dose tolerance limits outlined by AAPM Task Group 101 were given priority over treatment coverage [16]. The minimum dose to the most heavily irradiated 2 cc of OARs were also recorded. After plan approval and quality assurance checks, the patient is transported to the brachytherapy suite, where a ^{192}Ir source is delivered using an HDR remote afterloader unit. Upon completing treatment, both the coaxial needle and brachytherapy catheter(s) are removed, with placement of a resorbable hydrogel to seal the pleural site of entry.

Fig. 13.3 Brachytherapy catheter and coaxial needle are affixed to each other and to the patient's skin at the end of catheter implantation

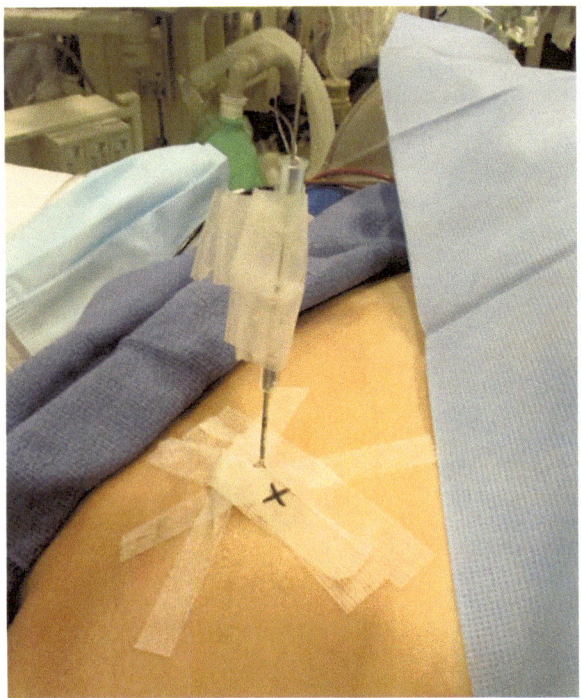

Clinical Cases

Case 1

A 51-year-old male with hepatocellular carcinoma secondary to hepatitis C treated by orthotopic liver transplantation presented to our clinic for possible brachytherapy for an enlarging lung metastasis. He developed several new lung nodules on surveillance CT chest in 2016, 3 years after his liver transplant. One dominant lung lesion located in the right middle lobe (RML) and in close proximity to the heart continued to enlarge throughout the year despite taking regorafenib.

During surveillance, the patient also developed chest pain due to myocardial infarction from stenosis in the mid-distal left anterior descending artery (LAD). Three bare metal stents were placed at the end of 2017. One month later, in 2018, he developed another stenosis in one of the diagonal branches of the LAD for which he underwent coronary angiography.

Meanwhile, the RML mass continued to enlarge, measuring 3.6 × 2.9 cm, and right pleural nodules consistent with pleural carcinomatosis developed (Fig. 13.4a). No other sites of metastatic disease in the abdomen or pelvis were noted. Aside from his recent myocardial infarction, the patient did not experience any pulmonary or airway-obstructive symptoms. Because systemic therapy options were limited for this patient in setting of his orthotopic liver transplant, a multi-disciplinary decision was made to switch systemic therapy to gain better systemic disease control while also to ablate the RML mass that had been refractory to prior systemic therapies. Given the tumor's ultra-central location, large size, and the patient's recent history of myocardial infractions, brachytherapy was recommended in a multi-disciplinary setting to treat this mass.

A single brachytherapy catheter was inserted into the tumor of interest during catheter implantation. The tumor was prescribed to 25 Gy in a single fraction. Figure 13.4b shows the isodose distribution of radiation treatment. The target volume measured 27.2 cc, and D90% = 101% (25.3 Gy). D2.0cc to normal ipsilateral lung (without CTV) was 193.7% (48.4 Gy). Likewise, D2.0cc of the heart was 20.0% (5 Gy). Serial follow-up CT scans of the chest with contrast were taken every 3 months. The nodule slowly decreased in size so that a year and a half after treatment the RML nodule measured 2.3 × 2.3 cm (Fig. 13.4c), which was consistent with partial response according to the Response Evaluation Criteria in Solid Tumours (RECIST).

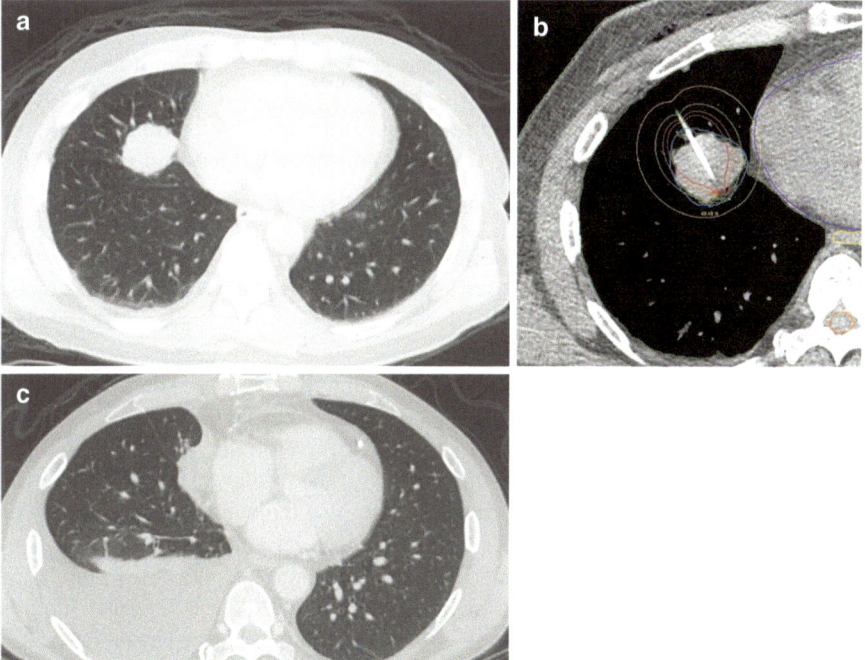

Fig. 13.4 A 51-year-old male with metastatic hepatocellular carcinoma. (**a**) Ultra-central lesion located in the right middle lobe before interstitial HDR brachytherapy. This lesion measured 3.6 × 2.9 cm. (**b**) Resultant isodose distribution from treatment planning. The target lesion was 27.2 cc and 25 Gy dose in a single fraction was prescribed. The 100% isodose line is shown in light green, encompassing the entire CTV while avoiding the heart. (**c**) Solid and linear consolidation consistent with evolving response to radiation a year and a half after treatment. This lesion decreased in size to 2.3 × 2.3 cm, which was consistent with partial response according to the Response Evaluation Criteria in Solid Tumours (RECIST)

The patient was followed every 3 months for a total of 15 months, and he did not experience any adverse sequelae of the radiation therapy. Unfortunately, he developed disease progression outside the irradiated area 3 months after brachytherapy treatment, and ultimately died 2 years later owing to respiratory failure from bilateral pleural effusions and multisystem organ failure. This case underscores the complexity of managing and palliating patients with metastatic disease. It also highlights the importance of a multi-disciplinary approach to management and the need for effective systemic therapies.

Case 2

A 65-year-old active smoker with medical history of early-stage renal cell carcinoma treated with nephrectomy and adrenalectomy developed multiple pulmonary metastasis soon after resection. Metastatic disease was temporarily controlled with pazopanib. Three years later disease progression was found, which manifested as increasing size of existing pulmonary nodules and a new left lower lobe interlobular septal thickening, raising concern of lymphangitic carcinomatosis. His systemic therapy was subsequently switched to nivolumab; and his pulmonary lesions remained stable for a year without additional sites of metastatic disease in the abdomen or pelvis. In light of the patient's stable disease state, his favorable response to immunotherapy, and the limited number of available systemic therapy options should immunotherapy stop being effective, it was decided in a multi-disciplinary setting to treat some of the largest pulmonary lesions aggressively with local therapy. The patient did not present any obstructive airway symptoms. He was referred to our clinic for interstitial HDR brachytherapy to ablate four of the largest lesions with radiation in a staged approach over 6 months.

One ultra-central pulmonary lesion measuring 1.6×1.4 cm was located in the left lower lobe (LLL) and was adjacent to an enlarged basilar segmental lymph node measuring 1.7×1.5 cm. Given the close proximity to critical normal structures (such as the posterior pericardium, thoracic aorta, and basilar segmental arteries and bronchi), percutaneous HDR brachytherapy was recommended. A coaxial needle and a single brachytherapy catheter were introduced posteriorly in order to traverse the least amount of lung tissue (Fig. 13.5a). The patient underwent CT simulation, and the treatment planned was a prescribed dose of 21 Gy in a single fraction. Figure 13.5b shows the isodose curve of the final treatment plan. The target volume was 7.2 cc, and 95% of CTV met received full prescription dose (V100% = 95%) which met planning goals. D90% to the target was 122%. The treatment plan also met acceptable constraints on the dose to nearby OAR as well. D2.0cc to the aorta was 66.6% (14.0 Gy), D2.0cc to the heart/pericardium was 45.8% (9.6 Gy), and D2.0cc to normal ipsilateral lung was 179% (37.6 Gy). A representative dose-volume histogram (DVH) from this treatment is shown in Fig. 13.6a. Both coaxial needles and catheters were subsequently removed after treatment on the same day as implantation.

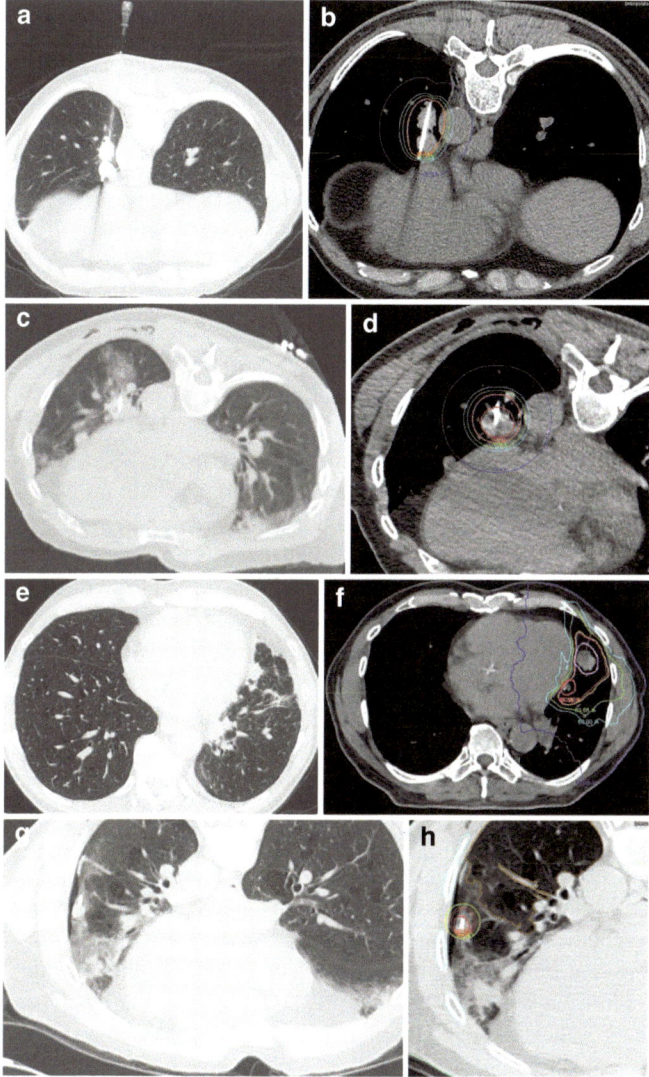

Fig. 13.5 A 65-year-old male with metastatic renal cell carcinoma. (**a**) Coaxial needle placement into an ultra-central lesion located in the left lower lobe (LLL) adjacent to posterior pericardium, thoracic aorta, and basilar segmental arteries and bronchi. (**b**) Representative isodose distribution. The target lesion was 7.2 cc and prescribed to 21 Gy in single fraction to the CTV surface. The 95%, 63.5%, and 50% isodose lines are shown in magenta (overlaps with yellow isodose line representing 91.6%), green, and light blue, respectively. (**c**) Coaxial needle placed in an ultra-central lesion located just superior to the first lesion. (**d**) Resultant isodose distribution. The volume measured was 7.6 cc, and 21 Gy in a single fraction was prescribed. The isodose distribution color scheme from (**b**) also applies here. (**e**) Two ultra-central lesions abutting the pericardium in the LLL treated with SBRT. (**f**) Isodose distribution resulting from SBRT prescribed to 50 Gy in 5 fractions. The isodose distribution color schema in (**b**) also applies here. (**g**) Coaxial needle placement into a peripheral LLL lesion in a previously irradiated area. (**h**) Resultant isodose distribution. The target was prescribed to receive 26 Gy in a single fraction. The thick red line outlines the clinical target volume. The 200% and 100% isodose lines are shown as thin red and green lines, respectively

A month later, a second LLL lesion just superior to the first treatment area measuring 3.2 × 2.6 cm was treated with interstitial HDR brachytherapy. This lesion was also in an ultra-central location, and adjacent to the descending thoracic aorta, pericardium, and left lower segmental arteries and bronchi. The lesion was prescribed to receive 21 Gy in a single dose to the CTV surface. Final treatment showed high conformality around the target lesion (Fig. 13.5c, d). The target volume was 7.6 cc, and planning goals for the CTV were also achieved: specifically, D90% was 102.5% to the target, D2.0cc = 41.7% (8.8 Gy) to the aorta, D2.0cc = 49.1% (10.3 Gy) to the heart/pericardium, and D2.0cc = 125.8% (26.4 Gy) to the ipsilateral normal lung. There was a small overlap from the first irradiated field occurring over a high-dose irradiated region.

A third large LLL ultra-central lesion that was more anteriorly positioned was targeted for brachytherapy a month later. However, the presence of calcifications in this particular nodule made placement of both coaxial needle and catheter difficult, and brachytherapy was aborted. Given its ultra-central location and tumor size, SBRT was considered to be the next best alternative. This lesion measured 1.7 × 1.1 cm, and an adjacent lesion measuring 1.0 × 0.7 cm lay just posterior to it (Fig. 13.5e). Both lesions were targeted during SBRT to a total of 50 Gy in 5 fractions (Fig. 13.5f). The total volume irradiated was 45.5 cc, which included additional margins added to the GTV to account for uncertainties in target location from respiratory motion, systematic patient set-up error, and random errors. All institutional and AAPM Task Group 101 OAR constraints for a 5-fraction SBRT regimen were met, including the V32Gy to the heart (2.4 cc) and V12.5Gy of normal lung (227.3 cc) (Fig. 13.6b).

Two months after SBRT, chest CT revealed new increased irregular airspace attenuation along the inferior aspect of the previously treated basilar left lower lobe nodule that was of concern for new regional pulmonary metastasis. After an additional month of close follow-up, the multi-disciplinary team believed that this area represented a new pulmonary lesion, and brachytherapy was pursued in order to spare as much normal lung tissue as possible since this area had been irradiated in the two previous brachytherapy procedures and SBRT. During brachytherapy catheter implantation, the patient developed a moderate pneumothorax in the left lung, requiring a chest tube insertion for 24 h. Despite this complication, the position of the single brachytherapy catheter was reconfirmed on CT. 26 Gy dose in a single fraction was prescribed for this lesion (Fig. 13.5g, h). CTV planning goals were met. CTV D90% was 138%. Dose constraints to OARs were also met: specifically, D2.0cc of normal left lung was 81.67% (21.2 Gy) and D2.0cc of adjacent rib was 24.3% (6.3 Gy).

Overall, the patient tolerated brachytherapy and SBRT well. Apart from the moderate pneumothorax that developed during one brachytherapy catheter placement, he did not experience any acute or long-term radiation-associated toxicities during 20 months of follow-up. On his 18-month post-treatment CT chest scan, there was mass-like consolidation, architectural distortion, and parenchymal bands in the area of the LLL basilar region from his first two brachytherapy treatments that were consistent with radiation-associated changes (Fig. 13.7a). The lesion treated with SBRT had a complete response and was replaced by patchy ground-glass opacifications (Fig. 13.7b). Finally, the fourth LLL lesion treated with brachytherapy also exhibited radiographic complete response with minimal surrounding pulmonary

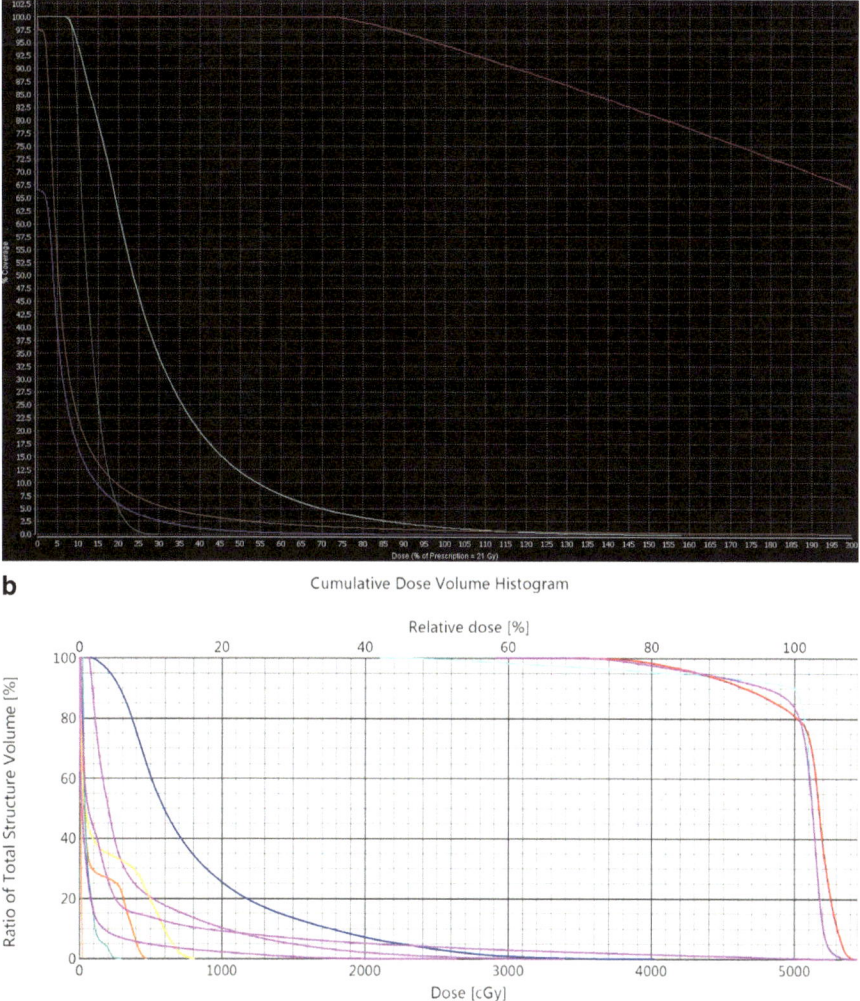

Fig. 13.6 Dose-volume histograms from (**a**) interstitial HDR brachytherapy treatment and (**b**) SBRT treatment. Both lesions were located in the left lower lobe, ultra-centrally

changes. No additional sites of metastatic disease developed, and the patient continues to be progression-free on maintenance nivolumab.

Case 3

A 38-year-old male was diagnosed with metastatic (yT3N1M1) rectal cancer. He underwent neoadjuvant chemoradiation to the pelvis and total mesorectal excision low anterior resection (TME-LAR). He subsequently developed disease progression with several metastatic liver and pulmonary nodules, and has since been on

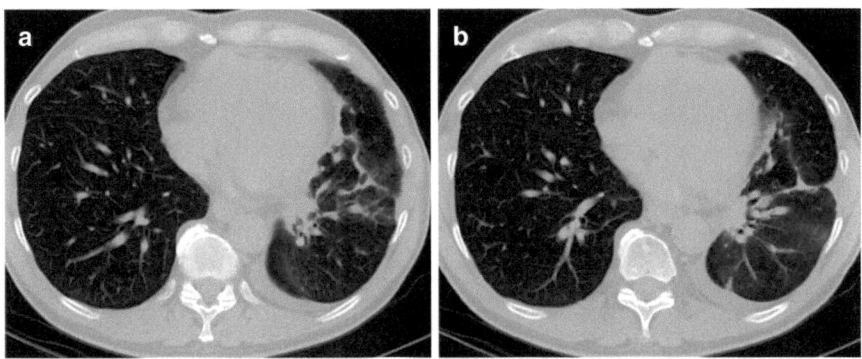

Fig. 13.7 Responses to radiation treatments 18 months after completion of radiation treatment. (**a**) Radiographic response following interstitial HDR brachytherapy treatments. There is a slowly evolving mass-like consolidation with architectural distortions and parenchymal bands consistent with radiation-associated changes. (**b**) Radiographic response after SBRT. The lesion is no longer seen and is replaced by patchy ground-glass opacifications

various lines of systemic chemotherapy. Pulmonary nodules were managed with several cryoablations and microwave ablations. He then presented at Radiation Oncology 5 years after his initial diagnosis for palliative treatment for a pulmonary lesion detected on surveillance CT causing right upper lobe (RUL) posterior segment airway occlusion that led to bronchial stenosis (Fig. 13.8a). Radiographic findings were associated clinically with productive cough and night sweats for several weeks.

The patient underwent bronchoscopy, which showed complete obstruction of the RUL posterior segment airway by tumor. After biopsies had been obtained, the obstructing mass was cryoresected and the airway was dilated. Pathology from biopsy specimens confirmed metastatic, moderately differentiated adenocarcinoma with mucinous features consistent with a colorectal primary. He was referred to Radiation Oncology to discuss palliative endobronchial HDR brachytherapy to minimize the risk of recurrence in this region. He was counseled about the limitations of this procedure and informed that it would not adequately treat the outer parenchymal component of the obstructing tumor. The patient expressed the wish to be as aggressive as possible with his treatment and desired to pursue endobronchial brachytherapy.

He began endobronchial brachytherapy treatment 2 weeks after his cryoresection. 20 Gy over 5 treatment fractions was administered to the post-cryoresection region in the RUL posterior segment airways. Figure 13.8b shows the resultant isodose lines from his last treatment fraction. Note that the 50% isodose line did not encompass the entire obstructing tumor, primarily at the superior and posterior tumor edges. The patient's cough soon resolved and he had no further issues with breathing. Within a few weeks, he resumed walking 6 miles per day and was able to go on vacation without any issues.

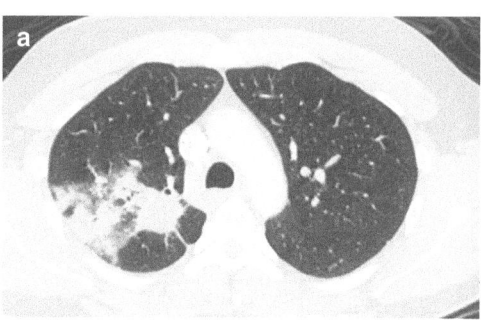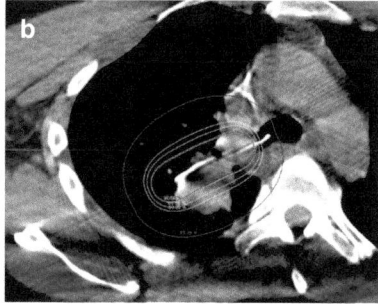

Fig. 13.8 A 38-year-old male with widely metastatic rectal adenocarcinoma who first underwent palliative endobronchial brachytherapy. (**a**) Right upper lobe lesion causing posterior segment airway obstruction in the background of radiographic changes from prior cryoablation. (**b**) Isodose distribution of endobronchial brachytherapy treatment. A dose of 20 Gy in 5 fractions was prescribed for the region. The 50% isodose line is represented in light blue

Unfortunately, subsequent surveillance scans showed increase in size of the RUL mass (measuring 4.0 × 3.6 cm) with persistent obliteration of the subsegmental airway and increased obstruction of the anterior and superior subsegmental airways. The patient again expressed the wish for aggressive treatment to optimize his quality of life. In multi-disciplinary discussion, it was agreed to palliate this persistently enlarging RUL mass with interstitial brachytherapy, given its close proximity to the right bronchus that was previously irradiated.

The patient underwent CT-guided interstitial HDR brachytherapy 8 months after his endobronchial brachytherapy. Owing to the size of the tumor and its close proximity to a previously irradiated critical structure, three brachytherapy catheters were implanted into the RUL mass (Fig. 13.9a). He was prescribed 21 Gy in a single fraction. This dose was kept lower than what was considered needed to achieve adequate tumor control in order to minimize the risk of damage from re-irradiation of surrounding normal structures. Figure 13.9b, c show the isodose curves and DVH from this treatment. The CTV shown in red is the achieved planning target goal (V95% = 110%). The CTV D90% was 126.4%. D2.0cc of the previously irradiated right bronchi was 49.3% (10.4 Gy).

Six months after interstitial brachytherapy treatment, postradiation changes were noted in surveillance CT scans. During this period, the patient had developed transient chest pain and nonproductive cough, with radiographic evidence of new airspace consolidation of the middle and lower margins of the irradiated area consistent with postradiation pneumonitis (Fig. 13.10a). He was treated with prednisone and symptoms resolved within a few weeks. Approximately 1 year after the brachytherapy, the patient's disease unfortunately progressed and he developed several new pulmonary and brain metastases. The RUL mass had continued to grow during this time and now extended to the right lower lobe and mediastinum. It was associated with satellite nodules extending into the right major fissure the right mainstem, upper and lower lobe airways (Fig. 13.10b). This case highlights the difficult

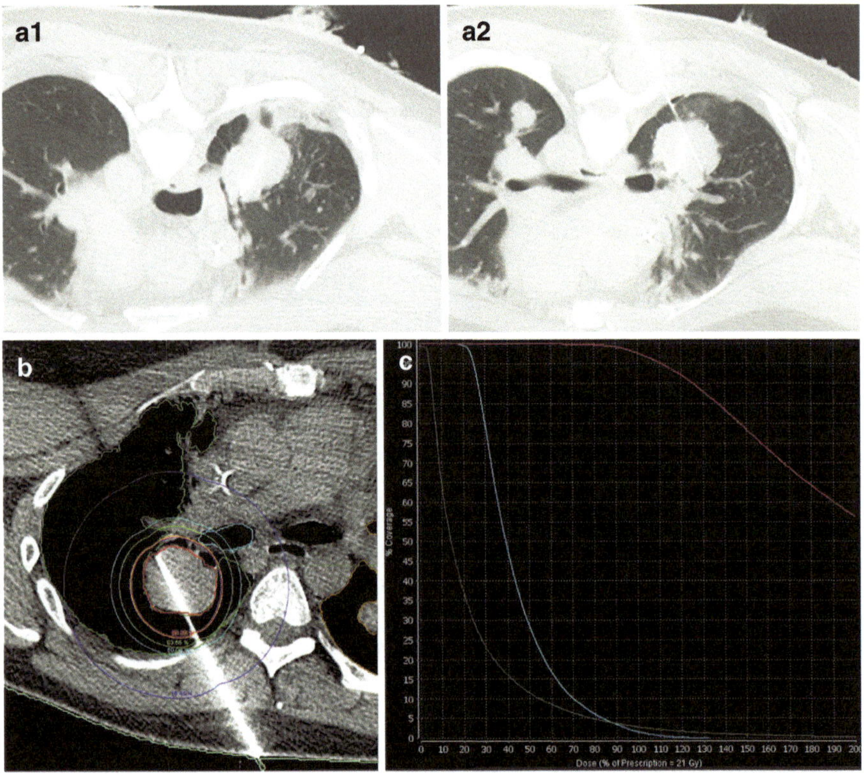

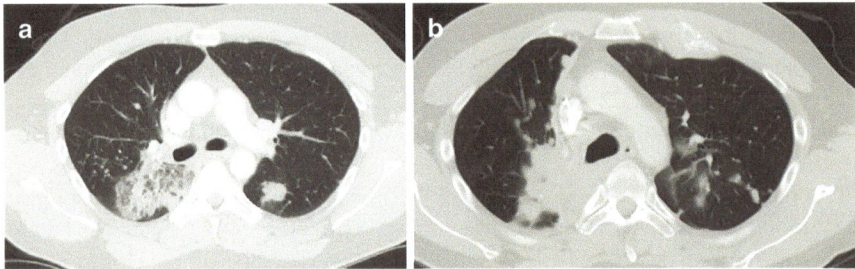

Fig. 13.9 A 38-year-old male with widely metastatic rectal adenocarcinoma who underwent palliative interstitial HDR brachytherapy for local tumor progression after endobronchial brachytherapy. (**a**) Three coaxial needles, and therefore brachytherapy catheters, were implanted in right upper lobe lung metastasis. (**b**) Isodose distribution. The lesion was prescribed to 21 Gy in a single fraction. (**c**) Dose-volume histogram of the resulting treatment. Red represents the CTV, blue is the right bronchus, and green is the right normal lung

Fig. 13.10 Follow-up scans after palliative interstitial HDR brachytherapy for a 38-year-old male with widely metastatic rectal adenocarcinoma. (**a**) Transient development of airspace consolidation near the irradiated site occurring 3 months after treatment. Findings were associated with chest pain and non-productive cough, altogether consistent with radiation pneumonitis. The patient was treated with prednisone, and symptoms resolved in a few weeks. (**b**) Radiographic findings 1 year after brachytherapy treatment. CT chest scan demonstrated slow interval disease progression, now involving portions of the right lower lobe, right main-/upper/lower lobe airways, and mediastinum. There are associated satellite nodules extending into the right major fissure

decisions that must be made during palliative interstitial brachytherapy treatments to balance optimum tumor control while minimizing normal tissue injury, especially in a location near previously irradiated tissue.

Clinical Outcomes

At our institution, 37 malignant lung lesions from 25 patients were treated with CT-guided interstitial HDR brachytherapy from September 2015 to August 2019. Common lung histologies were renal cell carcinoma (24%), NSCLC (20%), and soft-tissue sarcoma (20%). Twenty (80%) patients had received at least one prior treatment for their malignant lung lesion, including systemic therapy (72%), interventional procedure(s) such as cryoablation (32%), or radiotherapy (24%). Five (20%) patients had not received any prior therapy. Of the 37 treated lesions, 22 (88%) were metastatic lesions, 2 (8%) were primary NSCLC, and 1 (4%) was locally recurrent NSCLC. Altogether, 78% of lesions were located in either an ultracentral or a central location. Twenty-two (88%) of patients received a single fraction to a median total dose of 21.5 Gy (range 15–26 Gy). For the three patients (12%) receiving multi-fraction radiation treatment, the median dose was 24 Gy (range 20–25.5 Gy) with a range of 2–5 fractions.

After median follow-up of 19 months (range 3–48 months), 3 (14%), 9 (41%), and 9 (41%) patients experienced respectively complete response, partial response, and stable disease on follow-up imaging. Only one patient developed local progression of a right upper lobe lesion, as detailed in the previous section (Case 3). Two- and 3-year local control rates were both 90% on a per-patient basis, and 96% on a per-lesion basis. 52% of patients developed systemic disease progression outside the irradiated area after treatment. 80% of the patients were alive at last follow-up, and 2- and 3-year overall survival rates were both 67%. Four patients developed grade 1 and 2 acute toxicities: specifically, two patients developed grade 2 pneumonitis treated with steroids, and 1 patient developed a pneumothorax during catheter implantation which required an overnight chest tube insertion. No patient developed late treatment-related toxicities. One patient with metastatic colorectal cancer experienced mild dyspnoea on exertion 5 months after brachytherapy treatment, but the etiology was attributed to be multi-factorial given his smoking history and prior treatments (several resections and microwave ablations) for lung metastases.

Future Directions

Treatment paradigms for primary NSCLC and metastatic disease arising from many different primary sites are rapidly evolving. As newer systemic agents demonstrate improved efficacy in controlling advanced-stage solid tumors, locoregional therapies such as CT-guided interstitial HDR brachytherapy could play an increasing role in the future for the management of malignant pulmonary lesions. Further, understanding how local therapy interplays with systemic therapies will become increasingly important and can inform strategic combinations of these.

The immune system is widely recognized as playing a central role in cancer development, progression, and treatment. In particular, there has been increasing interest in the role of radiation as an in situ vaccination for immune activation, with numerous preclinical and clinical studies highlighting the importance of anti-tumor lymphocytes [51]. Indeed, absolute lymphocyte count has been found to correlate with clinical outcomes (i.e., survival) across various histologies [51].

In addition to the growing body of literature that supports immune-activating functions of radiation, radiation can act as a double-edged sword to exert immuno-suppression by several mechanisms, including depletion of lymphocytes by direct damage to DNA [52, 53]. Lymphocytes are known to be very radiosensitive, with doses as low as 1 Gy leading to destruction [53]. As a result, lymphocytes can be depleted by virtue of their transit through the vasculature of the irradiated field. This is of particular relevance in the context of the lung, where the neighboring heart circulates 100% of the total blood volume through the pulmonary vasculature [51, 54].

With increasing use of immunotherapy across various histologies in the up-front and salvage settings, lymphocyte preservation may be of increasing importance in optimizing the efficacy of immunotherapy [55, 56]. Numerous factors—such as lung V5, larger radiation portals, conventional fractionation, unintentional radiation to lymphoid organs, and the heart—can contribute to lymphopenia, suggesting that careful selection of radiation technique can help spare circulating lymphocytes [51, 54, 57–60].

Brachytherapy for lung lesions is well-positioned as a radiation modality to spare circulating lymphocytes, owing to its unique dosimetry, with sharp dose fall-off outside the target. There are limited studies evaluating brachytherapy compared with external-beam treatment, as it relates to lymphopenia, and studies by our group based on experience at UCLA are underway.

Conclusion

UCLA is one of the first institutions in the United States to gain experience with CT-guided interstitial HDR brachytherapy for the treatment and management of malignant lung lesions. Acquiring experience with this technique was made possible with the support of a multi-disciplinary team, including colleagues from interventional radiology, thoracic surgery, and medical oncology. Through this technique, we have been able to achieve high 2- and 3-year local tumor control rates of 96%, despite 78% of patients having central or ultra-central lesions. The majority of our patients did not develop any acute or late toxicities. Among those who developed acute toxicities, all adverse events were of grade 1–2 and self-limiting. Our experience with CT-guided interstitial HDR brachytherapy shows promising long-term safety and clinical efficacy. It can be an attractive treatment option to consider during the multi-disciplinary management of malignant lung lesions, especially for those in precarious locations close to critical organs or those that cannot be treated adequately with other alternative management options.

Key Points
- Management of malignant lung lesions is complex and should be done in a multi-disciplinary setting.
- There are several minimally invasive treatment options that are available for medically inoperable patients, but used under specific clinical conditions.
- CT-guided interstitial HDR brachytherapy is safe and effective.
- CT-guided interstitial brachytherapy should especially be considered for central or ultra-central lesions and for lesions located near previously irradiated areas.
- The role of locoregional therapies such as brachytherapy will expand in the future as treatment paradigms for advanced-stage solid cancers evolve.

References

1. Howlander N, Noone AM, Krapcho M, Miller D, Brest A, Yu M, Ruhl J, Tatalovich Z, Mariotto A, Lewis DR, Chen HS, Feuer EJ, Cronin KA. SEER cancer statistics review. https://seer.cancer.gov/csr/1975_2017/. Accessed 2020.
2. Molina JR, Yang P, Cassivi SD, Schild SE, Adjei AA. Non-small cell lung cancer: epidemiology, risk factors, treatment, and survivorship. Mayo Clin Proc. 2008;83(5):584–94.
3. Mohammed TL, Chowdhry A, Reddy GP, et al. ACR Appropriateness Criteria® screening for pulmonary metastases. J Thorac Imaging. 2011;26(1):W1–3.
4. Skowronek J. Brachytherapy in the treatment of lung cancer—a valuable solution. J Contemp Brachytherapy. 2015;7(4):297–311.
5. Gomez DR, Blumenschein GR Jr, Lee JJ, et al. Local consolidative therapy versus maintenance therapy or observation for patients with oligometastatic non-small-cell lung cancer without progression after first-line systemic therapy: a multicentre, randomised, controlled, phase 2 study. Lancet Oncol. 2016;17(12):1672–82.
6. Gomez DR, Tang C, Zhang J, et al. Local consolidative therapy vs. maintenance therapy or observation for patients with oligometastatic non-small-cell lung cancer: long-term results of a multi-institutional, phase II, randomized study. J Clin Oncol. 2019;37(18):1558–65.
7. Palma DA, Olson R, Harrow S, et al. Stereotactic ablative radiotherapy versus standard of care palliative treatment in patients with oligometastatic cancers (SABR-COMET): a randomised, phase 2, open-label trial. Lancet. 2019;393(10185):2051–8.
8. Reveiz L, Rueda JR, Cardona AF. Palliative endobronchial brachytherapy for non-small cell lung cancer. Cochrane Database Syst Rev. 2012;12:Cd004284.
9. Rosenzweig KE, Chang JY, Chetty IJ, et al. ACR appropriateness criteria nonsurgical treatment for non-small-cell lung cancer: poor performance status or palliative intent. J Am Coll Radiol. 2013;10(9):654–64.
10. Stewart A, Parashar B, Patel M, et al. American Brachytherapy Society consensus guidelines for thoracic brachytherapy for lung cancer. Brachytherapy. 2016;15(1):1–11.
11. Kelly JF, Delclos ME, Morice RC, Huaringa A, Allen PK, Komaki R. High-dose-rate endobronchial brachytherapy effectively palliates symptoms due to airway tumors: the 10-year M. D. Anderson cancer center experience. Int J Radiat Oncol Biol Phys. 2000;48(3):697–702.
12. Guarnaschelli JN, Jose BO. Palliative high-dose-rate endobronchial brachytherapy for recurrent carcinoma: the University of Louisville experience. J Palliat Med. 2010;13(8):981–9.

13. Armpilia CI, Dale RG, Coles IP, Jones B, Antipas V. The determination of radiobiologically optimized half-lives for radionuclides used in permanent brachytherapy implants. Int J Radiat Oncol Biol Phys. 2003;55(2):378–85.
14. Wernicke AG, Parikh A, Yondorf M, et al. Lung-conserving treatment of a pulmonary oligo-metastasis with a wedge resection and 131Cs brachytherapy. Brachytherapy. 2013;12(6): 567–72.
15. Mutyala S, Stewart A, Khan AJ, et al. Permanent iodine-125 interstitial planar seed brachy-therapy for close or positive margins for thoracic malignancies. Int J Radiat Oncol Biol Phys. 2010;76(4):1114–20.
16. Huo X, Wang H, Yang J, et al. Effectiveness and safety of CT-guided (125)I seed brachy-therapy for postoperative locoregional recurrence in patients with non-small cell lung cancer. Brachytherapy. 2016;15(3):370–80.
17. Fernando HC, Landreneau RJ, Mandrekar SJ, et al. Impact of brachytherapy on local recurrence rates after sublobar resection: results from ACOSOG Z4032 (Alliance), a phase III randomized trial for high-risk operable non-small-cell lung cancer. J Clin Oncol. 2014;32(23):2456–62.
18. Qiu H, Ji J, Shao Z, et al. The efficacy and safety of Iodine-125 brachytherapy combined with chemotherapy in treatment of advanced lung cancer: a meta-analysis. J Coll Physicians Surg Pak. 2017;27(4):237–45.
19. Wang Z-M, Lu J, Liu T, Chen K-M, Huang G, Liu F-J. CT-guided interstitial brachytherapy of inoperable non-small cell lung cancer. Lung Cancer. 2011;74(2):253–7.
20. Liu B, Wang Y, Tian S, Hertzanu Y, Zhao X, Li Y. Salvage treatment of NSCLC recurrence after first-line chemotherapy failure: Iodine-125 seed brachytherapy or microwave ablation? Thorac Cancer. 2020;11(3):697–703.
21. Ricke J, Wust P, Stohlmann A, et al. CT-guided interstitial brachytherapy of liver malignances alone or in combination with thermal ablation: phase I-II results of a novel technique. Int J Radiat Oncol Biol Phys. 2004;58(5):1496–505.
22. Ricke J, Wust P, Wieners G, et al. CT-guided interstitial single-fraction brachytherapy of lung tumors: phase I results of a novel technique. Chest. 2005;127(6):2237–42.
23. Peters N, Wieners G, Pech M, et al. CT-guided interstitial brachytherapy of primary and secondary lung malignancies: results of a prospective phase II trial. Strahlenther Onkol. 2008;184(6):296–301.
24. Tselis N, Ferentinos K, Kolotas C, et al. Computed tomography-guided interstitial high-dose-rate brachytherapy in the local treatment of primary and secondary intrathoracic malignancies. J Thorac Oncol. 2011;6(3):545–52.
25. Sharma DN, Rath GK, Thulkar S, Bahl A, Pandit S, Julka PK. Computerized tomography-guided percutaneous high-dose-rate interstitial brachytherapy for malignant lung lesions. J Cancer Res Ther. 2011;7(2):174–9.
26. Dupuy DE, Fernando HC, Hillman S, et al. Radiofrequency ablation of stage IA non-small cell lung cancer in medically inoperable patients: results from the American College of Surgeons Oncology Group Z4033 (Alliance) trial. Cancer. 2015;121(19):3491–8.
27. de Baère T, Aupérin A, Deschamps F, et al. Radiofrequency ablation is a valid treatment option for lung metastases: experience in 566 patients with 1037 metastases. Ann Oncol. 2015;26(5):987–91.
28. Zhu JC, Yan TD, Morris DL. A systematic review of radiofrequency ablation for lung tumors. Ann Surg Oncol. 2008;15(6):1765–74.
29. Lee JM, Jin GY, Goldberg SN, et al. Percutaneous radiofrequency ablation for inoperable non-small cell lung cancer and metastases: preliminary report. Radiology. 2004;230(1):125–34.
30. Huang L, Han Y, Zhao J, et al. Is radiofrequency thermal ablation a safe and effective procedure in the treatment of pulmonary malignancies? Eur J Cardiothorac Surg. 2011;39(3):348–51.
31. Jones GC, Kehrer JD, Kahn J, et al. Primary treatment options for high-risk/medically inoper-able early stage NSCLC patients. Clin Lung Cancer. 2015;16(6):413–30.
32. Simon CJ, Dupuy DE, Mayo-Smith WW. Microwave ablation: principles and applications. Radiographics. 2005;25(Suppl 1):S69–83.
33. Healey TT, March BT, Baird G, Dupuy DE. Microwave ablation for lung neoplasms: a retro-spective analysis of long-term results. J Vasc Interv Radiol. 2017;28(2):206–11.

34. Yashiro H, Nakatsuka S, Inoue M, et al. Factors affecting local progression after percutaneous cryoablation of lung tumors. J Vasc Interv Radiol. 2013;24(6):813–21.
35. Bi N, Shedden K, Zheng X, Kong F. Comparison of the effectiveness of radiofrequency ablation with stereotactic body radiation therapy in inoperable stage I non-small cell lung cancer: a systemic review and meta-analysis. Pract Radiat Oncol. 2013;3(2 Suppl 1):S19.
36. Hiraki T, Gobara H, Fujiwara H, et al. Lung cancer ablation: complications. Semin Interv Radiol. 2013;30(2):169–75.
37. Welch BT, Brinjikji W, Schmit GD, et al. A national analysis of the complications, cost, and mortality of percutaneous lung ablation. J Vasc Interv Radiol. 2015;26(6):787–91.
38. Ruggieri R, Naccarato S, Nahum AE. Severe hypofractionation: non-homogeneous tumour dose delivery can counteract tumour hypoxia. Acta Oncol (Stockholm, Sweden). 2010;49(8):1304–14.
39. Manning MA, Zwicker RD, Arthur DW, Arnfield M. Biologic treatment planning for high-dose-rate brachytherapy. Int J Radiat Oncol Biol Phys. 2001;49(3):839–45.
40. Onishi H, Shirato H, Nagata Y, et al. Hypofractionated stereotactic radiotherapy (HypoFXSRT) for stage I non-small cell lung cancer: updated results of 257 patients in a Japanese multi-institutional study. J Thorac Oncol. 2007;2(7 Suppl 3):S94–100.
41. Timmerman R, Paulus R, Galvin J, et al. Stereotactic body radiation therapy for inoperable early stage lung cancer. JAMA. 2010;303(11):1070–6.
42. Timmerman RD, Hu C, Michalski J, et al. Long-term results of RTOG 0236: a phase II trial of stereotactic body radiation therapy (SBRT) in the treatment of patients with medically inoperable stage I non-small cell lung cancer. Int J Radiat Oncol Biol Phys. 2014;90(1):S30.
43. Nguyen KNB, Hause DJ, Novak J, Monjazeb AM, Daly ME. Tumor control and toxicity after SBRT for ultracentral, central, and paramediastinal lung tumors. Pract Radiat Oncol. 2019;9(2):e196–202.
44. Timmerman R, McGarry R, Yiannoutsos C, et al. Excessive toxicity when treating central tumors in a phase II study of stereotactic body radiation therapy for medically inoperable early-stage lung cancer. J Clin Oncol. 2006;24(30):4833–9.
45. Tekatli H, Haasbeek N, Dahele M, et al. Outcomes of hypofractionated high-dose radiotherapy in poor-risk patients with "ultracentral" non-small cell lung cancer. J Thorac Oncol. 2016;11(7):1081–9.
46. Sebastian NT, Xu-Welliver M, Williams TM. Stereotactic body radiation therapy (SBRT) for early stage non-small cell lung cancer (NSCLC): contemporary insights and advances. J Thorac Dis. 2018;10(Suppl 21):S2451–s2464.
47. Li Q, Swanick CW, Allen PK, et al. Stereotactic ablative radiotherapy (SABR) using 70 Gy in 10 fractions for non-small cell lung cancer: exploration of clinical indications. Radiother Oncol. 2014;112(2):256–61.
48. Senthi S, Haasbeek CJ, Slotman BJ, Senan S. Outcomes of stereotactic ablative radiotherapy for central lung tumours: a systematic review. Radiother Oncol. 2013;106(3):276–82.
49. Murrell DH, Laba JM, Erickson A, Millman B, Palma DA, Louie AV. Stereotactic ablative radiotherapy for ultra-central lung tumors: prioritize target coverage or organs at risk? Radiat Oncol (London, England). 2018;13(1):57.
50. Bezjak A, Paulus R, Gaspar LE, et al. Safety and efficacy of a five-fraction stereotactic body radiotherapy schedule for centrally located non-small-cell lung cancer: NRG oncology/RTOG 0813 trial. J Clin Oncol. 2019;37(15):1316–25.
51. Venkatesulu BP, Mallick S, Lin SH, Krishnan S. A systematic review of the influence of radiation-induced lymphopenia on survival outcomes in solid tumors. Crit Rev Oncol Hematol. 2018;123:42–51.
52. Golden EB, Marciscano AE, Formenti SC. Radiation therapy and the in situ vaccination approach. Int J Radiat Oncol Biol Phys. 2020;108(4):891–8.
53. Sellins KS, Cohen JJ. Gene induction by gamma-irradiation leads to DNA fragmentation in lymphocytes. J Immunol (Baltimore, MD: 1950). 1987;139(10):3199–206.
54. Tang C, Liao Z, Gomez D, et al. Lymphopenia association with gross tumor volume and lung V5 and its effects on non-small cell lung cancer patient outcomes. Int J Radiat Oncol Biol Phys. 2014;89(5):1084–91.

55. Karantanos T, Karanika S, Seth B, Gignac G. The absolute lymphocyte count can predict the overall survival of patients with non-small cell lung cancer on nivolumab: a clinical study. Clin Transl Oncol. 2019;21(2):206–12.
56. Pike LRG, Bang A, Mahal BA, et al. The impact of radiation therapy on lymphocyte count and survival in metastatic cancer patients receiving PD-1 immune checkpoint inhibitors. Int J Radiat Oncol Biol Phys. 2019;103(1):142–51.
57. Crocenzi T, Cottam B, Newell P, et al. A hypofractionated radiation regimen avoids the lymphopenia associated with neoadjuvant chemoradiation therapy of borderline resectable and locally advanced pancreatic adenocarcinoma. J Immunother Cancer. 2016;4:45.
58. Wu G, Baine MJ, Zhao N, Li S, Li X, Lin C. Lymphocyte-sparing effect of stereotactic body radiation therapy compared to conventional fractionated radiation therapy in patients with locally advanced pancreatic cancer. BMC Cancer. 2019;19(1):977.
59. Chen D, Patel RR, Verma V, et al. Interaction between lymphopenia, radiotherapy technique, dosimetry, and survival outcomes in lung cancer patients receiving combined immunotherapy and radiotherapy. Radiother Oncol. 2020;150:114–20.
60. Liu J, Zhao Q, Deng W, et al. Radiation-related lymphopenia is associated with spleen irradiation dose during radiotherapy in patients with hepatocellular carcinoma. Radiat Oncol (London, England). 2017;12(1):90.
61. Yue TH, Xing W. (125)I Seed brachytherapy combined with single-agent chemotherapy in the treatment of non-small-cell lung cancer in the elderly: a valuable solution. Onco Targets Ther. 2020;13:10581–91.
62. Wang H, Lu J, Zheng X-T, et al. Oligorecurrence non-small cell lung cancer after failure of first-line chemotherapy: computed tomography-guided (125)I seed implantation vs. second-line chemotherapy. Front Oncol. 2020;10:470.

Brachytherapy of Renal and Adrenal Tumors

14

Robert Damm

Patient Management

Renal Tumors

Imaging

A typical imaging routine consists of thoracic/abdominal computed tomography (CT) and dedicated magnetic resonance imaging (MRI) of the kidneys. As benign neoplasms such as oncocytoma cannot be ruled out by either modality, imaging is carried out mainly to visualize the exact tumor location and to rule out lymphatic or distant metastases. As renal cell carcinoma and its metastases typically demonstrate strong arterial perfusion, contrast-enhanced imaging studies should always include an arterial phase as well as the typical portal or late venous phase.

CT scans may also include an excretion phase (delay after contrast injection >3 min) to depict the possible contact of a tumor with the renal pelvis. Furthermore, in MRI, T2-weighted sequences with and without fat saturation (e.g., T2 TSE or T2 single shot) provide good visualization and differentiation of any renal mass [1].

Ultrasound is not necessarily required, although catheter placement can in many patients be assisted by sonography guidance to reduce CT fluoroscopy time.

Renal Function Tests

As there are typically no other treatment options in patients with contralateral nephrectomy (beyond more invasive surgery), renal scintigraphy can be performed to monitor kidney function, but it typically has no impact on the treatment decision. Prior studies have confirmed a slow deterioration of ipsilateral renal function after

R. Damm (✉)
Department of Radiology and Nuclear Medicine, University Hospital Magdeburg, Magdeburg, Germany
e-mail: Robert.Damm@med.ovgu.de

© The Author(s), under exclusive license to Springer Nature Switzerland AG 2021
K. Mohnike et al. (eds.), *Manual on Image-Guided Brachytherapy of Inner Organs*, https://doi.org/10.1007/978-3-030-78079-1_14

image-guided HDR brachytherapy (see section "Safety and efficacy") but without a significant worsening of Kidney Disease Outcome Quality Initiative (KDOQI) stage. Individual cases of hemodialysis, years after brachytherapy, have so far only occurred in patients with contralateral nephrectomy and several local treatments (e.g., radiofrequency ablation and interstitial brachytherapy) of the ipsilateral kidney [2].

Routine laboratory tests should include creatinine serum levels with the calculation of the estimated glomerular filtration rate (eGFR), and the corresponding KDOQI stage should be documented.

Pretreatment Biopsy

Expert opinions differ on prior biopsy of renal tumors suspected to be renal cell carcinoma before a dedicated treatment. Overall, the prevalence of malignancy in renal masses is high (>80%), and many patients eligible for partial or radical nephrectomy will undergo surgery without prior histology. As patients with relevant comorbidities typically qualify for local-ablative treatment (thermal ablation, interstitial brachytherapy) or even active surveillance instead of surgery, the individual risk of malignancy should be considered. Small renal masses (<4 cm) are often found incidentally on cross-section imaging and often demonstrate a slow growth rate while imaging features cannot distinguish clearly between renal malignancies and benign masses such as oncocytoma [3]. Especially in patients with comorbidity that might entail an increased risk of complications, ultrasound- or CT-guided renal biopsy can aid decision-making. Furthermore, the efficacy of renal mass biopsy is high (>90%) and complication rates are low, while needle track seeding is reported in recent literature to be very low (<1%). Irrespective of whether the procedure is performed sequentially or directly before local ablation, a coaxial approach with an 18G core needle is recommended to avoid seeding and multiple needle engagements [4]. All in all, pretreatment biopsy is a valuable tool to identify patients for local ablation or active surveillance.

Patient Preparation

All patients must have laboratory values adequate for them to undergo interventional procedures (e.g., Quick >50%, thrombocyte count >50 Gpt/L, hemoglobin >6 mmol/L) and anticoagulation should be interrupted according to contemporary guidelines (e.g., Society of Interventional Radiology consensus guidelines). As often encountered in daily routine, intake of acetylsalicylic acid may be continued in patients with secondary prophylaxis. In renal masses with direct contact to the proximal ureter, pre-interventional placement of a double-J catheter by a urologist can prevent radiation-induced strictures and subsequent urinary congestion.

As interstitial brachytherapy is typically performed under conscious sedation (e.g., with midazolam and fentanyl), premedication with antiemetics (e.g., ondansetron 8 mg i.v. and dexamethasone 20 mg i.v. directly before catheter insertion) is recommended.

To enhance patient comfort in interstitial brachytherapies with longer duration of catheter implantation and/or irradiation, and to aid the detection of pelvic bleeding, a Foley catheter may be placed. Vital monitoring (noninvasive blood pressure, heart rate, oxygenation, and ECG) should be ensured during the intervention.

Follow-Up and Treatment Response

Cross-sectional imaging (preferably MRI) is recommended every 3–6 months for the first 2 years and every 6–12 months up to 5 years after interstitial brachytherapy of locally confined renal cell carcinoma (T1a, <4 cm), although many guidelines include longer intervals [5]. Additional or intermittent MRI can be performed, although an overall advantage in detecting local recurrences has so far not been demonstrated [6]. After stereotactic ablative body radiotherapy (SABR) of renal cell carcinoma, mild growth (up to 5 mm) of the overall mass up to 12 months after local therapy is reported in the literature [7]. From daily routine, this is also known to occur after interstitial brachytherapy, and it should be kept in mind when treatment response is being assessed. Also, contrast enhancement patterns after interstitial brachytherapy are variable, and overall enhancement need not necessarily decrease for the assessment to qualify as a treatment response. A typical case of local tumor control in renal cell carcinoma with long-term follow-up is depicted in Fig. 14.1.

Adrenal Tumors

Imaging

As most adrenal masses scheduled to undergo local treatment by interstitial brachytherapy will typically be distant metastases of various solid tumors (e.g., renal cell carcinoma, hepatocellular carcinoma, lung cancer), routine imaging will include thoracic/abdominal computed tomography (CT). However, additional MRI of the adrenal gland can be very helpful in distinguishing adrenal metastases from benign masses (e.g., angiomyolipoma or adrenal adenoma) if no imaging history is available. For this purpose, T2 TSE or single-shot sequences with and without fat suppression and T1 GRE in-phase and opposed-phase imaging (chemical shift MRI) are recommended [8].

Owing to the anatomical location of the adrenal glands, ultrasound imaging will be limited to special applications.

Pretreatment Biopsy

If CT or dedicated imaging with chemical shift MRI does not allow differentiation between benign and malignant masses, biopsy may be considered before ablation by interstitial brachytherapy. In many patients, imaging history strongly suggests a metastatic spread to one or more adrenal glands and biopsy may be obtained during catheter placement to confirm tumor involvement or to warrant mutational analyses. In either case, a coaxial approach should be preferred, as the placement of a brachytherapy catheter can be achieved through the coaxial needle directly after biopsy obtainment.

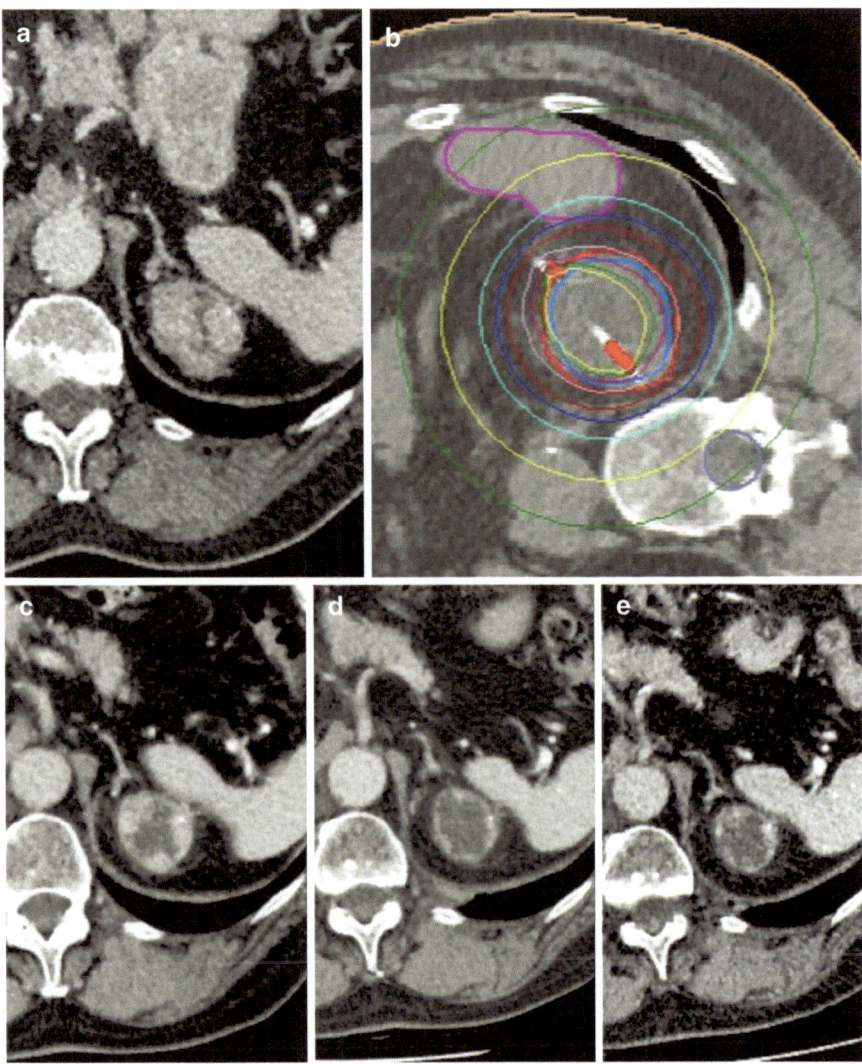

Fig. 14.1 Pretreatment CT imaging (**a**) and interstitial brachytherapy (**b**) in renal cell carcinoma. Follow-up imaging with typical reduction of vasculature and relatively low tumor shrinkage 3 months (**c**), 1 year (**d**), and 2 years (**e**) after treatment

Patient Preparation

Coagulation status must be sufficient for interventional procedures (e.g., Quick >50%, thrombocyte count >50 Gpt/L, hemoglobin >6 mmol/L) and anticoagulation should be paused according to contemporary guidelines (e.g., Society of Interventional Radiology consensus guidelines) and scientific literature [9, 10]. Intake of acetylsalicylic acid can be continued in patients with secondary prophylaxis after cardiovascular events.

If interstitial brachytherapy is performed as usual under conscious sedation (e.g., with midazolam and fentanyl), premedication with antiemetics (e.g., ondansetron 8 mg i.v. and dexamethasone 20 mg i.v. directly before catheter insertion) is recommended.

In interstitial brachytherapies with a longer duration of catheter implantation and/or irradiation, a Foley catheter may be placed to enhance patient comfort. During the intervention, continuous monitoring (noninvasive blood pressure, heart rate, oxygenation, and ECG) should be ensured.

Hormone Substitution

After unilateral irradiation by interstitial brachytherapy, substitution of corticosteroids is not usually necessary. In patients with contralateral adrenalectomy or bilateral tumors scheduled to undergo ablation, adrenocortical insufficiency must be expected. Hormone substitution should be prescribed in cooperation with an endocrinologist. As interstitial brachytherapy is usually well-tolerated and adrenocortical function decreases slowly, the following scheme may be applied in patients: Hydrocortisone 20 mg–0–10 mg orally starting the day after interstitial brachytherapy. If complications (e.g., bleeding, infection) occur, and in future situations of physical stress (e.g., surgery), intravenous administration of hydrocortisone 100 mg is recommended. Corresponding signs of adrenocortical insufficiency or insufficient dosages of hydrocortisone include nausea, hypotension, emesis, and abdominal pain.

All patients should also receive an emergency passport containing information about measures to be taken in an Addison's crisis.

Follow-Up

As most cases will involve patients with adrenal metastases, a follow-up interval of 3 months and imaging by computed tomography will be appropriate. MRI can be considered to enhance the detection of recurrences, although no scientific data are available on this topic.

Interventional Technique

Access Routes

Because of the location of the adrenal glands and kidneys, there are only a few patients for whom a supine position will allow direct access to the targeted tumor(s). Thus, a lateral or prone position will be necessary, and stable bedding on the CT bench is best achieved by utilizing a vacuum immobilization mat. To avoid a transhepatic approach or passing of the pleural recess, angulation of the needle (off-plane puncture) should be preferred in adrenal masses. Catheter paths can then be dorsolateral (between right liver lobe/spleen and kidney) or paravertebral (behind kidney, parallel to the spine); see Fig. 14.2. Depending on the location of renal masses, a transcostal or subcostal approach may be chosen. In larger or complex

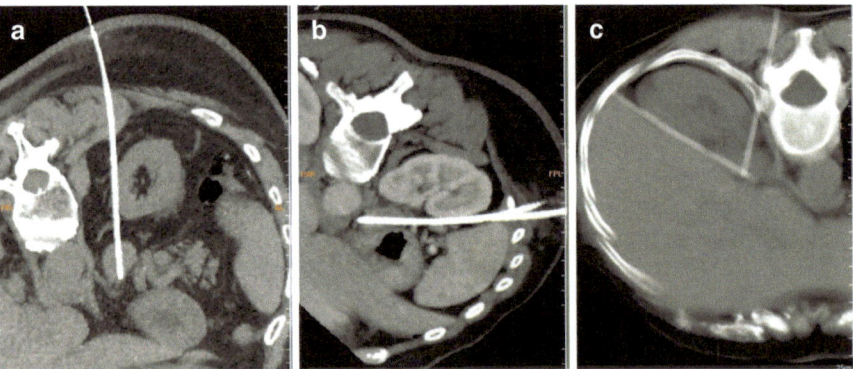

Fig. 14.2 Paravertebral (**a**) and dorsolateral (**b**) approach to the adrenal glands. In some situations, both access routes may be chosen (**c**). Images are oblique 5 mm MIP (**a**, **b**) or 40 mm Raysum (**c**) reconstructions of CT scans to reveal the catheter path

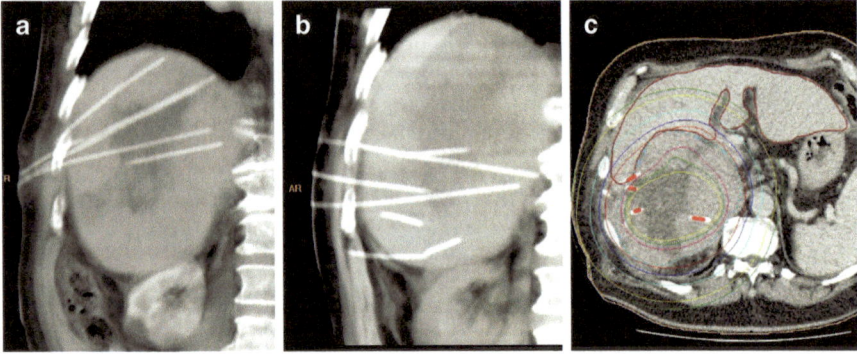

Fig. 14.3 Several catheters implanted to address a large lesion. Owing to its size (maximum diameter of 180 mm), two sessions (**a**, **b**) of interstitial brachytherapy were scheduled. Images are 40 mm Raysum reconstructions of CT scans (**a**, **b**) and treatment planning CT (**c**)

lesions, a combined arrangement of catheters is often required to achieve a sufficient geometry of the ablation zone. An example is depicted in Fig. 14.3.

Helpful Techniques

Especially in lean patients and in tumors located at the ventral aspect of the kidney, organs at risk (OAR) may be proximal to the target volume. In such cases, adjunctive interventional techniques can be mandatory to achieve a sufficient dose delivery to the PTV, e.g., implantation of angiographic balloon catheters to distance OAR from target lesions [11]. Typical techniques known from thermal ablation, such as hydrodissection, are limited by their volatile behavior over time—if image-guided HDR brachytherapy cannot be performed directly after catheter placement (e.g., different localization of departments), then the distancing of OAR can be reduced by redistribution of injected fluid leading to an incalculable dose exposure of adjacent organs.

In kidney tumors close to the renal pelvis or ureters, it might also be helpful to inject a small bolus of i.v. contrast agent (e.g., 20 mL, iodine concentration 300 mg/mL) at least 5 min before the intervention, as this will result in opacification of these structures during puncture/catheter insertion.

Catheter Removal

As adrenal and renal masses are typically hyperperfused (especially renal cell cancer), complications may arise from bleeding vessels in the catheter path after removal. Thus, it is highly recommended to perform catheter path embolization by applying a gelatine sponge through the catheter sheaths during stepwise retraction. Furthermore, a standardized follow-up is important for early detection of complications (e.g., dedicated sonography of the puncture site after 1–2 h) and routine monitoring (noninvasive blood pressure, heart rate, oxygenation, and ECG) should be ensured over at least 4 h.

Dose Considerations

Gross tumor volume (GTV) should be delineated in consensus between interventional radiology and the radiation oncologist. A safety margin of 5 mm should be included to create the clinical target volume (CTV). As respiratory motion can be neglected owing to the fixation of brachytherapy catheters within the tumor, the planning target volume (PTV) is identical to the CTV.

Renal Cell Carcinoma

Especially as small renal masses and early renal cell cancer often demonstrate slow tumor growth, and even active surveillance might be an option, dosage, and treatment-related risk should be balanced. In renal masses suspected or histologically proven to be renal cell cancer, a standard dose prescribed to the PTV of 15 Gy is recommended. In local recurrences, dose escalation to 20 Gy may be considered. Decisions on dosage should take into account clinical factors such as patient age and comorbidities, expected tumor biology, and renal function.

Adrenal and Renal Metastases

While adrenal malignancies scheduled to undergo interstitial brachytherapy are typically metastases from various primary cancers, metastases to the kidney are relatively infrequent. In any case, dose prescription should be based on clinical data available for the particular tumor entity. For the most common entities, the dose delivered to the PTV may be as follows: 15 Gy in hepatocellular carcinoma, lung cancer, breast cancer, and neuroendocrine tumors; 20 Gy in cholangiocarcinoma and gastric cancer; and 25 Gy in colorectal carcinoma [12, 13]. Additionally, factors such as other tumor locations, overall prognosis and concomitant systemic therapy should be considered.

Dose Constraints

Typical organs at risk (OAR) adjacent to the tumor site are the stomach and the small and large intestine. In recent literature, dose constraints were determined as follows: $D_{1CC} \leq 14$ Gy for stomach/small bowel and $D_{1CC} \leq 18$ Gy for large bowel [14, 15]. In most cases, exposure of the liver by interstitial brachytherapy of right adrenal or renal masses is very low. If a significant exposure of the liver parenchyma is expected, a volume-based dose constraint of $V_{5Gy} \leq 66\%$ is recommended.

Efficacy and Safety

Local Tumor Control and Survival

Scientific data on interstitial brachytherapy in renal and adrenal malignancies are, as yet, limited to smaller cohorts. On the basis of phase I study data, a local tumor control (LTC) of 85% can be anticipated in renal cell cancer (mean diameter 3.5 cm) after iridium-192 irradiation with a target dose (PTV) of 15 Gy. A dose prescription of 20 Gy can increase LTC to 95%, as suggested by a dose escalation in local recurrences [2]. During a follow-up period of up to 60 months, only one patient died of progression in an advanced renal cell carcinoma with hepatic metastases. No other cancer-related mortality occurred in the study cohort. Comparing the data with stereotactic ablative body-radiotherapy (SABR), a similar efficacy in local tumor control is seen, although randomized studies are lacking [16].

To date, only one study has been reported on the efficacy of interstitial brachytherapy with an iridium-192 source in adrenal masses [17], while another has utilized iodine-125 seeds [18]. In various tumor entities (e.g., lung cancer, hepatocellular carcinoma, colorectal carcinoma, and renal cell cancer), LTC was 88% and 95%, respectively. Median survival times were 11.4 months and 19 months, while overall survival in such cohorts is heavily influenced by the tumor entities and concomitant systemic therapies. Data on LTC after SABR as an alternative technique of high-conformal irradiation are consistent with these findings [19].

Peri-interventional Complications

The overall frequency of complications in CT-guided catheter placement for interstitial brachytherapy is low [20]. Morbidity in renal and adrenal brachytherapy typically arises from local bleeding and infections, which can usually be managed by transarterial embolization (e.g., coil embolization or particle embolization) and systemic administration of antibiotics. In rare cases of abscesses at the tumor site, CT-guided drainage may be indicated. The frequency of such events ranges from 3 to 6.3% in the scientific reports mentioned above and is similar to frequencies reported after thermal ablation (e.g., radiofrequency ablation) [21, 22].

Side Effects of Radiation

In interstitial brachytherapy of renal masses, deterioration of renal function is of very high concern. In a phase I study, mentioned above, renal function was investigated as a primary endpoint [2]. Regarding KDOQI stages of renal impairment, no significant decrease was found. Furthermore, a contralateral hypertrophy with an increase in tubular excretion was observed. In only one patient was hemodialysis required, 32 months after several local-ablative treatments in preexisting stage 4 renal insufficiency. Specific investigations of dose–response relationship in renal brachytherapy are in progress. The frequency of adverse events is also comparable between interstitial brachytherapy and SABR, while specific complications of invasive catheter placement are precluded in percutaneous irradiation techniques [23].

As function loss of adrenal glands after interstitial brachytherapy can be compensated for by administration of hydrocortisone, no relevant morbidity is to be expected. However, it is recommended that patients visit an endocrinologist on a regular basis. The same applies to SABR typically competing with interstitial brachytherapy [24].

Key Points
- CT-guided interstitial brachytherapy in renal cell carcinoma with a D100 of 15 Gy delivered to the planning target volume (PTV) yields a local tumor control (LTC) of 85%, while 20 Gy may result in an LTC of 95%.
- In adrenal gland malignancies, an LTC of >80% after 12 months can be expected.
- Efficacy after interstitial brachytherapy of renal and adrenal tumors is consistent with results achieved after stereotactic ablative body radiotherapy (SABR).
- Adjacent organs at risk (OAR) may require adjunctive techniques (e.g., interposition of balloon catheters) to achieve ablative irradiation doses to the target volume.

References

1. Wang ZJ, Westphalen AC, Zagoria RJ. CT and MRI of small renal masses. Br J Radiol. 2018;91(1087):20180131.
2. Damm R, Streitparth T, Hass P, Seidensticker M, Heinze C, Powerski M, Wendler JJ, Liehr UB, Mohnike K, Pech M, et al. Prospective evaluation of CT-guided HDR brachytherapy as a local ablative treatment for renal masses: a single-arm pilot trial. Strahlenther Onkol. 2019;195(11):982–90.
3. Sanchez A, Feldman AS, Hakimi AA. Current management of small renal masses, including patient selection, renal tumor biopsy, active surveillance, and thermal ablation. J Clin Oncol. 2018;36(36):3591–600.
4. Burruni R, Lhermitte B, Cerantola Y, Tawadros T, Meuwly JY, Berthold D, Jichlinski P, Valerio M. The role of renal biopsy in small renal masses. Can Urol Assoc J. 2016;10(1–2):E28–33.
5. Dabestani S, Marconi L, Kuusk T, Bex A. Follow-up after curative treatment of localised renal cell carcinoma. World J Urol. 2018;36(12):1953–9.
6. Patel U, Sokhi H. Imaging in the follow-up of renal cell carcinoma. AJR Am J Roentgenol. 2012;198(6):1266–76.
7. Sun MR, Brook A, Powell MF, Kaliannan K, Wagner AA, Kaplan ID, Pedrosa I. Effect of stereotactic body radiotherapy on the growth kinetics and enhancement pattern of primary renal tumors. AJR Am J Roentgenol. 2016;206(3):544–53.
8. Seo JM, Park BK, Park SY, Kim CK. Characterization of lipid-poor adrenal adenoma: chemical-shift MRI and washout CT. AJR Am J Roentgenol. 2014;202(5):1043–50.
9. Mohnike K, Sauerland H, Seidensticker M, Hass P, Kropf S, Seidensticker R, Friebe B, Fischbach F, Fischbach K, Powerski M, et al. Haemorrhagic complications and symptomatic venous thromboembolism in interventional tumour ablations: the impact of peri-interventional thrombosis prophylaxis. Cardiovasc Intervent Radiol. 2016;39(12):1716–21.
10. Patel IJ, Rahim S, Davidson JC, Hanks SE, Tam AL, Walker TG, Wilkins LR, Sarode R, Weinberg I. Society of Interventional Radiology Consensus Guidelines for the periprocedural management of thrombotic and bleeding risk in patients undergoing percutaneous image-guided interventions-part II: recommendations: endorsed by the Canadian Association for Interventional Radiology and the Cardiovascular and Interventional Radiological Society of Europe. J Vasc Interv Radiol. 2019;30(8):1168–1184.e1.
11. Hass P, Steffen IG, Powerski M, Mohnike K, Seidensticker M, Meyer F, Brunner T, Damm R, Willich C, Walke M, et al. First report on extended distance between tumor lesion and adjacent organs at risk using interventionally applied balloon catheters: a simple procedure to optimize clinical target volume covering effective isodose in interstitial high-dose-rate brachytherapy of liver malignomas. J Contemp Brachytherapy. 2019;11(2):152–61.
12. Bretschneider T, Ricke J, Gebauer B, Streitparth F. Image-guided high-dose-rate brachytherapy of malignancies in various inner organs—technique, indications, and perspectives. J Contemp Brachytherapy. 2016;8(3):251–61.
13. Ricke J, Wust P. Computed tomography-guided brachytherapy for liver cancer. Semin Radiat Oncol. 2011;21(4):287–93.
14. Mohnike K, Wolf S, Damm R, Seidensticker M, Seidensticker R, Fischbach F, Peters N, Hass P, Gademann G, Pech M, et al. Radioablation of liver malignancies with interstitial high-dose-rate brachytherapy : complications and risk factors. Strahlenther Onkol. 2016;192(5):288–96.
15. Streitparth F, Pech M, Bohmig M, Ruehl R, Peters N, Wieners G, Steinberg J, Lopez-Haenninen E, Felix R, Wust P, et al. In vivo assessment of the gastric mucosal tolerance dose after single fraction, small volume irradiation of liver malignancies by computed tomography-guided, high-dose-rate brachytherapy. Int J Radiat Oncol Biol Phys. 2006;65(5):1479–86.
16. Panje C, Andratschke N, Brunner TB, Niyazi M, Guckenberger M. Stereotactic body radiotherapy for renal cell cancer and pancreatic cancer : literature review and practice recommendations of the DEGRO Working Group on Stereotactic Radiotherapy. Strahlenther Onkol. 2016;192(12):875–85.

17. Mohnike K, Neumann K, Hass P, Seidensticker M, Seidensticker R, Pech M, Klose S, Streitparth T, Garlipp B, Benckert C, et al. Radioablation of adrenal gland malignomas with interstitial high-dose-rate brachytherapy: efficacy and outcome. Strahlenther Onkol. 2017;193(8):612–9.
18. Lin ZY, Yang JY, Chen J, Chen J. Evaluating the effectiveness of computed tomography-guided (125)I seed interstitial implantation in patients with secondary adrenal carcinoma. J Cancer Res Ther. 2019;15(4):813–7.
19. Toesca DAS, Koong AJ, von Eyben R, Koong AC, Chang DT. Stereotactic body radiation therapy for adrenal gland metastases: outcomes and toxicity. Adv Radiat Oncol. 2018;3(4):621–9.
20. Boning G, Buttner L, Jonczyk M, Ludemann WM, Denecke T, Schnapauff D, Wieners G, Wust P, Gebauer B. Complications of computed tomography-guided high-dose-rate brachytherapy (CT-HDRBT) and risk factors: results from more than 10 years of experience. Cardiovasc Intervent Radiol. 2020;43(2):284–94.
21. Zhou K, Pan J, Yang N, Shi HF, Cao J, Li YM, Zhang HZ, Wang KF, Chen SH. Effectiveness and safety of CT-guided percutaneous radiofrequency ablation of adrenal metastases. Br J Radiol. 2018;91(1085):20170607.
22. Zhou W, Arellano RS. Thermal ablation of T1c renal cell carcinoma: a comparative assessment of technical performance, procedural outcome, and safety of microwave ablation, radiofrequency ablation, and cryoablation. J Vasc Interv Radiol. 2018;29(7):943–51.
23. Pham D, Thompson A, Kron T, Foroudi F, Kolsky MS, Devereux T, Lim A, Siva S. Stereotactic ablative body radiation therapy for primary kidney cancer: a 3-dimensional conformal technique associated with low rates of early toxicity. Int J Radiat Oncol Biol Phys. 2014;90(5):1061–8.
24. Wardak Z, Meyer J, Ghayee H, Wilfong L, Timmerman R. Adrenal insufficiency after stereotactic body radiation therapy for bilateral adrenal metastases. Pract Radiat Oncol. 2015;5(3):e177–81.

Image-Guided HDR Brachytherapy of Abdominal Lymph Nodes, Pancreatic, and Peritoneal Neoplasms

15

Peter Hass

Introduction

Especially for abdominal malignancies, local control is a decisive prognostic factor. For pancreatic cancers and retroperitoneal sarcomas, surgically complete resection is considered the only therapy option with a curative chance [1, 2]. However, even after complete resection, there is a risk of local recurrence, depending on the tumor entity, its histology, and its location.

If resection with a sufficient safety margin is not successful, the risk of local failure is further increased [3, 4]. Therefore, it is important to have additive or alternative locally effective therapies available, especially in primary or secondary inoperability, in case of local recurrence. This applies both in the curative and in the palliative setting.

The available data show that radio-oncological concepts and techniques, alone or in combination with surgical procedures and simultaneous chemotherapy, improve local control in the treatment of pancreatic carcinomas, retroperitoneal sarcomas, abdominal cancer of unknown primary (CUP), and lymph-node metastases.

Improved local control can have a positive impact on OS [5, 6]. Prospective study results supporting this retrospective-analysis-based assumption are still rare.

Although radiotherapy for the treatment of malignant solid tumors was established as one of the important pillars of tumor therapy at the beginning of the last century, for a long time neither percutaneous radiation nor brachytherapy in the anatomical area between the diaphragm and small pelvis prevailed. The organs of the upper abdomen, especially the GI tract, react with inflammation, fistulas, or ulcerations, if excessive (i.e., by volume) doses are applied [7–9].

P. Hass (✉)

Department of Radiation Oncology, University Hospital Magdeburg, Magdeburg, Germany
e-mail: peter.hass@med.ovgu.de

© The Author(s), under exclusive license to Springer Nature
Switzerland AG 2021
K. Mohnike et al. (eds.), *Manual on Image-Guided Brachytherapy of Inner Organs*, https://doi.org/10.1007/978-3-030-78079-1_15

For a long time, this limited radiation tolerance of the organs at risk (OAR) prevented effective curative irradiation of abdominal primary tumors (e.g., pancreatic cancer) or metastases, since the technical possibilities did not allow high-precision external irradiation and the catheter-based minimally invasive procedures had not yet been developed.

Since 1925, various methods for implanting radioactive isotopes have been developed [10]. Today iodine seeds are used for LDR brachytherapy of, e.g., pancreatic carcinomas [11–13], but mainly with palliative intent. Since about 1976, intraoperative irradiation with electrons has been carried out; this makes possible high rates of local control [14].

In combination with percutaneous irradiation doses, a sustained curative effect can be sought, in addition to the purely palliative one.

Method

The publications researched in the PubMed database with the key terms "HDR brachytherapy," "abdominal lymph nodes," "peritoneal neoplasms," and "pancreatic tumor" were reviewed and the analyses, where relevant for this chapter, are presented in the Results section.

A total of 14 publications includes 1 review article, 3 case reports, 8 retrospective studies, 1 prospective study, and 1 technical report [15]. They describe both intraoperative application approaches with flexible brachytherapy catheters and CT-/MRI-based inserts of the BT catheters using the Seldinger technique, which was introduced already in 2004 by Ricke et al. for the treatment of liver malignancies [16].

While BT after intraoperative insertion was mainly realized fractionally, by using single doses of 1.8–5 Gy, the patients in the other studies mostly received single ablative doses between 8 and 20 Gy.

Technical Aspects for Single-Dose iBT

The workflow associated with the Seldinger technology is explained in detail in Chap. 5. Additionally, it is important to note that there are some special aspects regarding brachytherapy of the tumor entities described in this chapter.

First of all, it may be necessary to vary the patient's positioning. It is advisable to choose not the shortest route from the skin to the tumor, but the safest. For example, a lateral position can help to achieve a higher distance between the tumor and adjacent small or large intestine or larger blood vessels. A prone position should likewise be considered in this context.

Secondly, regarding lymph-node metastases, it is essential to avoid very close proximity between the catheter and surrounding nerve structures.

Finally, when a local recurrent pancreatic tumor is being treated there is a significantly increased risk of a liver abscess developing, if the patient has a biliodigestive

anastomosis. In such cases, it may be better to treat the patient by noninvasive irradiation, e.g., a hypofractionated EBRT or SBRT.

Figures 15.1 and 15.2 show representative planning images and a 3D reconstruction using the example of a large lymph-node metastasis in the liver hilum.

Results

Haage published a case report in 1987 [10], in which he described the combination
of percutaneous radiation (40.5 Gy) with interstitial LDR-BT (total dose 25 Gy,
dose rate 0.57 Gy/h) after intraoperative insertion of stiff BT needles in a non-
resectable but localized pancreatic head carcinoma. The procedure was uncompli-
cated, and the cumulative radiation dose could be significantly increased in

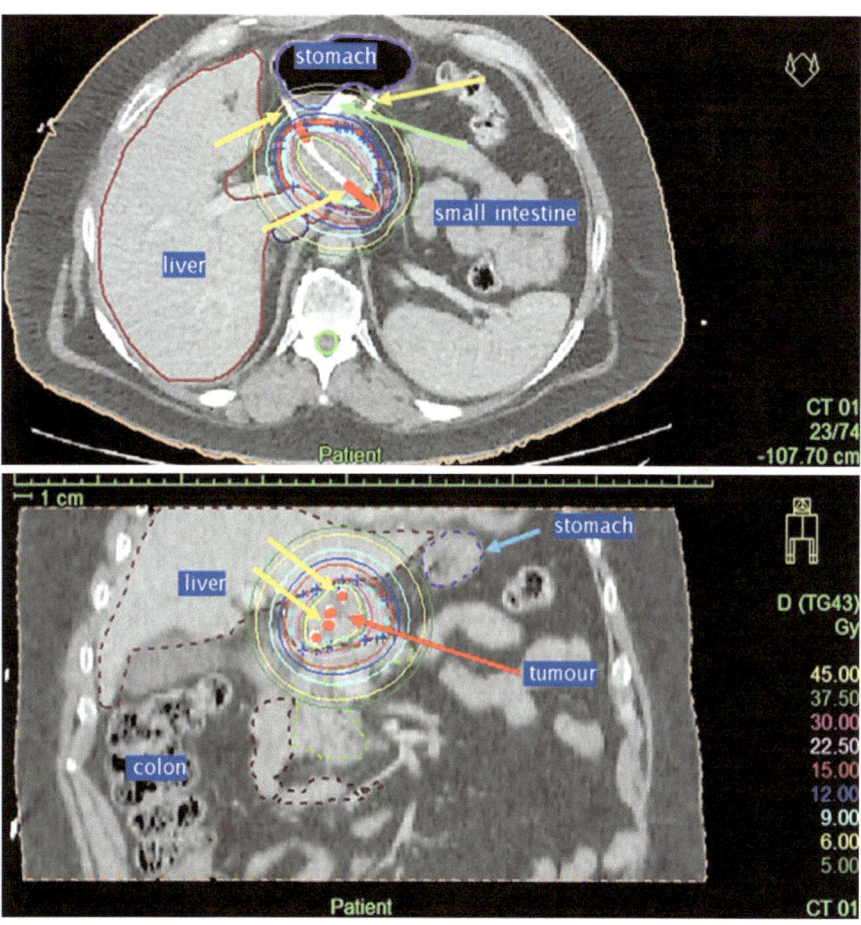

Fig. 15.1 CT-guided iBT of a lymph-node metastasis (red arrow) of NSCLC, with a prescribed
minimum dose of 15 Gy. Yellow arrows, BT catheters; green arrow, balloon for distancing

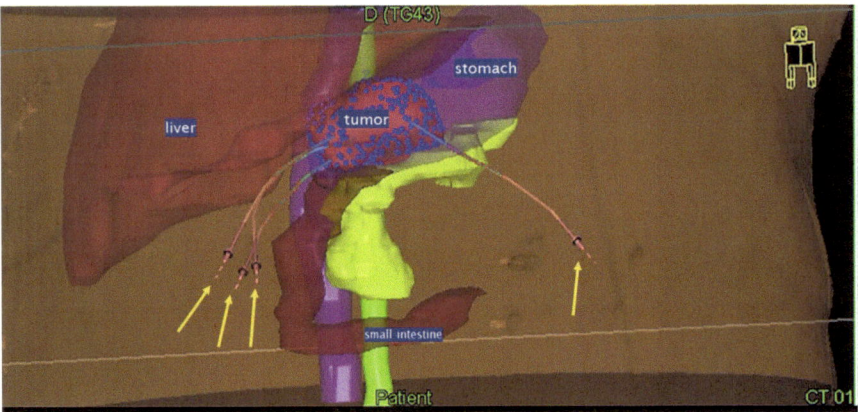

Fig. 15.2 3D reconstruction. Blue arrows, BT catheters

comparison with percutaneous radiation alone. The patient died after 14 months of liver and bone metastases, but the irradiated tumor was locally controlled. In 1992, Warzawski et al. [17–19] published their experience with a method developed in Würzburg for the intraoperative insertion of flexible BT catheters in inoperable pancreatic carcinomas, also for combined percutaneous/interstitial HDR radiation treatment. There were no severe side effects in a series of nine patients.

Pfreundner confirmed these good results in 1998 [20]; meanwhile, the size of the Würzburg patient cohort had grown to 19 patients, of whom nine received additional chemotherapy. Tolerability was good, and no serious side effects were observed. The LCR was 70% and the median OS was 6 months.

In a paper by Waniczek, a perioperative insert of brachytherapy catheters in non-resectable pancreatic head tumors was reported. The eight palliative patients received a biliodigestive or gastrointestinal bypass because of very severe pain. Immediately afterward, the BT catheters were implanted through specially developed cannulas and fixed into the tumor. On the sixth postoperative day, only four of the eight patients were able to start iBT with a single daily dose of 5–20 Gy [21]. Compared with a group without BT, the need for pain medications decreased, and the mean survival time was 6.7 months in the group with BT but only 4.4 months in the group that did not receive BT.

In 2006, Calvo described in a review article the results of intraoperative radiotherapy mainly for dose escalation. He concluded that an additional IORT can significantly improve local tumor control. Image-guided HDR brachytherapy is explicitly mentioned as a possible form of IORT [14].

In a prospective study conducted in 2006 at the Charité (Berlin), 19 patients with abdominal malignancies received a single-fraction iBT with PTV (planning target volume)-enclosing doses of 4–18 Gy [22]. Inter alia, two locally recurrent pancreatic carcinomas, six lymph-node metastases, and one mesogastric soft-tissue sarcoma were treated. Side effects of Grade ≥3 occurred in one case, the local control was 76.5%, and the PFS was 47% after 6 months.

Franck et al. report in a case collection on the results of a sequential chemo/iBT of three patients with locally recurrent pancreatic malignancies after primary resection and, in one case, after additional percutaneous RT. The patients received a single PTV-enclosing dose of respectively 15, 16, and 20 Gy. In each case, sufficient local control was achieved, and no complications occurred [23].

A retrospective analysis of the results after iBT in 24 patients with 47 retroperitoneal lymph-node metastases showed a high level of effectiveness and safety. Patients were given a median single dose of 14.9 Gy (range 4.5–20.6 Gy) prescribed to D99.9. The local control rate (LCR) was 95.7%, in one case, Grade 3 toxicity according to CTCAEv4 occurred. The cumulative median overall survival was 15.9 months [24].

Omari was able to show a local tumor control in 97.5% and 89% in two retrospective analyses with a total of ten peritoneal CTx-refractory GIST lesions as well as two pancreatic and five lymph-node metastases from gastric cancer after median iBT doses of 15 Gy, resulting in median overall survivals of respectively 37.5 [25] and 11.4 months [26].

Finally, a further case report published as an abstract showed that, by intraoperative insertion of an expandable tissue expander, risk structures can be distanced from the tumor bed, and thus a high ablative single dose is achievable [27].

Discussion

The few published data on iBT in abdominal lymph-node metastases, inoperable pancreatic cancers, pancreatic carcinoma recurrences, or retroperitoneal soft-tissue sarcomas reveal high local efficacy with good tolerability.

There is a consensus that perioperative radiation and/or chemotherapies improve the sustainability of surgical therapy, especially in pancreatic cancers and retroperitoneal sarcomas. This is stated to be because optimized local control can also extend the OS [5, 6].

Owing to the scarcity of data however the majority of leading oncology societies do not currently make any recommendations on the use of iBT in the abdominal tumor diseases specified in this chapter.

Therefore, to this end, some examples are given here.

- The NCCN (National Comprehensive Cancer Network) recommends radiation treatment by IORT, IMRT, or hypofractionated SBRT for the treatment of pancreatic cancer as a neoadjuvant or adjuvant option in curative or palliative therapy to stop tumor progression or to reduce symptoms such as pain or bleeding. The same applies to retroperitoneal soft-tissue sarcomas or CUP manifestations. On the other hand, the NCCN does not make an explicit recommendation for radiotherapeutic treatments of GIST, retroperitoneal lymph-node metastases, or aggressively growing lesions such as desmoid tumors. Brachytherapeutic procedures are not listed at all [28].

- The authors of the ESTRO-ACROP (the European Society for Radiotherapy and Oncology and the Advisory Committee on Radiation Oncology Practice) guidelines for pancreatic cancer are convinced that high-precision intraoperative [29] or percutaneous [30] radiation treatment has a place within multidisciplinary therapeutic concepts, although a potential role of BT is not discussed.
- Finally, the current ABS (American Brachytherapy Society) consensus guideline of 2019 [31] emphasizes that IORT can be discussed:
  - For the treatment of sarcomas with a narrow or positive resection hem, or
  - In cases of recurrence in combination with an EBRT for retroperitoneal sarcomas to improve local tumor control. LDR and HDR brachytherapy, electron radiation, and low-energy electronic are subsumed under the term IORT. A prospective study [32] documented the observation that supplementing postoperative EBRT with an IORT improved local control from 20 to 60%.
- Recommendations of the AWMF (Association of Scientific Medical Societies) for the treatment of pancreatic cancer [33] suggest that sequential radiochemotherapy is an option in patients with locally advanced inoperable tumors. In addition, in the case of isolated local recurrence, all possibilities of local therapy should be reviewed. Intraoperative radiotherapy (IORT, not specified) should not be carried out outside prospective, controlled studies.

With the technological advances of recent years, it is now also possible to place effective radiation doses in the tumor with high precision [34].

Therefore, SBRT has a high priority among the differentiated radiation-therapy concepts. However, although the upper abdominal organs, in particular, can be conserved much better than in comparable historical situations, the problem of closely adjacent OAR remains. Radiologically underdosed tumor components, as well as tight resection margins, can compromise local control.

Milickovic has pointed out the benefits of iBT. The steeper dose gradient compared with the SBRT can preserve the surrounding organs even better, with the additional possibility of a biologically effective dose escalation within the tumor [35].

In a study of 85 patients, the implemented iBT plans for liver malignancies were compared statistically with virtual SBRT calculations [36].

A significant advantage of the BT calculations with respect to the PTV parameters D99.9 and D90 as well as the V5 of the liver was found.

Furthermore, distancing OAR can make possible a more effective PTV-enclosing dose application [15, 27, 37].

In addition to the supposed disadvantage of invasiveness, brachytherapy obviously also has some advantages. However, the current results are at best hypotheses-generating. Without prospective comparative studies, it is difficult to determine predictive factors pro or contra iBT with respect to key endpoints such as LCR, PFS, or OS.

Conclusion

Initial results of the applications of iBT in abdominal lymph nodes and pancreatic and peritoneal neoplasms are promising. Image-guided HDR brachytherapy could occupy an important place within multidisciplinary concepts as a safe and highly effective radio-ablative option.

Key Points
- iBT is a feasible and effective radio-ablative method to treat the tumor entities described in this chapter.
- CT-/MRI-guided iBT is probably an alternative approach in the local treatment of abdominal lymph-node, pancreatic and peritoneal neoplasms, although the evidence level based on prospective studies is rather low at present.
- In the oligometastatic state, radio-ablation might be oncologically meaningful, in terms of possible improvement of the overall prognosis.
- In a palliative situation, interstitial brachytherapy is able to alleviate symptoms (e.g., pain).
- Preplanning, including positioning of the patient and dose calculation, is to be recommended owing to the presence of adjacent organs at risk in the upper abdomen.

Conflict of InterestP. Hass declares that he has no conflict of interest.

References

1. Doi R, Imamura M, Hosotani R, et al. Surgery versus radiochemotherapy for resectable locally invasive pancreatic cancer: final results of a randomized multi-institutional trial. Surg Today. 2008;38(11):1021–8.
2. Bonvalot S, Rivoire M, Castaing M, et al. Primary retroperitoneal sarcomas: a multivariate analysis of surgical factors associated with local control. J Clin Oncol. 2009;27:31–7.
3. Wagner M, Redaelli C, Lietz M, et al. Curative resection is the single most important factor determining outcome in patients with pancreatic adenocarcinoma. Br J Surg. 2004;91(5):586–94.
4. Esposito I, Kleeff J, Bergmann F, et al. Most pancreatic cancer resections are R1 resections. Ann Surg Oncol. 2008;15(6):1651–60.
5. Groot VP, van Santvoort HC, Rombouts SJ, et al. Systematic review on the treatment of isolated local recurrence of pancreatic cancer after surgery; re-resection, chemoradiotherapy and SBRT. HPB (Oxford). 2017;19(2):83–92.
6. Kelly KJ, Yoon SS, Kuk D, et al. Comparison of perioperative radiation therapy and surgery versus surgery alone in 204 patients with primary retroperitoneal sarcoma: a retrospective 2-institution study. Ann Surg. 2015;262(1):156–62.
7. Streitparth F, Pech M, Bohmig M, et al. In vivo assessment of the gastric mucosal tolerance dose after single fraction, small volume irradiation of liver malignancies by computed tomography-guided, high-dose-rate brachytherapy. Int J Radiat Oncol Biol Phys. 2006;65:1478–86.

8. Grimm J, LaCouture T, Croce R, et al. Dose tolerance limits and dose volume histogram evaluation for stereotactic body radiotherapy. J Appl Clin Med Phys. 2011;12(2):267–92.
9. Sterzing F, Brunner TB, Ernst I, Baus WW, Greve B, Herfarth K, Guckenberger M. Stereotactic body radiotherapy for liver tumors: principles and practical guidelines of the DEGRO Working Group on Stereotactic Radiotherapy. Strahlenther Onkol. 2014;190(10):872–81.
10. Haaga JR, Owens DB, Kellermeyer RW, et al. CT guided interstitial therapy of pancreatic carcinoma. J Comput Assist Tomogr. 1987;11(6):1077–8.
11. Fortner JG, D'Angio GJ, Hilaris BS, et al. Iodine 125 implantation for unresectable cancer of the pancreas. Postgrad Med. 1970;47(3):226–30.
12. Xiong J, Kwong Chian S, Li J, et al. Iodine-125 seed implantation for synchronous pancreatic metastases from hepatocellular carcinoma: a case report and literature review. Medicine. 2017;96(46):e8726.
13. Jia SN, Wen FX, Gong TT, et al. A review on the efficacy and safety of iodine-125 seed implantation in unresectable pancreatic cancers. Int J Radiat Biol. 2020;96(3):383–9.
14. Calvo FA, Meirino RM, Orecchia R. Intraoperative radiation therapy part 2: clinical results. Crit Rev Oncol Hematol. 2006;59(2):116–27.
15. Kishi K, Sonomura T, Shirai S, et al. Brachytherapy reirradiation with hyaluronate gel injection of paraaortic lymphnode metastasis of pancreatic cancer: paravertebral approach—a technical report with a case. J Radiat Res. 2011;52(6):840–4.
16. Ricke J, Wust P, Stohlmann A, et al. CT-guided interstitial brachytherapy of liver malignancies alone or in combination with thermal ablation: phase I-II results of a novel technique. Int J Radiat Oncol Biol Phys. 2004;58:1496–505.
17. Warszawski N, Pfreundner L, Bratengeier K, et al. HDR interstitial brachytherapy for pancreatic carcinoma. Activity J. 1992;6:90–4.
18. Warszawski N, Bratengeier K, Bohndorf W. Interstitial HDR afterloading therapy with flexible catheters. Aktuelle Radiol. 1993;3(3):177–81.
19. Warszawski N, Pfreundner L, Bratengeier K, et al. Combined isodose curves of high dose rate interstitial brachytherapy with external-beam radiation therapy in pancreatic carcinoma. Strahlenther Onkol. 1992;168:552–7.
20. Pfreundner L, Baier K, Schwab F, et al. 3D-Ct-planned interstitial HDR brachytherapy + percutaneous irradiation and chemotherapy in inoperable pancreatic carcinoma. Methods and clinical outcome. Strahlenther Onkol. 1998;174(3):133–41.
21. Waniczek D, Piecuch J, Rudzki M, et al. Perioperative high dose rate (HDR) brachytherapy in unresectable locally advanced pancreatic tumors. J Contemp Brachytherapy. 2011;3(2):84–90.
22. Wieners G, Pech M, Rudzinska M, et al. CT-guided interstitial brachytherapy in the local treatment of extrahepatic, extrapulmonary secondary malignancies. Eur Radiol. 2006;16(11):2586–93.
23. Franck C, Hass P, Malfertheiner P, et al. Combined systemic chemotherapy and CT-guided high-dose-rate brachytherapy for isolated local manifestation of pancreatic cancer after surgical resection. Digestion. 2018;98(2):69–74.
24. Heinze C, Omari J, Manig M, Hass P, Venerito M, Damm R, et al. Efficacy and safety of percutaneous computed tomography-guided high-dose-rate interstitial brachytherapy in treatment of oligometastatic lymph node metastases of retroperitoneal space. J Contemp Brachytherapy. 2019;11(5):436–2.
25. Omari J, Drewes R, Matthias M, et al. Treatment of metastatic, imatinib refractory, gastrointestinal stroma tumor with image-guided high-dose-rate interstitial brachytherapy. Brachytherapy. 2019;18(1):63–70.
26. Omari J, Drewes R, Orthmer M, Hass P, Pech M, Powerski M. Treatment of metastatic gastric adenocarcinoma with image-guided high-dose rate, interstitial brachytherapy as second-line or salvage therapy. Diagn Interv Radiol. 2019;25(5):360–7.
27. Hass P, Acciuffi S, Brunner T, et al. Retroperitoneale Sarkome: Optimierung der Dosisapplikation durch Vergrößerung des Abstandes zwischen Tumorbett und angrenzenden Darmschlingen durch Einlage eines expandierbaren Gewebe-Expanders: test of principle. Strahlenther Onkol. 2018;194(Suppl 1):P01–2.

28. NCCN clinical practice guidelines in oncology. https://www.nccn.org/professionals/.
29. Calvo FA, Krengli M, Asencio JM, et al. ESTRO IORT Task Force/ACROP recommendations for intraoperative radiation therapy in unresected pancreatic cancer. Radiother Oncol. 2020;148:57–64.
30. Brunner TB, Haustermans K, Huguet F, et al. ESTRO ACROP guidelines for target volume definition in pancreatic cancer. Radiother Oncol. 2021;154:60–9.
31. Tom MC, Joshi N, Vicini F, et al. The American Brachytherapy Society consensus statement on intraoperative radiation therapy. Brachytherapy. 2019;18:242–57.
32. Sindelar WF, Kinsella TJ, Chen PW, et al. Intraoperative radiotherapy in retroperitoneal sarcomas. Final results of a prospective, randomized, clinical trial. Arch Surg. 1993;128:402–10.
33. Seufferlein T, Porzner M, Becker T, et al. S3-guideline exocrine pancreatic cancer. Z Gastroenterol. 2013;51(12):1395–440.
34. Panje C, Andratschke N, Brunner TB, et al. Stereotactic body radiotherapy for renal cell cancer and pancreatic cancer: literature review and practice recommendations of the DEGRO Working Group on Stereotactic Radiotherapy. Strahlenther Onkol. 2016;192:875–85.
35. Milickovic N, Tselis N, Karagiannis E, et al. Iridium-Knife: another knife in radiation oncology. Brachytherapy. 2017;16(4):884–92.
36. Hass P, Mohnike K, Kropf S, Brunner TB, Walke M, Albers D, Petersen C, Damm R, Walter F, Ricke J, Corradini S. Comparative analysis between interstitial brachytherapy and stereotactic body irradiation for local ablation in liver malignancies. Brachytherapy. 2019;8(6):823–8.
37. Hass P, Steffen IG, Powerski M, et al. First report on extended distance between tumor lesion and adjacent organs at risk using interventionally applied balloon catheters: a simple procedure to optimize clinical target volume covering effective isodose in interstitial high-dose-rate-brachytherapy of liver malignomas. J Contemp Brachytherapy. 2019;11(2):152–61.

Interventional Image-Guided HDR Brachytherapy as a Salvage Treatment: Exclusive or in Combination with Other Local Therapies

16

Luca Tagliaferri, Andrea D'Aviero, Alessandro Posa, and Roberto Iezzi

Introduction

Interventional image-guided brachytherapy (iBT) represents a valid option in the repertoire of local treatments available for several oncological diseases. iBT allows the delivery of high doses to clinical targets with a steeply descending dose gradient to surrounding normal tissues, in the context not only of curative but also of salvage treatments [1].

The most frequently used percutaneous ablative treatments are radiofrequency thermal ablation (RFA), microwave ablation (MWA), and cryoablation (CA), while intra-arterial chemoembolization/chemoinfusion (TACE/IAC) and radioembolization (SIRT) are the most common endovascular options.

The development of interventional oncology centers (IOCs) and of multidisciplinary teams, based on close cooperation between radiotherapy (RT) and interventional radiology (IR) experts, has changed the spectrum of nonsurgical local procedures, providing optimum treatment options in the curative and salvage settings, also for elderly patients [2–4].

L. Tagliaferri · A. D'Aviero (✉)
U.O.C. di Radioterapia Oncologica, Dipartimento di Diagnostica per Immagini, Radioterapia Oncologica ed Ematologia, Fondazione Policlinico Universitario "A. Gemelli" IRCCS, Rome, Italy
e-mail: luca.tagliaferri@policlinicogemelli.it; andrea.daviero@guest.policlinicogemelli.it

A. Posa · R. Iezzi
U.O.C. di Radiologia Diagnostica e Interventistica Generale, Dipartimento di Diagnostica per Immagini, Radioterapia Oncologica ed Ematologia, Fondazione Policlinico Universitario "A. Gemelli" IRCCS, Rome, Italy
e-mail: alessandro.posa@guest.policlinicogemelli.it; roberto.iezzi@policlinicogemelli.it

K. Mohnike et al. (eds.), *Manual on Image-Guided Brachytherapy of Inner Organs*, https://doi.org/10.1007/978-3-030-78079-1_16

Liver

Patients affected by HCC or other liver malignancies, such as cholangiocarcinoma or metastases, can be deemed ineligible for surgical treatment if the tumor is not discovered at an early stage or if the patient has severe comorbidities that increase the surgical risk [5]. In these patients, systemic chemotherapy and/or supportive treatments are usually not very effective.

Interventional Radiotherapy (Brachytherapy)

Liver-directed high-dose-rate (HDR) interventional image-guided brachytherapy for primary and secondary malignancies represents a new field of interest, competing with stereotactic external beam techniques but requiring specific expertise [6, 7].

The rationale for iBT in treating liver malignancies can be related to the evidence that HDR ablation, in contrast to other focal therapies, is not limited by large tumor size, proximity to large vessels, central location or exophytic growth, or multiple foci [8, 9].

In liver iBT the radiation sources are temporarily inserted, in removable applicators, into the tissue under guidance by CT, ultrasound, or MR fluoroscopy.

iBT makes it possible to deliver a very high radiation dose to the target around the source positions while sparing normal tissues and structures on account of the rapid dose fall-off [10–13].

In order to estimate the correct number and pathway(s) of the catheters required, a CT or MRI preplan should be developed. The shape and size of the lesions, such as the local anatomy and the relationship with organs at risk (OAR), are the main factors influencing the arrangement and number of treatment catheters. The definition of the correct target volume can be improved by using PET-CT [14].

In cases of peripheral hepatic malignancies or critical proximity of OAR, during the CT-guided IRT catheter application, an interventional balloon catheter can be inserted at the tissue interface between the hepatic capsule and the OAR [15].

For the definition of target volumes in preparing the HDR-IRT plan, gross tumor volume (GTV) has to be defined as the volume enclosed by the visible tumor borders, including the enhancing rim, in contrast-enhanced CT. A 5 mm margin expansion should be added to the GTV in the definition of Clinical Target Volume (CTV). It is advisable to irradiate the path of the applicator catheters to avoid later intrahepatic metastatic spread [16].

There is no broad consensus on the minimum required dose, so the optimum dose to achieve tumor control should be defined on the basis of tumor histology and OAR constraints. The volume receiving more than 5 Gy should not exceed two-thirds of the normal liver tissue, in order to prevent liver damage [17].

In HCC, 15 Gy has been demonstrated to be adequate and well-tolerated for, e.g., liver metastases of breast cancer [16–18], while other tumor types require a minimum dose greater than 18 Gy.

iBT can be considered a valid option for liver tumors with a high risk of local failure, as a variety of experiences has demonstrated good local tumor control both in primary liver tumors and in liver metastases [9, 10].

In patients with primary hepatocellular carcinoma (HCC), iBT has been shown to achieve good rates of local control (LC) even in unresectable and large lesions. In 2015 Collettini et al. analyzed a cohort of 98 patients with unresectable HCC treated with CT-guided iBT with a local tumor progression rate of 8.5%, mean tumor diameter greater than 5 cm, and multifocal disease [19].

Other evidence has also underlined the potential role and efficacy of HDR-IRT in patients with poor prognosis HCC, such as a tumor diameter of >5 cm or where lesions are located in unfavorable anatomic sites (adjacent to the liver hilum, common bile duct, or hepatic bifurcation) [20–22]. In addition, a recent phase II trial showed a superior outcome (in terms of time to untreatable progression) of iBT compared with cTACE in HCC, in particular in patients with BCLC-B/BCLC-C [23].

Good control rates have also been demonstrated in liver metastasis compared with other local therapies [24]. iBT was also found to be an effective option for treating liver metastases close to critical structures such as the liver hilum [25].

Local Therapies (Interventional Radiology, IR)

Among interventional radiology therapies, the ones most commonly used in primary and secondary liver tumors are RFA, MWA, percutaneous ethanol injection (PEI), CA, irreversible electroporation (IRE), and endovascular treatments such as transarterial embolization (TAE), transarterial chemoembolization (TACE), and transarterial radioembolization (TARE), the latter also known as selective internal radiation therapy (SIRT). Depending on histology and disease stage at diagnosis, these treatments can be performed alone or in a multimodality approach (also with systemic options), with curative or palliative intent, to downstage inoperable diseases, for bridging to transplantation or surgical resection, or to prolong overall survival and quality of life [26–29].

Ablative percutaneous treatments are usually of great effectiveness in lesions up to 3 cm in size and are recommended in cases of paucinodular (<3) primary tumors or oligometastatic secondary liver tumors.

In patients deemed unfit for surgery or percutaneous ablative treatments because of comorbidities and/or multinodular disease, but with preserved liver function and absence of vascular invasion, TACE can represent the best treatment choice, for both primary and secondary liver lesions; it is an endovascular treatment based on the superselective embolization of the arterial supply to the target neoplastic lesions with microparticles and chemotherapeutic drug, sparing the surrounding healthy parenchyma [30–34].

However, TACE is relatively contraindicated in patients with portal-vein invasion, as the therapeutic embolization of the arterial vessels where there is a coexisting portal-vein thrombosis could potentially lead to liver failure. For these patients, as well as for patients who decline, or who are ineligible for, the systemic chemotherapeutic drug sorafenib, a particular variant of TACE which uses degradable starch microspheres (DSM-TACE) could be of great effectiveness; the starch microspheres are rapidly digested by liver enzymes and therefore exert only a limited ischaemic effect, while nonetheless granting an effective and safe superselective delivery of the chemotherapeutic drug with low systemic cytotoxic effects [35].

New emerging devices and techniques are expanding the role of TACE and widening its indications, in particular for secondary tumors, with a higher probability of achieving good curative results, also using combined treatments with percutaneous IRT and systemic options.

In contrast to TACE, another option in the endovascular treatment of liver malignancies is offered by SIRT, which acts mainly by irradiation using microspheres loaded with yttrium-90 (^{90}Y) or holmium-166 (^{166}Ho). SIRT can be performed in patients with impaired liver function, portal-vein thrombosis, or neoplastic invasion, as well as in cases of large neoplastic lesions [36, 37]. Recent literature has highlighted the role of dosimetry in predicting tumor response to treatment.

Combination Treatment

Combined treatments can help achieve greater tumor necrosis, enhancing the effects of the various techniques, and thus achieving greater rates of overall survival and disease control.

In primary hepatic lesions, such as hepatocellular carcinoma, the combination of ablative treatments (RFA and MWA) and TACE showed high efficacy and good safety, especially in patients with large (>3 cm) lesions, in which percutaneous ablation or TACE alone could not be of great effectiveness [38–40].

Combined treatments, such as ablation plus TACE, also help to overcome the contraindications of these two techniques, as lesions located in "complex" sites (subcapsular, near the gallbladder or the intestinal loops) or in "complex" patients (with high bleeding risk) can be safely treated in a single session, exploiting the advantages of both techniques [38].

Among combined treatments, the combination of endovascular brachytherapy and TACE has recently been investigated, with improved mean overall survival and progression-free survival rates as compared with TACE alone [41].

Lung

Primary lung cancer is the second most common cancer in both sexes and represents the leading cause of death by tumor worldwide, accounting for 1.37 million deaths per year (18% of all tumor-related deaths). The most common type of lung cancer is non-small-cell lung cancer (NSCLC), accounting for 85% of lung cancer diagnosis. Only in 20% of cases is it detected at an early stage (T1–T2).

The treatment of choice for patients with NSCLC is surgical resection: pulmonary lobectomy and local lymphadenectomy is the optimum therapy for early-stage cancer, affording 5-year survival rates of 60–92%. However, as many as 15% of these patients are excluded from surgical treatment owing to inadequate lung capacity, comorbidities or the patient's refusing surgery [42, 43].

For these patients it is mandatory to find a safe and effective alternative to resection; according to the National Comprehensive Cancer Network (NCCN) guidelines, alternative local therapies are stereotactic ablative radiotherapy (SABR or SBRT), and percutaneous treatments [42, 44, 45].

Interventional Radiotherapy (Brachytherapy)

Salvage iBT in lung cancer malignancies play a relevant role in the treatment of palliative airway obstruction and in overcoming breathing difficulties. Patients with endobronchial tumor growth, caused by a primary lung tumor or metastasis, may develop obstruction symptoms such as cough, dyspnoea, haemoptysis, and obstructive pneumonia.

In deciding on the correct approach, bronchoscopy is fundamental for defining the location and length of the target. Furthermore, bronchoscopy is used to estimate the diameter of the obstruction, and it provides the opportunity to perform biopsy.

The HDR-iBT applicators can be inserted through the working channel of the bronchoscope in the case of small applicators (5F or 6F) or by using a flexible guidewire inserted through an extra bronchoscopic tube; X-ray and fluoroscopy help to verify correct positioning. Even in palliative treatments, the use of CT allows better coverage of target volumes with the aim of reducing doses to OAR. Peripheral lesions not accessible by bronchoscopy can be reached by a percutaneous CT-guided interstitial approach.

CT scans and bronchoscopy findings help to assess the GTV defined as the macroscopic tumor, and a 20 mm longitudinal margin is usually added to define the CTV [46, 47].

A salvage palliative HDR-iBT dose can be delivered in single or in several fractions, usually in one to three sessions of 5–15 Gy; different schedules are used, as there is a lack of clear consensus [48, 49].

Evidence in the literature underlines the role of HDR-IRT in improving symptom relief and quality of life in patients with obstructive lung tumors [50–52].

A recent review showed that according to clinical experiences, a palliative effect is usually achieved within a few days, with reported amelioration of symptoms in 60–90% of patients and objective endoscopic regression in more than 60% of cases. In the series analyzed, cough and hemoptysis seemed more sensitive to endobronchial brachytherapy than dyspnoea or atelectasis [53].

Recently, good experience with CT-guided interstitial ^{125}I seed implantation was reported [54–56]; especially in the palliative setting, the use of ^{125}I seeds loaded stents offered better results compared with non-coated bronchus stents in the palliative treatment of malignant obstructions of the bronchus [57].

Locoregional Therapies (Interventional Radiology)

Percutaneous ablative therapies have shown good safety and efficacy in the treatment of unresectable primary early-stage tumors (less than 3 cm in size, with no lymph node or distant metastasis) in patients not amenable to surgical resection, and in oligometastatic cancers involving the lung (up to 3 ipsilateral nodules, or 5 nodules in total, with a total tumor diameter less than 3 cm) [58, 59].

RFA is the most commonly used technique to date, and has proven safe and effective in treating lesions up to 2 cm in size [60–65].

Major limitations upon its use in the lung are the insulating effect of the aerated lung parenchyma and the presence of large parenchymal vessels (heat-sink effect), which hinder the correct diffusion of the heat to the target lesion [66, 67].

On the other hand, MWA is a more recent technique, which overcomes the limitations of RFA, not being susceptible to insulation by air or limited by the heat-sink effect; it is not affected by the carbonization of adjacent tissues and therefore grants a greater and faster heat deposition, which yields a larger zone of tumor necrosis [59, 60, 68–74].

Cryoablation creates tumor necrosis using cold instead of heat: cycles of freezing and thawing cause cell death. CA is of great use in cases where "complex" primary and secondary lesions such as tumors adjacent to, or infiltrating, the chest wall or the mediastinum, or in cases of central parenchymal lesions near the pulmonary hilum [10, 75–77].

It has high efficacy in treating recurrent lesions after surgery or radiotherapy, which can grow in difficult locations deemed unsafe for other ablative treatments. Even if CA is limited by the ablative volume (a single probe is effective in lesions of less than 2 cm diameter), the multiprobe approach can ablate large volumes; however, the procedure time for CA (more than 30 min) is longer than for RFA or MWA (up to 12 min), and this must be taken into consideration during the pre-procedural evaluations and set-up (for example, it can be a factor for patients who cannot remain in a prone position for a long time) [75, 78, 79].

Salvage and palliative treatments can also be performed by percutaneous ablative techniques: local ablation can be performed in recurrent primary lung cancer (both small-cell and NSCLC) after surgical resection or radio-chemotherapy, and it can also be indicated in advanced stages to reduce tumor burden and relieve symptoms, Frequent examples are cases of malignant pleural effusion which cause dyspnoea, or local bone (rib, thoracic vertebrae) and nerve invasion leading to intractable pain [80].

Cryoablation is helpful in "complex" lesions and in addition, owing to the low procedural pain associated with it, it only requires mild sedation. It therefore has fewer anesthesiological contraindications and can be used in comorbid patients deemed ineligible for other procedures [75, 78, 79].

Palliative ablation treatment can also be performed in metastatic lesions of the lung, when the size and number of lesions exceed the curative indications [80].

Combination Treatment

Combining treatments in salvage settings for lung cancer could represent an effort to obtain improvement in life quality through symptom relief, also with the aim of obtaining greater rates of disease control. Only a little experience is available in exploring the role of the combination of local treatments; moreover, the sequence of treatments is not fully defined to date. The main evidence available regarding the combination of IRT-HDR with local techniques is from using the Nd-YAG laser, in patients with primary and secondary lung lesions with obstructive symptoms. In the palliative setting, this experience has confirmed the benefit of IRT in stabilizing the effect of laser debulking and prolonging the improvement of symptoms, as well as reducing the need for further endoscopic interventions [49, 81–83].

Further experiences have also been analyzed to investigate the combination of interstitial ^{125}I seed implantation and cryoablation. Single-center case series have demonstrated an advantage in adding IRT to cryoablation in terms of palliating the symptoms and improving overall survival compared with cryotherapy alone [84, 85].

Head and Neck

Head and neck carcinoma (HNC) accounts worldwide for more than 650,000 new cases and 330,000 deaths annually [86].

Local failure (LF) occurs in about 30% of patients with H&N cancer and is mostly diagnosed within 5 years after the end of treatment. LF is also responsible for about 85% of deaths attributable to disease progression [87, 88].

Interventional Radiotherapy (Brachytherapy)

Brachytherapy represents a proven therapeutic option for salvage treatments of neo-plasms of the head and neck [89].

The settings in which iBT can play a central role are the treatment of local, locoregional, or nodal recurrence of neck disease, mainly in re-irradiation of H&N tumors and in the treatment of primary lesions in regions previously irradiated. As reported in international guidelines, IRT is an acceptable treatment option in asso-ciation with surgery and other treatment approaches (EBRT, CTX) or in patients who are ineligible for salvage surgery because of the extent of disease and/or the anatomic relationship between the target and adjacent structures [90, 91].

In this context, the main contraindications to IRT are bone invasion, fistula, and limited life expectancy [92–96].

Salvage iBT (both remote afterloading and ^{125}I seeds) in H&N cancers is performed by following the same principles of primary treatments. Afterloading HDR is performed through interstitial RT and mold RT approaches: ^{125}I seeds are placed by personalized 3D template and CT-guided implantations. In interstitial HDR-iBT, fixed applicators with plastic and/or steel catheters are inserted around the CTV (Fig. 16.1). Mold implants are used for treatments involving fixed areas.

In the definition of proper IRT treatment at the H&N site, the risk of toxicity should be carefully considered [97].

Considering the anatomic relationship with adjacent structures, the toxicity profile includes neurological toxicity, dysphagia, carotid artery rupture, skin necrosis, fistulas, and osteoradionecrosis [97].

A recent review of experience in treating recurrent H&N cancers with IRT, in association with surgery or without surgery, showed encouraging rates of LC and OS. IRT in combination with salvage surgery showed a 2-year LR control rates ranging from 62 to 88% and OS rates between 38 and 65%. In cases of H&N recurrences not accessible to salvage surgery, BT alone showed LR control rates from 27 to 92% and 2-year OS rates from 18 to 43% [96].

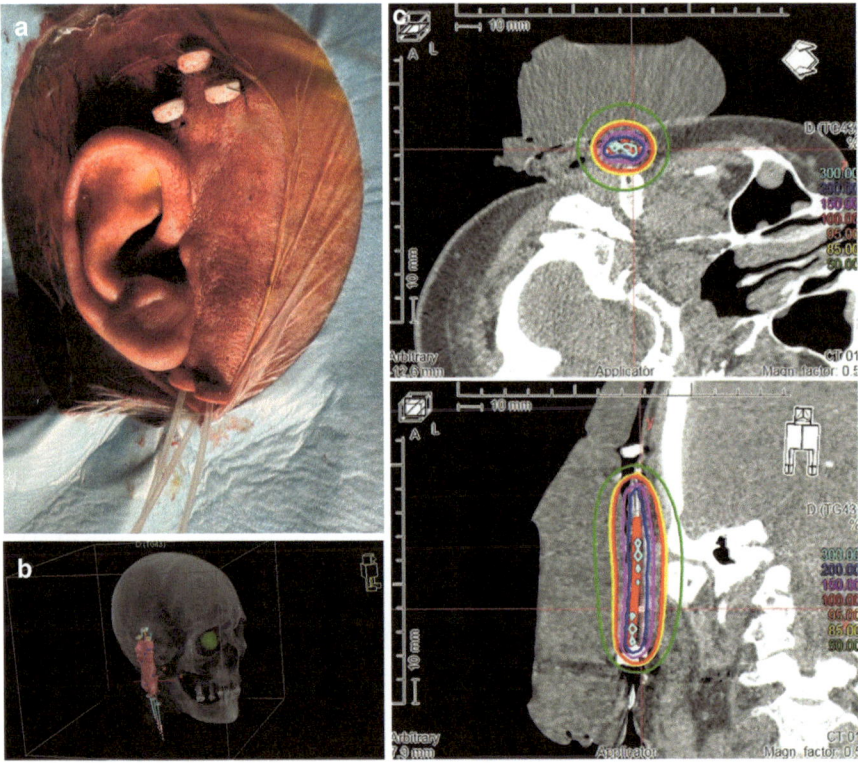

Fig. 16.1 iBT for head and neck cancer. (**a**) iBT implant. (**b**) Implant reconstruction. (**c**) Dose distribution

Local Therapies (Interventional Radiology)

There are still no guidelines on the use of percutaneous ablation techniques in head and neck lesions; however, experimental studies have shown promising results, and these procedures can be performed as palliative treatments in patients unsuitable for re-irradiation with RT or in association with RT [98, 99]. Ablative treatment showed improved quality of life and fewer complications than did repeated RT. RFA is the most common ablative treatment in this area. A few studies have described the use of MWA, mostly on thyroid lesions [100, 101]. In every therapeutic approach to the head and neck region, it is important to consider the proximity of the target lesion to cranial nerves, major arterial and venous vessels, the trachea and digestive tract structures; the risk of damage to adjacent structures must be explained clearly to the patient.

Various authors have reported the outcome of ablative therapy (RFA and MWA), before or after RT and chemotherapy, both on primary tumors and on neck recurrences and metastases located at various sites in the head and neck region, as a salvage treatment to improve quality of life and reduce pain. In patients with superficial lesions, conscious sedation was indicated, and normal tissues adjacent to the target lesion can be protected from the heat by using moist gauze or throat packing [102, 103]. Ablative treatment increased overall survival, and at 6-month follow-up after ablative and RT treatment the quality-of-life indicators showed a significant improvement in pain, speech, senses, swallowing, social eating and contact, and sexuality) [103–106].

When one is dealing with complications of head and neck tumors, the risk of hemorrhage must be taken into account: this complication occurs in up to 10% of patients with advanced disease and could be related to tumor growth or recurrence, or to radiation necrosis, which can go so far as to include rupture of the carotid artery [107–112]. In such cases, prompt endovascular embolization or stent placement can be life-saving [107, 113–119].

Intra-arterial chemotherapy (IAC) can represent an effective tool in the treatment of head and neck cancers, particularly for squamous-cell carcinoma; it is performed through a common femoral artery and grants superselective infusion of the chemotherapeutic drug. IAC has been performed alone or in combination with radiation treatment, even though it has not been shown to be better than intravenous chemotherapy [120–122].

Cryoablation can be of great value in head and neck tumors, both for pain relief and for functional status preservation, although there are few reports in the literature: CA can preserve nerves, vessels, and other structures adjacent to the tumor, with low morbidity, and owing to ice-ball formation the area of ablation can be directly visualized by MRI and CT, making possible real-time modification of the probe position [106, 123].

Combination Treatment

As regards treatment combining IRT and locoregional interventional radiology, there are no current literature data. However, owing to the importance of the head and neck region in social interactions and to the aggressiveness of tumors in this region, combined salvage treatment aimed at debulking large or infiltrative lesions, or for pain relief, can be of great help.

Key Points
- iBT in liver malignancies can be an option for large lesions, central location, exophytic growth, or multiple foci.
- iBT plays a relevant role in the treatment of palliative airway obstruction and in overcoming breathing difficulties for lung cancer malignancies.
- Unresectable primary early-stage tumors in patients not amenable to surgical resection, and oligometastatic cancers involving the lung, are main areas of application for ablative percutaneous treatments.
- iBT in H&N cancers plays a relevant role in the treatment of primary or secondary lesions not amenable for surgery, in areas irradiated previously or in combination with surgery. Palliative IR ablation treatments in H&N lesions have been investigated only in experimental studies.

References

1. Autorino R, et al. A national survey of AIRO (Italian Association of Radiation Oncology) brachytherapy (Interventional Radiotherapy) study group. J Contemp Brachytherapy. 2018;10:254–9. https://doi.org/10.5114/jcb.2018.76981. Termedia Publishing House Ltd.
2. Kovács G, et al. TURKISH JOURNAL of ONCOLOGY interventional oncology: should interventional radiotherapy (brachytherapy) be integrated into modern treatment procedures? J Oncol. 2019b;34:16–22. https://doi.org/10.5505/tjo.2019.4.
3. Kovács G, Tagliaferri L, Valentini V. Is an Interventional Oncology Center an advantage in the service of cancer patients or in the education? The Gemelli Hospital and INTERACTS experience. J Contemp Brachyther. 2017a;9:497–8. https://doi.org/10.5114/jcb.2017.72603. Termedia Publishing House Ltd.
4. Lancellotta V, et al. Age is not a limiting factor in interventional radiotherapy (brachytherapy) for patients with localized cancer. Biomed Res Int. 2018;2018:2178469. https://doi.org/10.1155/2018/2178469. Hindawi Limited.
5. Bruix J, Reig M, Sherman M. Evidence-based diagnosis, staging, and treatment of patients with hepatocellular carcinoma. Gastroenterology. 2016;150:835–53. https://doi.org/10.1053/j.gastro.2015.12.041. W.B. Saunders.
6. Dionisi F, et al. Radiotherapy in the multidisciplinary treatment of liver cancer: a survey on behalf of the Italian Association of Radiation Oncology. Radiol Med. 2016;121(9):735–43. https://doi.org/10.1007/s11547-016-0650-5. Springer-Verlag Italia s.r.l.
7. Hass P, Mohnike K, et al. Comparative analysis between interstitial brachytherapy and stereotactic body irradiation for local ablation in liver malignancies. Brachytherapy. 2019a;18(6):823–8. https://doi.org/10.1016/j.brachy.2019.08.003. Elsevier Inc.

8. Kieszko D, et al. Treatment of hepatic metastases with computed tomography-guided interstitial brachytherapy. Oncol Lett. 2018;15(6):8717–22. https://doi.org/10.3892/ol.2018.8415. Spandidos Publications.

9. Vogel A, et al. Hepatocellular carcinoma: ESMO Clinical Practice Guidelines for diagnosis, treatment and follow-up. Ann Oncol. 2018;29(Suppl 4):iv238–55. https://doi.org/10.1093/annonc/mdy308. Oxford University Press.

10. Kovács A, et al. Critical review of multidisciplinary non-surgical local interventional ablation techniques in primary or secondary liver malignancies. J Contemp Brachytherapy. 2019a;11:589–600. https://doi.org/10.5114/jcb.2019.90466. Termedia Publishing House Ltd.

11. Ricke J, Wust P. Computed tomography-guided brachytherapy for liver cancer. Semin Radiat Oncol. 2011;21:287–93. https://doi.org/10.1016/j.semradonc.2011.05.005.

12. Schnapauff D, et al. Computed tomography-guided interstitial HDR brachytherapy (CT-HDRBT) of the liver in patients with irresectable intrahepatic cholangiocarcinoma'. Cardiovasc Interv Radiol. 2012;35(3):581–7. https://doi.org/10.1007/s00270-011-0249-0. Springer New York LLC.

13. Schnapauff D, et al. Activity-based cost analysis of hepatic tumor ablation using CT-guided high-dose rate brachytherapy or CT-guided radiofrequency ablation in hepatocellular carcinoma. Radiat Oncol. 2016;11(1):26. https://doi.org/10.1186/s13014-016-0606-x. BioMed Central Ltd.

14. Steffen IG, et al. Value of combined PET/CT for radiation planning in CT-guided percutaneous interstitial high-dose-rate single-fraction brachytherapy for colorectal liver metastases. Int J Radiat Oncol Biol Phys. 2010;77(4):1178–85. https://doi.org/10.1016/j.ijrobp.2009.06.047.

15. Hass P, Steffen IG, et al. First report on extended distance between tumor lesion and adjacent organs at risk using interventionally applied balloon catheters: a simple procedure to optimize clinical target volume covering effective isodose in interstitial high-dose-rate brachytherapy of liver malignomas. J Contemp Brachytherapy. 2019b;11(2):152–61. https://doi.org/10.5114/jcb.2019.84798. Termedia Publishing House Ltd.

16. Collettini F, Golenia M, et al. Percutaneous computed tomography-guided high-dose-rate brachytherapy ablation of breast cancer liver metastases: initial experience with 80 lesions. J Vasc Interv Radiol. 2012a;23(5):618–26. https://doi.org/10.1016/j.jvir.2012.01.079.

17. Mohnike K, et al. Computed tomography-guided high-dose-rate brachytherapy in hepatocellular carcinoma: safety, efficacy, and effect on survival. Int J Radiat Oncol Biol Phys. 2010;78(1):172–9. https://doi.org/10.1016/j.ijrobp.2009.07.1700. Elsevier.

18. Wieners G, et al. Treatment of hepatic metastases of breast cancer with CT-guided interstitial brachytherapy—a phase II-study. Radiother Oncol. 2011;100(2):314–9. https://doi.org/10.1016/j.radonc.2011.03.005.

19. Collettini F, et al. CT-gesteuerte Hochdosis-Brachytherapie beim inoperablen hepatozellulären Karzinom. Strahlenther Onkol. 2015;191(5):405–12. https://doi.org/10.1007/s00066-014-0781-3. Urban und Vogel GmbH.

20. Collettini F, Schnapauff D, et al. Hepatocellular carcinoma: computed-tomography-guided high-dose-rate brachytherapy (CT-HDRBT) ablation of large (5-7 cm) and very large (>7 cm) tumours. Eur Radiol. 2012b;22(5):1101–9. https://doi.org/10.1007/s00330-011-2352-7.

21. Denecke T, et al. CT-guided interstitial brachytherapy of hepatocellular carcinoma before liver transplantation: an equivalent alternative to transarterial chemoembolization? Eur Radiol. 2015;25(9):2608–16. https://doi.org/10.1007/s00330-015-3660-0. Springer.

22. Ricke J, et al. Liver malignancies: CT-guided interstitial brachytherapy in patients with unfavorable lesions for thermal ablation. J Vasc Interv Radiol. 2004;15(11):1279–86. https://doi.org/10.1097/01.RVI.0000141343.43441.06. Lippincott Williams and Wilkins.

23. Mohnike K, et al. Radioablation by image-guided (HDR) brachytherapy and transarterial chemoembolization in hepatocellular carcinoma: a randomized phase II trial. Cardiovasc Interv Radiol. 2019;42(2):239–49. https://doi.org/10.1007/s00270-018-2127-5. Springer New York LLC.

24. Wieners G, et al. CT-guided high-dose-rate brachytherapy in the interdisciplinary treatment of patients with liver metastases of pancreatic cancer. Hepatobiliary Pancreat Dis Int.

2015;14(5):530–8. https://doi.org/10.1016/S1499-3872(15)60409-X. Elsevier (Singapore) Pte Ltd.

25. Collettini F, et al. Computed-tomography-guided high-dose-rate brachytherapy (CT-HDRBT) ablation of metastases adjacent to the liver hilum. Eur J Radiol. 2013;82(10):e509–14. https://doi.org/10.1016/j.ejrad.2013.04.046. Elsevier Ireland Ltd.

26. Becker G, et al. Combined TACE and PEI for palliative treatment of unresectable hepatocellular carcinoma. World J Gastroenterol. 2005;11(39):6104–9. https://doi.org/10.3748/wjg.v11.i39.6104. WJG Press.

27. Katsanos K, et al. Comparative effectiveness of different transarterial embolization therapies alone or in combination with local ablative or adjuvant systemic treatments for unresectable hepatocellular carcinoma: a network meta-analysis of randomized controlled trials. PLoS One. 2017;12(9):e0184597. https://doi.org/10.1371/journal.pone.0184597. Public Library of Science.

28. Pitton MB, et al. Randomized comparison of selective internal radiotherapy (SIRT) versus drug-eluting bead transarterial chemoembolization (DEB-TACE) for the treatment of hepatocellular carcinoma. Cardiovasc Interv Radiol. 2015;38(2):352–60. https://doi.org/10.1007/s00270-014-1012-0. Springer New York LLC.

29. Wang YB, et al. Quality of life after radiofrequency ablation combined with transcatheter arterial chemoembolization for hepatocellular carcinoma: comparison with transcatheter arterial chemoembolization alone. Qual Life Res. 2007;16(3):389–97. https://doi.org/10.1007/s11136-006-9133-9.

30. Van Cutsem E, et al. ESMO consensus guidelines for the management of patients with metastatic colorectal cancer. Ann Oncol. 2016;27(8):1386–422. https://doi.org/10.1093/annonc/mdw235. Oxford University Press.

31. Iezzi R, Kovacs A, et al. Transarterial chemoembolisation of colorectal liver metastases with irinotecan-loaded beads: what every interventional radiologist should know. Eur J Radiol Open. 2020b;7:100236. https://doi.org/10.1016/j.ejro.2020.100236. Elsevier Ltd.

32. Llovet JM, et al. EASL-EORTC clinical practice guidelines: management of hepatocellular carcinoma. J Hepatol. 2012;56(4):908–43. https://doi.org/10.1016/j.jhep.2011.12.001. Elsevier.

33. Llovet JM, Brú C, Bruix J. Prognosis of hepatocellular carcinoma: the BCLC staging classification. Semin Liver Dis. 1999;19(3):329–37. https://doi.org/10.1055/s-2007-1007122. Thieme Medical Publishers, Inc.

34. Pereira PL, et al. The CIREL cohort: a prospective controlled registry studying the real-life use of irinotecan-loaded chemoembolisation in colorectal cancer liver metastases: interim analysis. Cardiovasc Interv Radiol. 2020;44(1):50–62. https://doi.org/10.1007/s00270-020-02646-8. Springer.

35. Iezzi R, et al. TACE with degradable starch microspheres (DSM-TACE) as second-line treatment in HCC patients dismissing or ineligible for sorafenib. Eur Radiol. 2019;29(3):1285–92. https://doi.org/10.1007/s00330-018-5692-8. Springer.

36. Smits MLJ, et al. Holmium-166 radioembolization for the treatment of patients with liver metastases: design of the phase i HEPAR trial. J Exp Clin Cancer Res. 2010;29(1):70. https://doi.org/10.1186/1756-9966-29-70.

37. Wang EA, et al. Treatment options for unresectable HCC with a focus on SIRT with Yttrium-90 resin microspheres. Int J Clin Pract. 2017. https://doi.org/10.1111/ijcp.12972. Blackwell Publishing Ltd.

38. Iezzi R, et al. Combined locoregional treatment of patients with hepatocellular carcinoma: state of the art. World J Gastroenterol. 2016;22:1935–42. https://doi.org/10.3748/wjg.v22.i6.1935. Baishideng Publishing Group Co., Limited.

39. Kim JW, et al. Hepatocellular carcinomas 2-3 cm in diameter: transarterial chemoembolization plus radiofrequency ablation vs. radiofrequency ablation alone. Eur J Radiol. 2012;81(3):e189–93. https://doi.org/10.1016/j.ejrad.2011.01.122.

40. Sheta E, et al. Comparison of single-session transarterial chemoembolization combined with microwave ablation or radiofrequency ablation in the treatment of hepatocellular carcinoma:

a randomized-controlled study. Eur J Gastroenterol Hepatol. 2016;28(10):1198–203. https://doi.org/10.1097/MEG.0000000000000688. Lippincott Williams and Wilkins.

41. Luo JJ, et al. Endovascular brachytherapy combined with stent placement and TACE for treatment of HCC with main portal vein tumor thrombus. Hepatol Int. 2016;10(1):185–95. https://doi.org/10.1007/s12072-015-9663-8. Springer.

42. Abtin FG, et al. Radiofrequency ablation of lung tumors: imaging features of the postablation zone. Radiographics. 2012;32(4):947–69. https://doi.org/10.1148/rg.324105181.

43. Zhang Y, et al. Meta-analysis of lobectomy, segmentectomy, and wedge resection for stage I non-small cell lung cancer. J Surg Oncol. 2015;111(3):334–40. https://doi.org/10.1002/jso.23800. Wiley.

44. Chheang S, et al. Imaging features following thermal ablation of lung malignancies. Semin Interv Radiol. 2013;30(2):157–68. https://doi.org/10.1055/s-0033-1342957. Thieme Medical Publishers, Inc.

45. Lencioni R. Quality of life as an endpoint of treatment efficacy in malignant lung tumours—author's reply. Lancet Oncol. 2008:821–2. https://doi.org/10.1016/S1470-2045(08)70220-1. Elsevier.

46. Van Limbergen E, et al. THE GEC ESTRO HANDBOOK OF BRACHYTHERAPY, Part II Clinical Practice Version 1 - 30/04/2017.

47. Stewart A, et al. American Brachytherapy Society consensus guidelines for thoracic brachytherapy for lung cancer. Brachytherapy. 2016;15(1):1–11. https://doi.org/10.1016/j.brachy.2015.09.006. Elsevier Inc.

48. Skowronek J, et al. HDR endobronchial brachytherapy (HDRBT) in the management of advanced lung cancer—comparison of two different dose schedules. Radiother Oncol. 2009;93(3):436–40. https://doi.org/10.1016/j.radonc.2009.09.005.

49. Skowronek J. Brachytherapy in the treatment of lung cancer—a valuable solution. J Contemp Brachytherapy. 2015;7(4):297–311. https://doi.org/10.5114/jcb.2015.54038. Termedia Publishing House Ltd.

50. Chang LFL, et al. High dose rate afterloading intraluminal brachytherapy in malignant airway obstruction of lung cancer. Int J Radiat Oncol Biol Phys. 1994;28(3):589–96. https://doi.org/10.1016/0360-3016(94)90183-X.

51. Macha HN, et al. Endobronchial radiation therapy for obstructing malignancies: ten years' experience with iridium-192 high-dose radiation brachytherapy afterloading technique in 365 patients. Lung. 1995;173(5):271–80. https://doi.org/10.1007/BF00176890. Springer.

52. Soror T, et al. Salvage treatment with sole high-dose-rate endobronchial interventional radiotherapy (brachytherapy) for isolated endobronchial tumor recurrence in non–small-cell lung cancer patients: a 20-year experience. Brachytherapy. 2019;18(5):727–32. https://doi.org/10.1016/j.brachy.2019.04.271. Elsevier Inc.

53. Hennequin C, et al. Endoluminal brachytherapy: bronchus and oesophagus. Cancer Radiother. 2018;22:367–71. https://doi.org/10.1016/j.canrad.2017.11.013.

54. Ji Z, et al. Safety and efficacy of CT-guided radioactive iodine-125 seed implantation assisted by a 3D printing template for the treatment of thoracic malignancies. J Cancer Res Clin Oncol. 2020;146(1):229–36. https://doi.org/10.1007/s00432-019-03050-7. Springer.

55. Jiang AG, Lu HY, Ding ZQ. Implantation of 125I radioactive seeds via c-TBNA combined with chemotherapy in an advanced non-small-cell lung carcinoma patient. BMC Pulm Med. 2019;19(1):205. https://doi.org/10.1186/s12890-019-0974-8. BioMed Central Ltd.

56. Zhao J, et al. Efficacy and safety of CT-guided 125I brachytherapy in elderly patients with non-small cell lung cancer. Oncol Lett. 2020;20(1):183–92. https://doi.org/10.3892/ol.2020.11550. Spandidos Publications.

57. Wang Y, et al. A novel tracheobronchial stent loaded with 125I seeds in patients with malignant airway obstruction compared to a conventional stent: a prospective randomized controlled study. EBioMedicine. 2018;33:269–75. https://doi.org/10.1016/j.ebiom.2018.06.006. Elsevier B.V.

58. Jiang B, et al. Efficacy and safety of thermal ablation of lung malignancies: a network meta-analysis. Ann Thorac Med. 2018;13(4):243–50. https://doi.org/10.4103/atm.ATM_392_17. Wolters Kluwer Medknow Publications.

59. Prud'homme C, et al. Image-guided lung metastasis ablation: a literature review. Int J Hyperthermia. 2019;36:37–45. https://doi.org/10.1080/02656736.2019.1647358. Taylor and Francis Ltd.

60. Aufranc V, et al. Percutaneous thermal ablation of primary and secondary lung tumors: comparison between microwave and radiofrequency ablation. Diagn Interv Imaging. 2019;100(12):781–91. https://doi.org/10.1016/j.diii.2019.07.008. Elsevier Masson SAS.

61. Brace CL. Radiofrequency and microwave ablation of the liver, lung, kidney, and bone: what are the differences? Curr Probl Diagn Radiol. 2009;38:135–43. https://doi.org/10.1067/j.cpradiol.2007.10.001. NIH Public Access.

62. Curley SA, et al. Radiofrequency ablation of unresectable primary and metastatic hepatic malignancies: results in 123 patients. Ann Surg. 1999;230(1):1–8. https://doi.org/10.1097/00000658-199907000-00001.

63. Louis Hinshaw J, et al. Percutaneous tumor ablation tools: microwave, radiofrequency, or cryoablation-what should you use and why? Radiographics. 2014;34(5):1344–62. https://doi.org/10.1148/rg.345140054. Radiological Society of North America Inc.

64. Palussière J, Catena V, Buy X. Percutaneous thermal ablation of lung tumors—radiofrequency, microwave and cryotherapy: where are we going? Diagn Interv Imaging. 2017;98:619–25. https://doi.org/10.1016/j.diii.2017.07.003. Elsevier Masson SAS.

65. Xiong L, Dupuy DE. Lung ablation: whats new? Journal of Thoracic Imaging. 2016;31:228–37. https://doi.org/10.1097/RTI.0000000000000212. Lippincott Williams and Wilkins.

66. Goldberg SN, Dupuy DE. Image-guided radiofrequency tumor ablation: challenges and opportunities-part I. J Vasc Interv Radiol. 2001;12:1021–32. https://doi.org/10.1016/S1051-0443(07)61587-5.

67. Nemcek AA. Complications of radiofrequency ablation of neoplasms. Semin Interv Radiol. 2006;23:177–87. https://doi.org/10.1055/s-2006-941448. Thieme Medical Publishers.

68. Belfiore G, et al. Patients' survival in lung malignancies treated by microwave ablation: our experience on 56 patients. Eur J Radiol. 2013;82(1):177–81. https://doi.org/10.1016/j.ejrad.2012.08.024.

69. Dupuy DE. Science to practice: microwave ablation compared with radiofrequency ablation in lung tissue—is microwave not just for popcorn anymore? Radiology. 2009;251:617–8. https://doi.org/10.1148/radiol.2513090129.

70. Iezzi R, Cioni R, et al. Standardizing percutaneous microwave ablation in the treatment of lung tumors: a prospective multicenter trial (MALT study). Eur Radiol. 2020a;31(4):2173–82. https://doi.org/10.1007/s00330-020-07299-2. Springer Science and Business Media Deutschland GmbH.

71. Palussiere J, et al. Percutaneous lung thermal ablation of non-surgical clinical N0 non-small cell lung cancer: results of eight years' experience in 87 patients from two centers. Cardiovasc Interv Radiol. 2015;38(1):160–6. https://doi.org/10.1007/s00270-014-0999-6. Springer New York LLC.

72. Tsakok MT, et al. Local control, safety, and survival following image-guided percutaneous microwave thermal ablation in primary lung malignancy. Clin Radiol. 2019;74(1):80.e19–26. https://doi.org/10.1016/j.crad.2018.09.014. W.B. Saunders Ltd.

73. Vogl TJ, et al. Microwave ablation therapy: clinical utility in treatment of pulmonary metastases. Radiology. 2011;261(2):643–51. https://doi.org/10.1148/radiol.11101643.

74. Yuan Z, et al. A meta-analysis of clinical outcomes after radiofrequency ablation and microwave ablation for lung cancer and pulmonary metastases. J Am Coll Radiol. 2019;16(3):302–14. https://doi.org/10.1016/j.jacr.2018.10.012. Elsevier B.V.

75. Aarts BM, et al. Cryoablation and immunotherapy: an overview of evidence on its synergy. Insights Imaging. 2019. Springer. https://doi.org/10.1186/s13244-019-0727-5.

76. Duan H, et al. Cryoablation for advanced non-small cell lung cancer: a protocol for a systematic review. BMJ Open. 2020. BMJ Publishing Group. https://doi.org/10.1136/bmjopen-2019-033460.

77. Sun M, et al. A multicenter randomized controlled trial to assess the efficacy of cancer green therapy in treatment of stage IIIb/IV non-small cell lung cancer. Medicine. 2020;99(33):e21626. https://doi.org/10.1097/MD.0000000000021626. NLM (Medline).

78. Callstrom MR, et al. Multicenter study of metastatic lung tumors targeted by interventional cryoablation evaluation (SOLSTICE). J Thorac Oncol. 2020;15:1200–9. https://doi.org/10.1016/j.jtho.2020.02.022.

79. Das SK, et al. Comparing cryoablation and microwave ablation for the treatment of patients with stage IIIB/IV non-small cell lung cancer. Oncol Lett. 2020;19(1):1031–41. https://doi.org/10.3892/ol.2019.11149. Spandidos Publications.

80. Liu BD, et al. Expert consensus on image-guided radiofrequency ablation of pulmonary tumors: 2018 edition. Thorac Cancer. 2018;9(9):1194–208. https://doi.org/10.1111/1759-7714.12817. Wiley.

81. Freitag L, et al. Sequential photodynamic therapy (PDT) and high dose brachytherapy for endobronchial tumour control in patients with limited bronchogenic carcinoma. Thorax. 2004;59:790–3. https://doi.org/10.1136/thx.2003.013599.

82. Ornadel D, et al. Defining the roles of high dose rate endobronchial brachytherapy and laser resection for recurrent bronchial malignancy. Lung Cancer. 1997;16(2–3):203–13. https://doi.org/10.1016/S0169-5002(96)00630-7. Elsevier.

83. Patelli M, Trisolini R. La terapia endoscopica palliative. In: Pneumologia interventistica. Milan: Springer; 2008. p. 425–33. https://doi.org/10.1007/978-88-470-0556-3_41.

84. Wang H, et al. Cryosurgery combined with radioactive seeds and release-controlled chemical drugs implantation for the treatment of lung carcinoma. Zhongguo Fei Ai Za Zhi. 2009;12(5):408–11. https://doi.org/10.3779/j.issn.1009-3419.2009.05.006.

85. Zhou H, et al. Cryosurgery combined with Iodine-125 seed implantation in the treatment of unresectable lung cancer. Chin J Lung Cancer. 2008;11(6):780–3. https://doi.org/10.3779/j.issn.1009-3419.2008.06.06.

86. Bray F, et al. Global cancer statistics 2018: GLOBOCAN estimates of incidence and mortality worldwide for 36 cancers in 185 countries. CA Cancer J Clin. 2018;68(6):394–424. https://doi.org/10.3322/caac.21492. Wiley.

87. Bayman E, et al. Patterns of failure after intensity-modulated radiotherapy in head and neck squamous cell carcinoma using compartmental clinical target volume delineation. Clin Oncol. 2014;26(10):636–42. https://doi.org/10.1016/j.clon.2014.05.001. Elsevier Ltd.

88. Due AK, et al. Recurrences after intensity modulated radiotherapy for head and neck squamous cell carcinoma more likely to originate from regions with high baseline [18F]-FDG uptake. Radiother Oncol. 2014;111(3):360–5. https://doi.org/10.1016/j.radonc.2014.06.001. Elsevier Ireland Ltd.

89. Bussu F, et al. HDR interventional radiotherapy (brachytherapy) in the treatment of primary and recurrent head and neck malignancies. Head Neck. 2019;41(6):1667–75. https://doi.org/10.1002/hed.25646. Wiley.

90. Tagliaferri L, et al. Endoscopy-guided brachytherapy for sinonasal and nasopharyngeal recurrences. Brachytherapy. 2015;14(3):419–25. https://doi.org/10.1016/j.brachy.2014.11.012. Elsevier Inc.

91. Tagliaferri L, et al. Perioperative HDR brachytherapy for reirradiation in head and neck recurrences: single-institution experience and systematic review. Tumori. 2017;103:516–24. https://doi.org/10.5301/tj.5000614. Wichtig Publishing Srl.

92. Bhalavat R, et al. High-dose-rate interstitial brachytherapy in recurrent head and neck cancer: an effective salvage option. J Contemp Brachytherapy. 2018;10(5):425–30. https://doi.org/10.5114/jcb.2018.78995. Termedia Publishing House Ltd.

93. Kovács G, et al. GEC-ESTRO ACROP recommendations for head & neck brachytherapy in squamous cell carcinomas: 1st update—improvement by cross sectional imaging based

treatment planning and stepping source technology. Radiother Oncol. 2017b;122(2):248–54. https://doi.org/10.1016/j.radonc.2016.10.008. Elsevier Ireland Ltd.

94. Narayana A, et al. High-dose-rate interstitial brachytherapy in recurrent and previously irra-diated head and neck cancers-preliminary results. Brachytherapy. 2007;6(2):157–63. https://doi.org/10.1016/j.brachy.2006.12.001.

95. Puthawala A, et al. Interstitial low-dose-rate brachytherapy as a salvage treatment for recurrent head-and-neck cancers: long-term results. Int J Radiat Oncol Biol Phys. 2001;51(2):354–62. https://doi.org/10.1016/S0360-3016(01)01637-6. Elsevier.

96. Rodin J, et al. A systematic review of treating recurrent head and neck cancer: a reintroduc-tion of brachytherapy with or without surgery. J Contemp Brachytherapy. 2018;10(5):454–62. https://doi.org/10.5114/jcb.2018.79399. Termedia Publishing House Ltd.

97. García-Consuegra A, et al. Dose volume histogram constraints in patients with head and neck cancer treated with surgery and adjuvant HDR brachytherapy: a proposal of the head and neck and skin GEC ESTRO Working group. Radiother Oncol. 2021;154:128–34. https://doi.org/10.1016/j.radonc.2020.09.015. Elsevier Ireland Ltd.

98. Goldstein DP, et al. Outcomes following reirradiation of patients with heap and neck cancer. Head Neck. 2008;30(6):765–70. https://doi.org/10.1002/hed.20786.

99. Sulman EP, et al. IMRT reirradiation of head and neck cancer-disease control and morbid-ity outcomes. Int J Radiat Oncol Biol Phys. 2009;73(2):399–409. https://doi.org/10.1016/j.ijrobp.2008.04.021.

100. Brook AL, et al. CT-guided radiofrequency ablation in the palliative treatment of recurrent advanced head and neck malignancies. J Vasc Interv Radiol. 2008;19(5):725–35. https://doi.org/10.1016/j.jvir.2007.12.439.

101. Wang L, et al. Ultrasonography-guided percutaneous radiofrequency ablation for cervical lymph node metastasis from thyroid carcinoma. J Cancer Res Ther. 2014;10:C144–9. https://doi.org/10.4103/0973-1482.145844. Medknow Publications.

102. Owen RP, et al. Techniques for radiofrequency ablation of head and neck tumors. Arch Otolaryngol Head Neck Surg. 2004;130(1):52–6. https://doi.org/10.1001/archotol.130.1.52.

103. Owen RP, et al. Radiofrequency ablation of advanced head and neck cancer. Arch Otolaryngol Head Neck Surg. 2011;137(5):493–8. https://doi.org/10.1001/archoto.2011.62.

104. Ahmed M, et al. Principles of and advances in percutaneous ablation. Radiology. 2011;258:351–69. https://doi.org/10.1148/radiol.10081634.

105. Belfiore MP, et al. Preliminary results in unresectable head and neck cancer treated by radio-frequency and microwave ablation: feasibility, efficacy, and safety. J Vasc Interv Radiol. 2015;26(8):1189–96. https://doi.org/10.1016/j.jvir.2015.05.021. Elsevier Inc.

106. Guenette JP, et al. Percutaneous image-guided cryoablation of head and neck tumors for local control, preservation of functional status, and pain relief. Am J Roentgenol. 2017;208(2):453–8. https://doi.org/10.2214/AJR.16.16446. American Roentgen Ray Society.

107. Amin M, Wilson JA. Radical neck dissection: a 19-year experience. J Laryngol Otol. 1989;103(8):760–4. https://doi.org/10.1017/S002221510011000X.

108. Chen YF, et al. Transarterial embolization for control of bleeding in patients with head and neck cancer. Otolaryngol Head Neck Surg. 2010;142(1):90–4. https://doi.org/10.1016/j.otohns.2009.09.031.

109. Christison-Lagay E. Complications in head and neck surgery. Semin Pediatr Surg. 2016;25(6):338–46. https://doi.org/10.1053/j.sempedsurg.2016.10.007. W.B. Saunders.

110. Mccall JW, Whitaker CW, Hendershot EL. Rupture of the common carotid artery following radical neck surgery in radiated cases. AMA Arch Otolaryngol. 1959;69(4):431–4. https://doi.org/10.1001/archotol.1959.00730030441009. American Medical Association.

111. McCready RA, et al. Radiation-induced arterial injuries. Surgery. 1983;93(2):306–12. https://doi.org/10.5555/URI:PII:0039606083903501. Elsevier.

112. Minion DJ, et al. Pseudoaneurysm of the external carotid artery following radical neck dis-section and irradiation: a case report and review of the literature. Vascular. 1994;2(5):607–11. https://doi.org/10.1177/096721099400200513. Sage Publications UK: London, England.

113. Gemmete JJ, et al. Preliminary experience with the percutaneous embolization of juvenile angiofibromas using only ethylene-vinyl alcohol copolymer (Onyx) for preoperative devascularization prior to surgical resection. AJNR Am J Neuroradiol. 2012;33(9):1669–75. https://doi.org/10.3174/ajnr.A3043.
114. Kim HS, et al. Life-threatening common carotid artery blowout: rescue treatment with a newly designed self-expanding covered nitinol stent. Br J Radiol. 2006;79(939):226–31. https://doi.org/10.1259/bjr/66917189.
115. Lesley WS, et al. Preliminary experience with endovascular reconstruction for the management of Carotid Blowout syndrome. AJNR Am J Neuroradiol. 2003; 24: 975-81. PMID: 12748106; PMCID: PMC7975806.
116. Morrissey DD, et al. Endovascular management of hemorrhage in patients with head and neck cancer. Arch Otolaryngol Head Neck Surg. 1997;123(1):15–9. https://doi.org/10.1001/archotol.1997.01900010017002. American Medical Association.
117. Patsalides A, et al. Endovascular treatment of carotid blowout syndrome: who and how to treat. J Neurointerv Surg. 2010;2(1):87–93. https://doi.org/10.1136/jnis.2009.001131.
118. Sesterhenn AM, et al. Acute haemorrhage in patients with advanced head and neck cancer: value of endovascular therapy as palliative treatment option. J Laryngol Otol. 2006;120:117–24. https://doi.org/10.1017/S0022215105003178.
119. Shah H, et al. Acute life-threatening hemorrhage in patients with head and neck cancer presenting with carotid blowout syndrome: follow-up results after initial hemostasis with covered-stent placement. AJNR Am J Neuroradiol. 2011;32(4):743–7. https://doi.org/10.3174/ajnr.A2379.
120. Rasch CRN, et al. Intra-arterial versus intravenous chemoradiation for advanced head and neck cancer: results of a randomized phase 3 trial. Cancer. 2010;116(9):2159–65. https://doi.org/10.1002/cncr.24916.
121. Robbins KT, et al. A targeted supradose cisplatin chemoradiation protocol for advanced head and neck cancer. Am J Surg. 1994;168(5):419–22. https://doi.org/10.1016/S0002-9610(05)80089-3.
122. Robbins KT, et al. Efficacy of targeted supradose cisplatin and concomitant radiation therapy for advanced head and neck cancer: the Memphis experience. Int J Radiat Oncol Biol Phys. 1997;38(2):263–71. https://doi.org/10.1016/S0360-3016(97)00092-8.
123. Dar SA, et al. CT-guided cryoablation for palliation of secondary trigeminal neuralgia from head and neck malignancy. J Neurointerv Surg. 2013;5(3):258–63. https://doi.org/10.1136/neurintsurg-2012-010265.

Konrad Mohnike and Stefanie Corradini

Procedural and Radiotherapy Complications

From a technical perspective, interstitial brachytherapy (iBT) combines the minimally invasive interventional puncture and catheter placement, usually by the Seldinger technique, with a specialized form of radiation therapy.

Brachytherapy of inner organs has two special features. First, it does not have a homogeneous dose distribution as in external beam radiotherapy (EBRT); on the contrary, the distribution is highly inhomogeneous, with very high doses close to the radiation source and a very steep dose fall-off. Second, it can be applied as a single-fraction treatment with single doses between 15 and 25 Gy, without the need for fractionation.

After completion of the treatment, when the catheters are removed, the puncture tract cannot be coagulated as in thermal ablation techniques. Therefore, in iBT, the use of an angiography sheath as a "catheter-in-catheter" technique was introduced, with the brachytherapy catheter inside. This allows the puncture tract to be filled with gelatine-sponge plugs after removal of the brachytherapy catheter. This procedure helps to avoid major bleeding complications. However, in thermal ablation the puncture tract is also coagulated to avoid tumor seeding and metastasis within the

---

K. Mohnike (✉)
Department of Diagnostics, Department of Interventional Oncology & Radionuclide Therapy, Diagnostic Therapeutic Center Berlin, Berlin, Germany

Department of Radiology and Nuclear Medicine, University Hospital Magdeburg, Magdeburg, Germany
e-mail: konrad.mohnike@berlin-dtz.de

S. Corradini
Department of Radiation Oncology, Ludwig Maximilian University (LMU) Hospital Munich, Munich, Germany
e-mail: stefanie.corradini@med.uni-muenchen.de

puncture tract. The same effect can be achieved with iBT by irradiation of the puncture tract at ~5 Gy.

For these reasons, procedural complications that may arise from the invasiveness of the intervention should be distinguished from the toxicity of the radiation itself.

These aspects have been addressed in a comprehensive study. A total of 192 patients who had undergone 343 hepatic iBT interventions were analyzed. Baseline patient and treatment characteristics are shown in Tables 17.1 and 17.2. Major complications (Grade ≥ 3 according to version 3.0 of the *Common Terminology Criteria for Adverse Events*, CTCAE) were reported for fewer than 5% of the interventions (15/343) [1]. These major adverse events comprised 5 cases of Grade 3/4 bleeding, treated mostly by embolization or by administration of erythrocyte concentrates (see patient example, Fig. 17.1). Other toxicities included one case of Grade 3 ascites; three cases of gastroduodenal ulcerations; four cases of liver abscesses; one case of hemorrhagic bile-duct obstruction, which was treated by temporary stenting; and one case of nonclassical RILD. Two patients died within 30 days of treatment: one of the deaths was caused by oesophageal variceal hemorrhage and the other by neutropenic sepsis during chemotherapy. Previous publications have reported a purely quantitatively higher 30-day mortality for patients with hepatocellular carcinoma and liver cirrhosis (3.6%, 3/83) than for patients with colorectal liver metastases (0%, 0/73) [2, 3].

Among the minor complications reported were pleural effusion, ascites, subcapsular hematoma of Grade ≤ 2, and pneumothorax. Classical RILD did not occur. One patient with hepatocellular carcinoma and hepatitis C, who received the first iBT 22 months after partial liver resection, developed an atypical form of RILD, with ascites and an icteric elevation of hepatic enzymes (bilirubin, transaminases, and alkaline phosphatase) 7 weeks after the last of four iBT treatments. However, under treatment corresponding to RILD prophylaxis, the changes resolved completely after 7 months and the patient died 2 years after the last iBT treatment. In an earlier study of 83 patients with hepatocellular carcinoma only two atypical, possible RILD cases were observed.

A subgroup of 48 patients was investigated in more detail by using standardized questionnaires concerning somatic discomfort. Overall, Grade 1–2 nausea and vomiting occurred in 37% of these patients. Severe pain was significantly correlated with the occurrence of a bleeding event (reported in 3/5 patients with a major bleeding event and 4/338 without; $p < 0.001$). Female patients reported nausea and vomiting significantly more frequently than males ($p = 0.049$ for nausea and $p = 0.016$ for vomiting).

In this study, major bleeding complications occurred exclusively in interventions in patients with liver cirrhosis (5/89 patients with cirrhosis and 0/254 without; $p = 0.001$) and, among these patients, predominantly in the group with moderately to severely impaired liver function (Child–Pugh stage B 3/13, stage A 2/230; $p < 0.001$). This confirmed the results of the pilot studies in patients with hepatocellular carcinoma or colorectal liver metastases [2, 3]. Here the pre-therapeutic platelet count was found to be a predisposing factor, at significance level for bleeding events ($p = 0.043$), while the number of inserted catheters, prothrombin time, portal

Table 17.1 Baseline patient characteristics, Mohnike et al., 2016

$N = 192$ patients; no. of patients (%) are shown except where otherwise stated	
Age (mean ± SD)	66.08 (± 10.2)
Male	111 (57.8)
Tumor entity	
Colorectal carcinoma	84 (43.8)
Hepatocellular carcinoma	50 (26.0)
Cholangial carcinoma	16 (8.3)
Mamma carcinoma	13 (6.7)
Lung carcinoma	8 (4.2)
Others[a]	21 (10.9)
Diameter of the largest lesion	
<5 cm	105 (54.7)
5–10 cm	66 (34.4)
>10 cm	12 (6.3)
Diffuse tumor spread	9 (4.7)
More than one lesion to treat	79 (41.1)
Previous chemotherapy	114 (59.4)
First line	38 (33.3)
Second line or more	76 (66.7)
Previous liver resection	52 (22.4)
Previous tumor ablation[b]	51 (26.6)
RFA or LITT	23 (45.1)
TACE	13 (25.5)
Ibt	15 (29.4)
Stereotactic radiation	1 (2.0)
Previous other therapies[c]	12 (6.3)
Liver cirrhosis	50 (26.0)
Child–Pugh class	44 (88.0)
A (76 interventions)	
B (12 interventions)	6 (12.0)
Portal vein thrombosis (30 interventions)[d]	15 (7.8)
Karnofsky index ≥70%	188 (97.9)

[a]Leiomyosarcoma of the vena cava, urinary bladder cancer, gastric cancer, renal cell cancer, jejunal cancer, adenocarcinoma of unknown primary (two each) and oesophageal cancer, pancreatic cancer, gastrointestinal stroma tumor, cervical cancer, thyroid cancer, anal cancer, hypopharyngeal cancer, choroidal melanoma, prostate cancer (one each)
[b]*RFA* radiofrequency ablation, *LITT* laser-induced thermotherapy, *TACE* transarterial chemoembolization, *iBT* interstitial-HDR brachytherapy
[c]Additional hormone- or tyrosine-kinase-inhibitor therapy
[d]Thrombosis in the main, right, or left hemi-liver portal vein

vein thrombosis, and age were not. The relationship between the maximum dose (usually defined as D1 cm^3 or D0.1 cm^3) and the development of radiogenic gastro-duodenal ulcers has been described previously [4]. The overall frequency of major complications, reported for <5% of iBT procedures, has recently been confirmed by another group [5].

Table 17.2 Treatment characteristics, Mohnike et al., 2016

Interventional/radiotherapeutic characteristics and follow-up
($N = 343$ interventions)

Variable	Value	No. with available data (%)
Guiding imaging		343 (100)
CT [n (%)]	284 (82.8)	
MRI [n (%)]	59 (17.2)	
Number of catheters [n (IQR; maximum)]	4.0 (2.0–5.0; 9)	342 (99.7)
Target dose per lesion [in Gy (± SD)]	17.3 (± 3.1)	337 (98.3)
CTV[a] [in cm³ (IQR; maximum)]	36.7 (13.0–78.8; 796.0)	317 (92.4)
LV[b] [in cm³ (± SD)]	1352.3 (± 413.5)	295 (86.0)
(CTV/LV) × 100 [% (IQR; maximum)]	2.7 (1.1–6.1; 61.2)	291 (84.8)
(5 Gy/LV) × 100[c] [% (IQR; maximum)]	22.5 (13.8–34.7; 87.9)	293 (85.4)

Attendance for follow-up was as follows: nominally 3 days (actually 2.9 ± 0.9 days, appointments kept by patients representing 343/343 interventions); 6 weeks (42 ± 12 days, appointments kept by patients representing 269/288 interventions); 3 months (85 ± 12 days, 139/196); 6 months (147 ± 29 days, 113/144); 9 months (215 ± 34 days, 85/106); 12 months (293 ± 33 days, 56/60); 15 months (386 ± 39 days, 42/45); 18 months (484 ± 41 days, 37/37); 21 months (611 ± 49 days, 20/20); 24 months (712 ± 58 days, 9/9)
[a]Clinical target volume
[b]Liver volume
[c]5 Gy-volume of total tumor-free liver volume

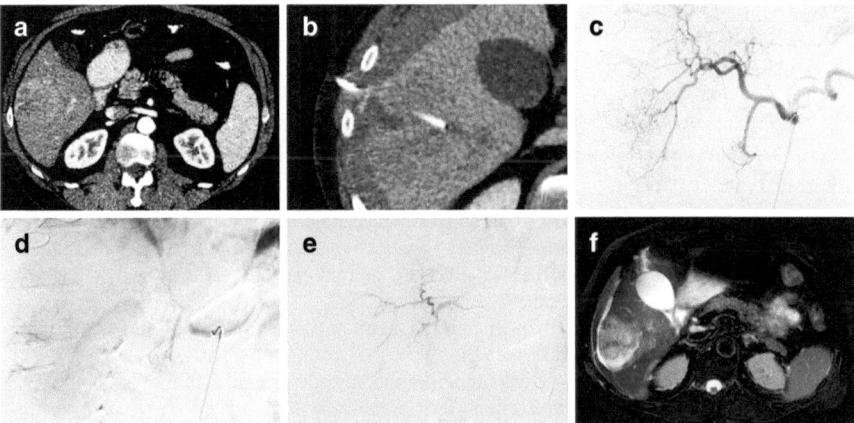

Fig. 17.1 Hemorrhage during catheter placement. (**a**) CT before iBT. (**b**) Subcapsular hematoma and arterial blush supporting active arterial bleeding in the CE-CT. (**c, d**) Subsequent angiography over the A. hepatica with a peripheral bleeding blush corresponding to the CT. (**e**) Angiography after embolization with Gelaspon and coils. (**f**) T2-weighted MRI after embolization

Interstitial Brachytherapy in the Context of Biliodigestive Anastomosis

There is evidence that the presence of a biliodigestive anastomosis increases the risk of post-interventional abscesses (see patient example Fig. 17.2), as is known to be the case for transarterial chemoembolization (TACE) and transarterial embolization (TAE) [6–8]. This is supported by the results of a study at our center (data not yet published) on the treatment of cholangiocellular carcinomas by iBT in combination with systemic therapy. Similarly, retrospective studies indicate that radioembolization (RE) with yttrium-90 in the presence of biliodigestive anastomosis carries a lower risk of abscess formation than other interventions do.

Peri-interventional Prophylaxis of Thrombosis with Low-Molecular-Weight Heparins: Risk of Bleeding and Thrombosis

In contrast to the dose-dependent effect of radiation therapy, the risk of (possibly severe) bleeding complications used to be difficult to predict. However, there is now good evidence that allows assessment of the individual risk in advance of the invasive procedure. In the study summarized above, an association between cirrhosis-related impairment of liver function and the risk of bleeding was demonstrated.

When invasive procedures are performed in hospitalized cancer patients, patients frequently receive low-molecular-weight heparin (LMWH) for thromboprophylaxis. This is because these patients are predisposed to thromboembolic events (venous thromboembolism, VTE), which are indeed more frequent than in hospitalized non-oncological patients [9, 10]. It has long been postulated that

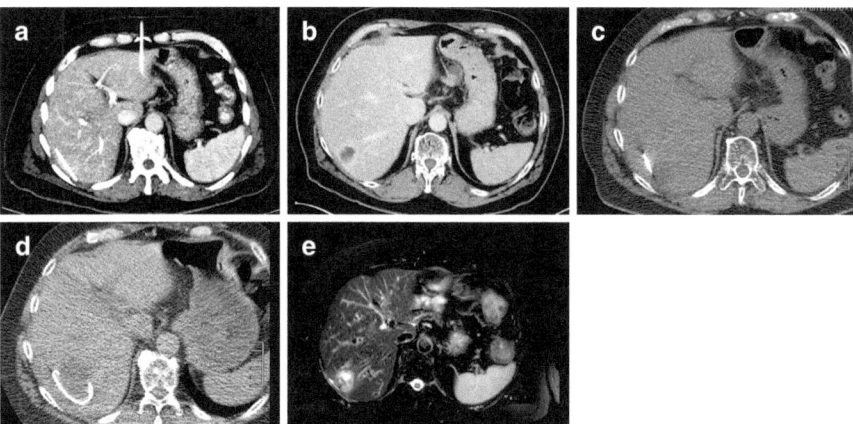

Fig. 17.2 Liver abscess after iBT following a recent papillotomy. (**a**) Implanted catheters. (**b**) CE-CT with the suspicion of abscess formation. CT fluoroscopy, (**c**) puncture, (**d**) subsequent drainage, and (**e**) Later examination, T2-weighted MRI

VTE-associated mortality and morbidity can be effectively reduced by the administration of LMWH [11–13]. However, a recent meta-analysis of 16,000 oncological and non-oncological patients did not find any significant reduction in the incidence of deep vein thrombosis, pulmonary embolism, or mortality associated with the use of LMWH [14]. The administration of LMWH is associated with an elevated risk of bleeding events following hepatopancreatobiliar surgery [15]. It is regrettable that the current guidelines do not include any recommendations concerning thrombo-prophylaxis in cancer patients who are treated by minimally invasive therapies [16].

An analysis of 446 cancer patients who were treated with a total of 781 tumor ablations (iBT, $N = 669$; RFA, $N = 112$) compared the impact of peri-interventional LMWH administration ($N = 260$ with LMWH and 521 without). Tumor locations were the liver, lung, kidney, lymph nodes, and other locations. Baseline patient and treatment characteristics are shown in Table 17.3. A total of 63 bleeding events of all severities were observed during these interventions, and bleeding was significantly more frequent among the patients with thromboprophylaxis than in those without (for all interventions 11.7% versus 6.3%, $p = 0.0127$; for hepatic interventions 12.7 versus 7.1%, $p = 0.0416$). Moreover, bleeding events were significantly more frequent with RFA than with iBT (overall, 14.3 versus 7.0%, $p = 0.0149$; for hepatic interventions, 19.6% versus 7.7%, $p = 0.0054$). The proportions of patients receiving thromboprophylaxis were well balanced: 33% in the iBT group and 34.8% in the RFA group ($p = 0.710$). Overall, the number of major bleedings (CTCAE Grade ≥ 3) was greater by a factor of 2.6 in the prophylaxis group (4.6% versus 1.7%; $p = 0.0243$); while for hepatic interventions the corresponding factor was 3.3

Table 17.3 Patients and treatment characteristics, Mohnike et al., 2017

Patients	$N = 446$
Interventions	$N = 781$ (100.0%)
Primary cancer	$n = 308$ (39.4%)
Colorectal cancer	$n = 104$ (13.3%)
Hepatocellular carcinoma	$n = 96$ (12.3%)
Cholangiocellular cancer	$n = 50$ (6.4%)
Breast cancer	$n = 50$ (6.4%)
Renal cell cancer	$n = 30$ (3.8%)
Liver cancer	$n = 24$ (3.1%)
Gastroenteropancreatic neuroendocrinal tumor Other	$n = 119$ (15.2%)
Clotting disorders	$n = 22$ (2.9%)
Thrombopenic	$n = 14$ (1.8%)
Thrombophilic	$n = 8$ (1.0%)
Cirrhosis	$n = 98$ (12.5%)
Child–Pugh stage B	$n = 21$ (2.7%)
Padua score < 4	$n = 229$ (29.3%)
Padua score ≥ 4	$n = 552$ (70.7%)
RFA	$n = 112$ (14.3%)
iBT	$n = 669$ (85.8%)
Peri-interventional LMWH dosing	$n = 260$ (33.3%)
Hospital stay	4.8 days (95% CI 4.6–5.1, range 2–15)

(5.2% versus 1.5%; $p = 0.028$). The treatment modality (iBT or RFA) did not show any significant influence. In uni- und multivariate analyses of the study, the administration of LMWH was the only independent factor associated with the frequency of bleeding occurrence (see Table 17.4). Regardless of the subsequent therapy for bleeding (angiographic embolization or surgical resection), the 30- and 90-day mortalities were significantly higher among the patients with major bleeding events (23.1% and 38.5%) than among those with no or moderate (Grade ≤ 2) bleeding events (0.5% and 2.3%; in both cases $p < 0.0001$). However, post-interventional administration of LMWH did not influence the occurrence of bleeding events. Overall, symptomatic VTE (pulmonary embolism) occurred only in one patient 2 months after iBT; this patient had not received LMWH. No other symptomatic thrombotic or thromboembolic events were observed [17].

These results allow us to draw major conclusions:

1. In terms of mortality, a bleeding event of CTCAE Grade ≥ 3 is the most serious complication, in both iBT and other tumor-ablation techniques such as RFA. Regardless of timely measures and hemostasis, secondary complications after a major bleeding event are common, and events such as hypovolemia or secondary infection of the hematoma with subsequent sepsis can be fatal [17].
2. Patients with advanced liver cirrhosis are predisposed for the occurrence of severe bleeding.
3. Regardless of the abovementioned factors, peri-interventional administration of LMWH is the most important risk factor for bleeding. The morbidity and mortality associated with LMWH administration are significantly higher than those associated with thromboembolic events among cancer patients treated by minimally invasive interventions requiring only a short period of immobilization. Therefore, LMWH cannot be generally recommended; in fact, in the absence of thrombogenic comorbidities it is contraindicated.
4. The closure of the puncture tract(s) with gelatine-sponge plugs is effective. Thus, in this respect iBT is not inferior to RFA, which offers the possibility of thermal coagulation. On the contrary, in a large patient cohort the incidence of bleeding of any grade was lower for patients treated by iBT than for those treated by RFA [17].

The Risk of Needle-Tract Metastases

The risk of seeding of malignant tumor cells during diagnostic or therapeutic puncture is well known and has been extensively studied, particularly in hepatocellular carcinoma. In a meta-analysis that included diagnostic puncture and local ablations the rate of occurrence of extrahepatic puncture-tract metastasis (PTM) was 1.27% [18]. Early studies of RFA reported a per-patient PTM rate of up to 12.5%, highlighting the need for ablation of the puncture channel [19]. In more recent reports of RFA or microwave ablation (MWA) the rate was reduced to 0.61–1.6% [20, 21]. In iBT, thermal puncture-tract ablation is not possible, so the problem of PTM was investigated in the following study.

Table 17.4 Severe hemorrhagic complications

Covariate	Mean value (95% CI)	Bleeding rate: Interaction between peri-interventional LMWH dosing and covariate, p value		Influence of peri-interventional LMWH dosing on bleeding rate adjusted for covariate, p value		Influence of covariate on bleeding rate adjusted for peri-interventional LMWH dosing, p value		Influence of covariate only, p value	
		All	Liver	All	Liver	All	Liver	All	Liver
Interventions:									
Modality (RFA/iBT)	n.a.	0.4563	0.9079	**0.0248**	**0.0281**	0.5669	0.2469	0.5351	0.2357
Number of catheters (iBT)	2.71 (1–9)	0.4867	0.8657	**0.0241**	**0.0281**	0.8403	0.8923	0.8041	0.8778
Thrombocytes [Gpt/L, 176–391]	212 (204–220)	0.2422	0.5330	**0.0216**	**0.0224**	0.1773	0.1658	0.1987	0.2095
Hemoglobin [mmol/L, 7.2–9.6]	8.04 (7.95–8.14)	0.6401	0.5974	**0.0247**	**0.0284**	0.8841	0.9593	0.8203	0.8552
Hematocrit [L/L, 0.35–0.45]	0.39 (0.39–0.39)	0.7044	0.7844	**0.0243**	**0.0279**	0.9896	0.9443	0.9902	0.9895
Prothrombin time [>70%]	108 (106–109)	0.1718	0.2555	**0.0202**	0.1680	0.4277	0.8612	0.2738	0.9942
Creatinine [µmol/L]	89 (82–95)	0.8958	0.5906	**0.0146**	**0.0144**	0.7404	0.5808	0.8160	0.7184
Cirrhosis	n.a.	0.7635	0.7331	**0.0245**	**0.0287**	0.8350	0.7809	0.8083	0.7212
Cirrhosis Child–Pugh B	n.a.	0.7364	0.9234	**0.0262**	**0.0274**	*0.0871*	0.4657	*0.0707*	0.4853

Generalized linear mixed model. Interaction between peri-interventional LMWH dosing and different covariates. Influence of LMWH adjusted for covariates and vice versa and of covariates alone. p values <0.05 (bold letters) indicate statistical significance. p values at the border of significance ($p < 0.1$) are in italics

In a total of 100 patients, 233 hepatocellular carcinoma (HCC) lesions were treated by iBT. This involved the placement of a total of 588 catheters, resulting in an average of 5.9 catheters per patient. For PTM assessment, iBT planning imaging, including dosimetry, was image-fused with the follow-up sectional imaging (CT or MRI). After a mean follow-up of 5.5 months (range 4.8–6.2 months) overall nine PTMs (seven intrahepatic, two peritoneal) were found, corresponding to a per-catheter PTM rate of 1.5% (1.2% intrahepatic, 0.3% extrahepatic), a per-lesion rate of 3.9% and a per-patient rate of 9%. Tumor seeding was observed more frequently for smaller HCC lesions, although not at the level of significance ($p = 0.09$). Other factors as liver cirrhosis, etiology, pseudo-capsulation, in-body catheter path, catheter insertion beyond the tumor, the D100, and subsequent treatment with sorafenib did not affect the PTM rate. Eight of nine PTMs were subsequently treated successfully by iBT. There was no relevant difference in median OS between patients with and without PTM (25 vs. 20 months).

A unique feature of this study was the fact that the comparison of the iBT treatment-planning images to the follow-up imaging allowed also to identify intrahepatic PTM, whereas other studies in this area have only considered extrahepatic tumor seeding. Thus, the extrahepatic PTM rates per-catheter and per-patient were 0.2% and 2% respectively, without ablation of the puncture tract. This proportion is lower or similar to that encountered in RFA and MWA. This low PTM rate confirms the results of a study in a small patient cohort, in which iBT was performed as a bridging therapy for hepatocellular carcinoma before liver transplantation [22]. In earlier studies of iBT, adverse effects such as local recurrence or PTM had not affected overall survival. This may be due to the repeatability of iBT, in view of its almost unrestricted applicability in terms of location and tumor size. In fact, almost all PTMs of patients with colorectal liver metastases in this study, and local recurrences in the study mentioned elsewhere [23], were retreated by repeated iBT [3].

According to this analysis, the puncture tract is now irradiated routinely at most centers, irrespective of the cancer entity: this is done either by using a default dwell-time approach (with 0.5–1 s per dwell position) or by using a dose prescription (with about 5 Gy at the surface of the catheter) [23].

Organs at Risk: Bile Ducts, Stomach, Duodenum, Kidney, Pancreas

The liver as an organ at risk in large- or small-volume intrahepatic iBT and the monitoring of post-therapeutic liver function after iBT are discussed in detail in Chap. 11.

In iBT of centrally located liver tumors, the common, left and right bile ducts are frequently exposed to high single doses of radiation. Changes in the adjacent bile ducts are frequently observed during follow-up, such as, for example, an irregular widening of bile ducts on imaging. However, only a minority of cases show changes in clinic or laboratory values that are typical of cholestasis. The following study was aimed at investigating to what extent these bile-duct changes correlate with iBT dose distribution and reach clinical relevance.

A total of 102 patients with various hepatic malignancies were analyzed retrospectively. Each patient had received a maximum dose to the central bile-duct structures of at least 1 Gy. Twenty-two of these patients (22%) developed morphological dilation of the bile ducts after a median interval of 17 (range 3–54) months. Eighteen of these were treated by percutaneous or endoscopic drainage. The median bile-duct point dose was 24.8 Gy (range 4.4–80 Gy) in patients with bile-duct dilation compared with 14.2 Gy (range 1.8–61.7 Gy) for those without ($p = 0.028$). The calculated cut-off value was 20.8 Gy ($p = 0.028$; sensitivity 59%, specificity 24%). Secondary occurrence of abscesses and cholangitis were rare, but were nonetheless seen in both groups, and significantly more frequently in the group with morphological cholestasis (4/22 vs. 2/80; $p = 0.029$). However, median overall survival did not differ between the two groups (43 versus 36 months, $p = 0.571$) [24].

The wide distribution of maximum doses in both groups and the low sensitivity and very low specificity of the calculated cut-off value make it difficult to derive recommendations for dose constraints in clinical routine. On the one hand, individual patients developed a morphological cholestasis at very low doses of 4.4 Gy, while others did not develop any cholestasis despite a dose exposure of up to 61.7 Gy. At first glance, this suggests two possible explanations: one is that each patient has an individual bile-duct dose tolerance value. As this seems unlikely, another possible explanation is that morphological cholestasis is less a consequence of the reaction of the healthy bile-duct wall than a sign of response to iBT of the infiltrated bile-duct wall, which responds by developing scar tissue.

Taken together, clinically relevant complications in iBT administered to central liver tumors are rare and many patients also tolerate very high maximum doses administered to the central bile-duct structures. To date, unfortunately, we still have no clear dose constraint in this respect. The excellent response of central liver tumors is a unique feature of iBT as compared with other local-therapeutic procedures, including surgical resection. Therefore, the risk of a post-interventional cholestasis can be considered acceptable, since this complication does not reduce life expectancy. However, the awareness of these side effects must be present and the patient must be appropriately informed.

Other clinically important organs at risk (OARs) include the stomach and the duodenum. In the early years of iBT, a small but relevant number of radiation-induced gastric or duodenal ulcerations were observed, especially in left-hepatic interventions, so that increased scientific attention was given to developing constraints for these OARs.

In the study described above, overall 192 patients underwent 343 CT- or MRI-guided iBT procedures for various cancer entities. A total of 57 patients received a dose exposure of the stomach or duodenum in 72 interventions, defined as a dose of more than 1 Gy to 1 cm^3. Among these patients, gastroduodenal ulcers were identified following three interventions (3/72; 4%). Patients in whom the gastroduodenal ulceration could be correlated to the dose distribution of iBT (because of the localization of the ulcer or by pathology) had received a significantly higher D1 cm^3 to the stomach or duodenal wall as such without ulceration (15.8 ± 2.5 vs. 10.0 ± 4.1 Gy;

$p = 0.020$). The cut-off dose for the development of gastroduodenal ulcers was a D1 cm^3 of 14 Gy [4].

This supports the results of an earlier study with a smaller patient cohort (33 patients who received iBT in liver segments 2 or 3). In this study, borderline values for symptomatic gastrointestinal toxicity and the development of gastroduodenal ulcers of D1 cm^3 of 11 and 15.5 Gy, respectively, were found [25].

The extent to which a pre- or post-interventional systemic therapy that includes ulcerogenic substances such as bevacizumab reinforces these dose effects has not yet been scientifically studied.

In clinical routine, proton-pump inhibitors are prescribed for 3–6 months if a relevant dose exposure to the gastric or duodenal wall of 8–10 Gy D1 cm^3 has been administered [4]. However, dose exposures above a D1 cm^3 of 14–16 Gy should be avoided. In these cases, dose coverage of the target lesion must be compromised, or the treatment must be fractionated. This challenge led to the development of a new technique to increase the distance between the liver and the stomach or bowel wall, and thus distancing the OAR from radiation. For this purpose, angiography occlusion balloons are inserted as a spacer.

In a study of 31 patients receiving iBT, occlusion balloons were introduced between the stomach and the liver during the placing of the iBT catheter. For each patient, the calculated point dose without the balloons was compared on a virtual iBT plan (created from a native CT-scan performed immediately before catheter insertion and fused with the iBT treatment plan) with the actual point dose at the organ at risk after insertion of the balloon. It was found that the treatment plans with the balloon resulted in a mean D1 cm^3 of 12.6 Gy to the organ at risk, compared with 16 Gy without the balloon ($p < 0.001$). This result is relevant because without a significant reduction in dose exposure of the OAR, the much more invasive balloon technique would be highly questionable. Nevertheless, it allows the effective, unfractionated treatment of left-hepatic malignomas [26].

The Lung as a Treatment Target and OAR

Yoon et al. report in their chapter of this book "CT-guided interstitial HDR brachytherapy for malignant lung lesions: Experience from University of California Los Angeles" about iBT of 37 malignant lung lesions in 25 patients. Common lung histologies were renal cell carcinoma (24%), NSCLC (20%), and soft-tissue sarcoma (20%). Of the 37 lesions treated, 22 (88%) were metastatic lesions, 2 (8%) were primary NSCLC, and 1 (4%) was locally recurrent NSCLC. Altogether, 78% of lesions were located in either an ultra-central or a central location. Twenty-two patients (88%) received a single-fraction iBT at a median total dose of 21.5 Gy (range 15–26 Gy). For the three patients (12%) receiving a multi-fraction radiation treatment, the median dose was 24 Gy (range 20–25.5 Gy) with a range of 2–5 fractions.

After a median follow-up of 19 months (range 3–48 months), 62% of patients did not develop acute or late toxicities following brachytherapy, while 33% of patients developed Grade 1 and 2 acute toxicities. More specifically, four patients experienced Grade 1 chest wall pain, two patients developed Grade 2 pneumonitis (treated with steroids), and one patient developed a pneumothorax during catheter implantation which required an overnight chest tube insertion. No patient developed late treatment-related toxicities. One patient with metastatic colorectal cancer experienced mild dyspnoea on exertion 5 months after brachytherapy treatment, but the etiology was considered to be multi-factorial given his prior smoking history and treatments (several resections and microwave ablations) for lung metastases.

Hass et al. reported outcomes and safety of lung iBT in a retrospective study of 174 patients; this was presented at the ESTRO37 conference in Barcelona analyzing 156 patients with lung metastases and 18 patients with primary NSCLC [27]. A total of 359 lesions were treated, in 276 mostly single-fraction CT-guided iBT procedures. Local bleedings occurred in six cases (2.2%) which were quickly resolved by angiographic coiling. In 60 treatments (21.8%) a mild pneumothorax (<1 cm) could be observed; among these cases, seven patients (2.5%) needed a temporary chest tube drainage to address the complication. In five patients (2%) pneumonitis was associated with typical radiological findings; among them, two patients were given anti-inflammatory medication.

Similarly, in the study by Peters et al, 30 consecutive patients with 83 primary or secondary pulmonary malignancies were treated by lung iBT. Minor complications included nausea (three reports, 6% of treatments) and discrete pneumothorax (six reports, 12%) which were treated conservatively and showed complete regression after 24 h. One major pneumothorax was treated with a chest tube. Two patients had a history of previous lung surgery of the respective lobe of the lung, and a total of six patients demonstrated diminished lung function before brachytherapy with a vital capacity (VC) of <85% (minimum 40%, 20% of patients) and an FEV1/VC of <70% (minimum 17%, 20% of patients). No significant changes in VC or FEV1 were noted during follow-up [28].

Kidney, Pancreas, and Adrenal Glands as Treatment Targets and/or OARs

Frequently, the kidney is an OAR with relevant dose exposure in iBT. In the treatment of renal cell carcinomas or the rare renal metastases from other primaries, adrenal gland malignancies or segment 6 liver iBT, the kidney is often not only involved as a target organ but also as an OAR at the same time.

In one study, the functional outcome of iBT in 18 patients with renal cell carcinomas and two renal metastases was analyzed. The primary endpoint was loss of renal function after 12 months. A planned dose of 15 Gy (20 Gy in local recurrences) was applied. Serum creatinine, estimated glomerular filtration rate (eGFR), and other values were measured 3 days, 3 months, 6 months, and 12 months after iBT. Also, a technetium-99m-MAG3 kidney sequence scintigraphy of both kidneys was performed (with separate assessment for each kidney) directly after iBT and 3, 6, and 12 months later. A reduction in median eGFR was observed, from 71 mL/min (range 26–125 mL/min) to 58 mL/min (range 23–88 mL/min) after 12 months, without statistical significance.

After 12 months, the tubular extraction rate (TER, determined by scintigraphy) decreased ipsilaterally in the kidney treated by iBT, from a median value of 52 mL/min (range 37–100 mL/min) to 33 mL/min (range 5–100 mL/min). At the same time the median contralateral TER had risen from 51 mL/min to 95 mL/min; in neither case was statistical significance achieved. Overall median TER of both kidneys decreased from 156 mL/min (range 97–340 mL/min) to 108 mL/min (range 108–142 mL/min).

However, it should be noted that, on account of the study design, complications with late onset (more than a year after iBT) were not recorded for all of the patients. The comprehensive follow-up with image-guided monitoring lasted for a median of 22.5 months. During follow-up, only one patient required hemodialysis, with onset approximately 2.5 years after iBT. However, this patient had bilateral disease, diabetes, and preexisting renal insufficiency. In summary, within the limitations of this study, iBT could safely be performed without significant functional impairment [29].

Another organ that is frequently at risk is the pancreas, either because of its proximity to irradiated areas in the liver, lymph nodes, kidneys, or adrenal glands or because of the treatment of the pancreas itself. In a study of pancreatic iBT performed in 13 patients (8 metastases and 5 primary tumors, of which 2 were locally recurrent), with a median tumor diameter of 3 cm and a D100 of 15.3 Gy, no toxicity of CTCAE $\geq$ Grade 3 was observed. Only one patient developed mild acute pancreatitis, which resolved spontaneously within a week [30].

Regarding adrenal glands, a recent study report described the outcome of 37 patients with adrenal gland metastases from different primary tumors treated by iBT. Overall, 11 toxicities of Grade 1 or 2 occurred (29%) including pain, nausea, vomiting, and fatigue. One Grade 3 event occurred (bleeding requiring angiographic embolization, 3%). Owing to decreased function, two patients required ongoing cortisone substitution after treatment, while one patient required intermittent cortisone substitution for 1 month after treatment [31]. Special attention is required if both adrenal glands are treated.

Key Points
- Interstitial brachytherapy (iBT) is a procedure that allows substantial sparing of healthy liver tissue. Classical radiation-induced liver disorders (RILDs) have not been reported in the literature; only atypical cases have been reported in individual instances.
- For large, centrally located liver tumors, clinically relevant biliary duct complications are rare and have not been associated with a reduction in overall survival in available study reports. The excellent treatability of central liver tumors is a unique feature of iBT as compared with other local-therapeutic procedures, including surgical resection.

- In addition to the liver, clinically important organs at risk are the stomach and the duodenum, which are at risk of gastroduodenal ulceration. In clinical routine, this implies that proton-pump inhibitors are prescribed at a relevant gastroduodenal dose exposure. Furthermore, angiographic occlusion balloons can be placed between the stomach wall and the liver to avoid a significant dose exposure of the stomach.
- There is evidence of a strong correlation between severe bleeding events and (1) the secondary diagnosis of an advanced liver cirrhosis, e.g., in patients with hepatocellular carcinoma, and (2) the peri-interventional administration of low-molecular-weight heparin. In terms of mortality, a bleeding event of CTCAE Grade ≥ 3 is overall very rare but remains a serious complication with a potentially fatal outcome.
- There is evidence that a history of biliodigestive anastomosis or papillotomy are risk factors for post-interventional development of cholangitis or liver abscesses.
- Lung iBT is associated with a low rate of severe adverse events, whereas mild pneumothorax without the need for a chest tube placement is reported in up to 20% of treatments.
- iBT of the kidneys, the adrenal glands, and the pancreas seems to be safe for the vast majority of patients, although the reported evidence on safety and outcome is still limited.
- The overall risk of extrahepatic puncture-tract metastases is very low, and in case of a puncture-tract recurrence after iBT, it does not affect overall survival. Moreover, in appropriately designed studies, iBT has been successfully used for treating local recurrences.

References

1. Trotti A, Colevas AD, Setser A, et al. CTCAE v3.0: development of a comprehensive grading system for the adverse effects of cancer treatment. Semin Radiat Oncol. 2003;13:176–81.
2. Mohnike K, Wieners G, Schwartz F, et al. Computed tomography-guided high-dose-rate brachytherapy in hepatocellular carcinoma: safety, efficacy, and effect on survival. Int J Radiat Oncol Biol Phys. 2010;78:172–9.
3. Ricke J, Mohnike K, Pech M, et al. Local response and impact on survival after local ablation of liver metastases from colorectal carcinoma by computed tomography-guided high-dose-rate brachytherapy. Int J Radiat Oncol Biol Phys. 2010;78:479–85.
4. Mohnike K, Wolf S, Damm R, et al. Radioablation of liver malignancies with interstitial high-dose-rate brachytherapy: complications and risk factors. Strahlenther Onkol. 2016;192:288–96.
5. Boning G, Buttner L, Jonczyk M, et al. Complications of computed tomography-guided high-dose-rate brachytherapy (CT-HDRBT) and risk factors: results from more than 10 years of experience. Cardiovasc Intervent Radiol. 2020;43:284–94.
6. Wieners G, Schippers AC, Collettini F, et al. CT-guided high-dose-rate brachytherapy in the interdisciplinary treatment of patients with liver metastases of pancreatic cancer. Hepatobiliary Pancreat Dis Int. 2015;14:530–8.

7. Huang SF, Ko CW, Chang CS, Chen GH. Liver abscess formation after transarterial chemoembolization for malignant hepatic tumor. Hepatogastroenterology. 2003;50:1115–8.
8. Kim W, Clark TW, Baum RA, Soulen MC. Risk factors for liver abscess formation after hepatic chemoembolization. J Vasc Interv Radiol. 2001;12:965–8.
9. Barbar S, Noventa F, Rossetto V, et al. A risk assessment model for the identification of hospitalized medical patients at risk for venous thromboembolism: the Padua Prediction Score. J Thromb Haemost. 2010;8:2450–7.
10. Stein PD, Beemath A, Meyers FA, Skaf E, Sanchez J, Olson RE. Incidence of venous thromboembolism in patients hospitalized with cancer. Am J Med. 2006;119:60–8.
11. Anderson FA Jr, Wheeler HB, Goldberg RJ, Hosmer DW, Forcier A, Patwardhan NA. Physician practices in the prevention of venous thromboembolism. Ann Intern Med. 1991;115:591–5.
12. Clagett GP, Anderson FA Jr, Heit J, Levine MN, Wheeler HB. Prevention of venous thromboembolism. Chest. 1995;108:312S–34S.
13. Group LGCotTc. Risk of and prophylaxis for venous thromboembolism in hospital patients. Thromboembolic Risk Factors (THRIFT) Consensus Group. BMJ. 1992;305(6853):567–74.
14. Spencer A, Cawood T, Frampton C, Jardine D. Heparin-based treatment to prevent symptomatic deep venous thrombosis, pulmonary embolism or death in general medical inpatients is not supported by best evidence. Intern Med J. 2014;44:1054–65.
15. Doughtie CA, Priddy EE, Philips P, Martin RC, McMasters KM, Scoggins CR. Preoperative dosing of low-molecular-weight heparin in hepatopancreatobiliary surgery. Am J Surg. 2014;208:1009–15; discussion 15.
16. Farge D, Frere C, Connors JM, et al. 2019 international clinical practice guidelines for the treatment and prophylaxis of venous thromboembolism in patients with cancer. Lancet Oncol. 2019;20:e566–e81.
17. Mohnike K, Sauerland H, Seidensticker M, et al. Haemorrhagic complications and symptomatic venous thromboembolism in interventional tumour ablations: the impact of peri-interventional thrombosis prophylaxis. Cardiovasc Intervent Radiol. 2016;39:1716–21.
18. Stigliano R, Marelli L, Yu D, Davies N, Patch D, Burroughs AK. Seeding following percutaneous diagnostic and therapeutic approaches for hepatocellular carcinoma. What is the risk and the outcome? Seeding risk for percutaneous approach of HCC. Cancer Treat Rev. 2007;33:437–47.
19. Llovet JM, Vilana R, Bru C, et al. Increased risk of tumor seeding after percutaneous radiofrequency ablation for single hepatocellular carcinoma. Hepatology. 2001;33:1124–9.
20. Yu J, Liang P, Yu XL, Cheng ZG, Han ZY, Dong BW. Needle track seeding after percutaneous microwave ablation of malignant liver tumors under ultrasound guidance: analysis of 14-year experience with 1462 patients at a single center. Eur J Radiol. 2012;81:2495–9.
21. Zhong-Yi Z, Wei Y, Kun Y, et al. Needle track seeding after percutaneous radiofrequency ablation of hepatocellular carcinoma: 14-year experience at a single centre. Int J Hyperth. 2017;33:454–8.
22. Denecke T, Stelter L, Schnapauff D, et al. CT-guided interstitial brachytherapy of hepatocellular carcinoma before liver transplantation: an equivalent alternative to transarterial chemoembolization? Eur Radiol. 2015;25:2608–16.
23. Damm R, Zorkler I, Rogits B, et al. Needle track seeding in hepatocellular carcinoma after local ablation by high-dose-rate brachytherapy: a retrospective study of 588 catheter placements. J Contemp Brachytherapy. 2018;10:516–21.
24. Powerski M, Penzlin S, Hass P, et al. Biliary duct stenosis after image-guided high-dose-rate interstitial brachytherapy of central and hilar liver tumors: a systematic analysis of 102 cases. Strahlenther Onkol. 2019;195:265–73.
25. Streitparth F, Pech M, Bohmig M, et al. In vivo assessment of the gastric mucosal tolerance dose after single fraction, small volume irradiation of liver malignancies by computed tomography-guided, high-dose-rate brachytherapy. Int J Radiat Oncol Biol Phys. 2006;65:1479–86.
26. Hass P, Steffen IG, Powerski M, et al. First report on extended distance between tumor lesion and adjacent organs at risk using interventionally applied balloon catheters: a simple proce-

dure to optimize clinical target volume covering effective isodose in interstitial high-dose-rate brachytherapy of liver malignomas. J Contemp Brachytherapy. 2019;11:152–61.

27. Hass P, Sieber F, Willich C, et al. CT-guided interstitial BT of pulmonary malignomas. Retrospecticve analysis of 174 patients. ESTRO37. Barcelona; 2018.

28. Peters N, Wieners G, Pech M, et al. CT-guided interstitial brachytherapy of primary and secondary lung malignancies: results of a prospective phase II trial. Strahlenther Onkol. 2008;184:296–301.

29. Damm R, Streitparth T, Hass P, et al. Prospective evaluation of CT-guided HDR brachytherapy as a local ablative treatment for renal masses: a single-arm pilot trial. Strahlenther Onkol. 2019;195(11):982–90.

30. Omari J, Heinze C, Wilck A, et al. Efficacy and safety of CT-guided high-dose-rate interstitial brachytherapy in primary and secondary malignancies of the pancreas. Eur J Radiol. 2019;112:22–7.

31. Mohnike K, Neumann K, Hass P, et al. Radioablation of adrenal gland malignomas with interstitial high-dose-rate brachytherapy: efficacy and outcome. Strahlenther Onkol. 2017;193:612–9.

Radiological Interventions in the Age of Immunotherapy, Molecular Diagnostics, and Liquid Biopsy

Jens Ricke and Konrad Mohnike

Cancer is the second most common cause of death worldwide, with both incidence and mortality increasing dramatically over the past 100 years [1]. Globally, the number of cancer cases increased by 33% between 2005 and 2015, corresponding to the increase in world population and an increase in life expectancy [2]. The disease-specific mortality rate, in contrast, has declined over the past 20 years, which can primarily be attributed to advances in therapeutic methods. It is by no means unreasonable to assume that the evolution of procedures for local therapy has also played a part in this [3–5]. Nevertheless, cancer represents an immense problem in medical and health policy, owing to its high frequency, and it is therefore also a major challenge for health systems.

It is notable that Europe, with 9% of the world's population, records as many as 25% of global cancer cases. In 2018, 3.91 million new cancer cases were reported in Europe, and 1.93 million persons died as a result of cancer. The most common were breast cancer (ca. 523,000 cases), colorectal cancer (500,000), lung cancer (470,000), and pancreatic cancer (450,000). Regarding disease-related mortality, lung cancer was the most prominent (ca. 388,000 deaths), followed by colorectal (243,000), breast (138,000), and pancreatic (128,000) carcinomas [6].

J. Ricke
Department of Radiology, Ludwig Maximilian University (LMU) Hospital Munich, Munich, Germany
e-mail: Jens.Ricke@med.uni-muenchen.de

K. Mohnike (✉)
Department of Diagnostics, Department of Interventional Oncology & Radionuclide Therapy, Diagnostic Therapeutic Center Berlin, Berlin, Germany

Department of Radiology and Nuclear Medicine, University Hospital Magdeburg, Magdeburg, Germany
e-mail: konrad.mohnike@berlin-dtz.de

© The Author(s), under exclusive license to Springer Nature Switzerland AG 2021
K. Mohnike et al. (eds.), *Manual on Image-Guided Brachytherapy of Inner Organs*, https://doi.org/10.1007/978-3-030-78079-1_18

Recent progress of drug-based tumor therapy and its sometimes impressive achievements have continued to raise the prominence of systemic treatment of numerous tumor entities in the metastatic stage [7]. The most recent quantum leap has been the introduction of immuno-oncology including checkpoint inhibitors and CAR T cell therapy [8]. The immense increase in the number of new regimens for treating cancer is making it increasingly difficult to compare local and locoregional therapeutic concepts with systemic therapy in clinical studies. Identifying appropriate study formats and relevant clinical endpoints is challenging. It is worth mentioning that access to financial resources to support clinical trials is more difficult in device studies or surgery than in studies that are of interest to pharmaceutical companies.

The metastatic stage of solid tumors is generally regarded as the systemic stage of the disease, calling for systemic treatment concepts. Cure remains exceptional in the inoperable metastatic disease stages, and the number of possible therapies is limited. Moreover, systemic therapies may often provoke considerable systemic toxicity, which limits applicability for patients with comorbidities and almost invariably leads to a reduction in quality of life [9–11].

Limited metastatic spread may still offer potential for curative outcomes after local therapies or surgery. In recent years, observation of long-term survival after local treatments has led to establishing the concept of oligometastatic disease, accountable for all solid tumor entities (i.e., the possibility of curative treatment of metastatic-stage patients by local therapies) [12–15]. However, depending on the underlying tumor entity, only a small fraction of patients meet the criteria of oligometastatic disease, and technical limitations of surgical techniques have reduced the number of amenable patients even further [16, 17]. Data on surgical resection of colorectal liver metastasis demonstrates high recurrence rates of 50–75%. The shorter the interval between operation and recurrence, the worse is the patient's prognosis [18–22]. The cause of postsurgical tumor progression is multifactorial. There are indications that regeneration of the liver following surgical resection favors tumor progression [23]. Immune response, angiogenesis, lymphangiogenesis, the epithelial-to-mesenchymal transition, and the remodeling of the extracellular matrix may all play a part in this and are therefore preferred targets of various antibody and inhibitor therapies [24]. These phenomena are certainly present in image-guided, minimally invasive local procedures, too. However, final proof of their impact on recurrences and prognosis is still under scrutiny.

The possibilities offered by modern radiological techniques have led to the development of minimally invasive therapies, such as *radio-frequency ablation* (RFA), which today is the most widely used of these and is supported by strongest evidence. In early and very early stages of hepatocellular carcinoma, RFA has become a standard procedure, especially in patients with cirrhosis, and the CLOCC study of colorectal liver metastases, with very broad inclusion criteria, has revealed a significant advantage in OS for patients adding RFA (sometimes complementing resection) to chemotherapy compared with those treated by chemotherapy alone [5, 25–27]. Among the locoregional techniques in liver-dominant, diffuse metastasis, radioembolization (RE) with yttrium-90 has gained increasing importance in recent years [28–31]. However, randomized trials in both colorectal liver metastasis or advanced HCC have failed to demonstrate survival benefit, despite strong indications for improved outcomes in per protocol treated subgroups [27–30].

RFA and other thermoablative local therapies, such as MWA, are technically limited with respect to the location and size of the tumor to be treated. Local recurrence rates increase with size, the threshold likely to be around 3 cm; large blood vessels nearby restrict applicability by cooling effects and reduction of therapeutic efficacy [32]. Moreover, the proximity of thermosensitive structures such as the liver hilum or the gallbladder may prohibit the conduct of both MWA and RFA [33, 34].

Radiotherapeutic techniques, such as percutaneous stereotactic irradiation (SBRT) or CT-guided interstitial brachytherapy, overcome these limitations in various ways. However, as in thermoablation, a maximum is set to the size of lesions that can be effectively treated, here some 4–5 cm; the number of lesions that can be treated during a single intervention is limited [35, 36]. Above these limits, the efficacy of SBRT appears to decline substantially [37, 38].

In contrast, iBT provides greater flexibility in terms of lesion size and number, with satisfactory local tumor control up to 12 cm in some studies [39].

A long-term observational study of the use of RFA in treating colorectal liver metastases has shown impressive results in terms of overall survival of inoperable patients, as compared with published outcomes after surgery [40]. In other studies, radio-frequency ablation was found to be clearly inferior to resection; although this may have been due to the well-known size limitation in thermoablative procedures, it may also have been influenced by selection bias, as inoperable patients inevitably represent a patient population with comorbidities [32]. One way or another, high-quality prospective and randomized studies, ones that allow genuine comparison between the RFA-treated and surgically treated patient cohorts, have not been reported, and the idea of performing such studies is even rejected in some quarters on the basis of (sometimes questionable) ethical reservations, even though from a scientific and ethical viewpoint there is in fact an acute need for such studies [41]. Provisionally, one may retreat to the viewpoint that in clinical routine these two procedures do not so much compete with as complement one another [42–44].

It would be useful to debate the local and locoregional level of tumor therapy, with reference to the concept of oligometastasis—the stage between local and systemic disease, which despite (limited) formation of metastases is considered to be treatable locally with curative intent [45–47]. This is a recognized concept and is relevant for all local procedures, be they based on resection, stereotactic irradiation, thermoablation, or interstitial brachytherapy.

As a basic principle, the choice of treatment for metastases or for liver-specific tumors should be directed by consideration of the individual oncological situation, including the patient's age, comorbidities, and previous therapy, as well as taking account of the best possibilities for tumor control and the treatment's tolerability. This choice should reflect the available evidence for, and clinical experience with, a given method; surgery, including liver transplantation, generally has a (presumable or ascertained) lead in terms of supporting evidence.

The acquisition of evidence is a challenging task in all local and technical procedures for tumor treatment, for various reasons. Randomized, multicentric clinical studies constitute the acknowledged gold standard of evidence-based medicine; however, they may be outside financial reach, unless they are backed by the pharmaceutical industry. Central cancer registers, as established in Germany at the *Robert-Koch-Institut* presumably by the end of 2021, may one day significantly impact therapy standards by enhanced inclusion of real-world evidence. Finally, the clinical study endpoint overall survival (OS) has also been critically questioned. Multimodal therapy directed at metastases, even if not curative, may increase the duration of palliation in many patients, which means that the cohort size needed to demonstrate a statistical advantage in overall survival may become unrealistically large [48]. Therefore, there is a need to define new endpoints for the stratification and assessment of initial response to therapy. "Depth of response" has recently been proven as a surrogate for survival in systemic therapy of selected colorectal cancer patients [49]. Potential study endpoint proving benefit of local therapies could also include, for example, the quantification of biomarkers, such as circulating tumor DNA, obtained by liquid biopsy [50–54].

Key Points
- Progress in drug-based tumor therapy in recent years has continued to raise the importance of systemic treatment for a range of tumor entities at the metastatic stage.
- Metastasis-directed local tumor therapy has been demonstrated to be effective in a number of studies.
- Observation of long-term survival after local treatment has led to the concept of oligometastatic disease. Limited metastatic spread may offer potential for curative outcomes after local therapies or surgery.
- The possibilities offered by modern radiological techniques have led to the development of minimally invasive therapies, such as *radio-frequency ablation* (RFA), which today is the most widely used of these and is supported by the strongest evidence.
- Multimodal therapy directed at metastases is curatively successful with many patients, and when unsuccessful it is today achieving an increasingly long duration of palliation, which means that the cohort size needed to demonstrate an advantage in OS is becoming unrealistically large.
- There is a need to define new endpoints for the stratification and assessment of initial response to therapy, including the quantification of biomarkers, such as circulating tumor DNA, obtained by liquid biopsy.

References

1. Ferlay J, Soerjomataram I, Dikshit R, et al. Cancer incidence and mortality worldwide: sources, methods and major patterns in GLOBOCAN 2012. Int J Cancer. 2015;136:E359–86.
2. Global Burden of Disease Cancer Collaboration, Fitzmaurice C, Akinyemiju TF, et al. Global, regional, and national cancer incidence, mortality, years of life lost, years lived with disability,

and disability-adjusted life-years for 29 cancer groups, 1990 to 2016: a systematic analysis for the global burden of disease study. JAMA Oncol. 2018;4:1553–68.

3. Niesen W, Hank T, Buchler M, Strobel O. Local radicality and survival outcome of pancreatic cancer surgery. Ann Gastroenterol Surg. 2019;3:464–75.

4. Palma DA, Olson R, Harrow S, et al. Stereotactic ablative radiotherapy versus standard of care palliative treatment in patients with oligometastatic cancers (SABR-COMET): a randomised, phase 2, open-label trial. Lancet. 2019;393:2051–8.

5. Ruers T, Van Coevorden F, Punt CJ, et al. Local treatment of unresectable colorectal liver metastases: results of a randomized phase II trial. J Natl Cancer Inst. 2017;109:djx015.

6. Ferlay J, Colombet M, Soerjomataram I, et al. Cancer incidence and mortality patterns in Europe: estimates for 40 countries and 25 major cancers in 2018. Eur J Cancer. 2018;103:356–87.

7. Falzone L, Salomone S, Libra M. Evolution of cancer pharmacological treatments at the turn of the third millennium. Front Pharmacol. 2018;9:1300.

8. Christofi T, Baritaki S, Falzone L, Libra M, Zaravinos A. Current perspectives in cancer immunotherapy. Cancers (Basel). 2019;11:1472.

9. Funaioli C, Longobardi C, Martoni AA. The impact of chemotherapy on overall survival and quality of life of patients with metastatic colorectal cancer: a review of phase III trials. J Chemother. 2008;20:14–27.

10. Herman JM, Narang AK, Griffith KA, et al. The quality-of-life effects of neoadjuvant chemoradiation in locally advanced rectal cancer. Int J Radiat Oncol Biol Phys. 2013;85:e15–9.

11. Hunter KU, Schipper M, Feng FY, et al. Toxicities affecting quality of life after chemo-IMRT of oropharyngeal cancer: prospective study of patient-reported, observer-rated, and objective outcomes. Int J Radiat Oncol Biol Phys. 2013;85:935–40.

12. Fong Y, Cohen AM, Fortner JG, et al. Liver resection for colorectal metastases. J Clin Oncol. 1997;15:938–46.

13. Kopetz S, Chang GJ, Overman MJ, et al. Improved survival in metastatic colorectal cancer is associated with adoption of hepatic resection and improved chemotherapy. J Clin Oncol. 2009;27:3677–83.

14. Robertson DJ, Stukel TA, Gottlieb DJ, Sutherland JM, Fisher ES. Survival after hepatic resection of colorectal cancer metastases: a national experience. Cancer. 2009;115:752–9.

15. Simmonds PC, Primrose JN, Colquitt JL, Garden OJ, Poston GJ, Rees M. Surgical resection of hepatic metastases from colorectal cancer: a systematic review of published studies. Br J Cancer. 2006;94:982–99.

16. Khatri VP, Chee KG, Petrelli NJ. Modern multimodality approach to hepatic colorectal metastases: solutions and controversies. Surg Oncol. 2007;16:71–83.

17. Germer CT. [Hepatic metastases: an interdisciplinary therapy approach is desirable]. Chirurg. 2010;81:505–6.

18. Karanjia ND, Lordan JT, Fawcett WJ, Quiney N, Worthington TR. Survival and recurrence after neo-adjuvant chemotherapy and liver resection for colorectal metastases: a ten year study. Eur J Surg Oncol. 2009;35:838–43.

19. Malik HZ, Gomez D, Wong V, et al. Predictors of early disease recurrence following hepatic resection for colorectal cancer metastasis. Eur J Surg Oncol. 2007;33:1003–9.

20. Saiura A, Yamamoto J, Hasegawa K, et al. Liver resection for multiple colorectal liver metastases with surgery up-front approach: bi-institutional analysis of 736 consecutive cases. World J Surg. 2012;36:2171–8.

21. Takahashi S, Konishi M, Nakagohri T, Gotohda N, Saito N, Kinoshita T. Short time to recurrence after hepatic resection correlates with poor prognosis in colorectal hepatic metastasis. Jpn J Clin Oncol. 2006;36:368–75.

22. Yamashita Y, Adachi E, Toh Y, et al. Risk factors for early recurrence after curative hepatectomy for colorectal liver metastases. Surg Today. 2011;41:526–32.

23. Harun N, Nikfarjam M, Muralidharan V, Christophi C. Liver regeneration stimulates tumor metastases. J Surg Res. 2007;138:284–90.

24. Riddiough GE, Fifis T, Muralidharan V, Perini MV, Christophi C. Searching for the link; mechanisms underlying liver regeneration and recurrence of colorectal liver metastasis post partial hepatectomy. J Gastroenterol Hepatol. 2019;34:1276–86.
25. Cucchetti A, Piscaglia F, Cescon M, et al. An explorative data-analysis to support the choice between hepatic resection and radiofrequency ablation in the treatment of hepatocellular carcinoma. Dig Liver Dis. 2014;46:257–63.
26. de Lope CR, Tremosini S, Forner A, Reig M, Bruix J. Management of HCC. J Hepatol. 2012;56(Suppl 1):S75–87.
27. Ruers T, Punt C, Van Coevorden F, et al. Radiofrequency ablation combined with systemic treatment versus systemic treatment alone in patients with non-resectable colorectal liver metastases: a randomized EORTC Intergroup phase II study (EORTC 40004). Ann Oncol. 2012;23:2619–26.
28. Garlipp B, Gibbs P, Van Hazel GA, et al. Secondary technical resectability of colorectal cancer liver metastases after chemotherapy with or without selective internal radiotherapy in the randomized SIRFLOX trial. Br J Surg. 2019;106(13):1837–46.
29. Ricke J, Klumpen HJ, Amthauer H, et al. Impact of combined selective internal radiation therapy and sorafenib on survival in advanced hepatocellular carcinoma. J Hepatol. 2019;71(6):1164–74.
30. van Hazel GA, Heinemann V, Sharma NK, et al. SIRFLOX: randomized phase III trial comparing first-line mFOLFOX6 (plus or minus bevacizumab) versus mFOLFOX6 (plus or minus bevacizumab) plus selective internal radiation therapy in patients with metastatic colorectal cancer. J Clin Oncol. 2016;34:1723–31.
31. Wasan HS, Gibbs P, Sharma NK, et al. First-line selective internal radiotherapy plus chemotherapy versus chemotherapy alone in patients with liver metastases from colorectal cancer (FOXFIRE, SIRFLOX, and FOXFIRE-Global): a combined analysis of three multicentre, randomised, phase 3 trials. Lancet Oncol. 2017;18:1159–71.
32. Tanis E, Nordlinger B, Mauer M, et al. Local recurrence rates after radiofrequency ablation or resection of colorectal liver metastases. Analysis of the European Organisation for Research and Treatment of Cancer #40004 and #40983. Eur J Cancer. 2014;50:912–9.
33. Kunzli BM, Abitabile P, Maurer CA. Radiofrequency ablation of liver tumors: actual limitations and potential solutions in the future. World J Hepatol. 2011;3:8–14.
34. Rhim H, Lim HK. Radiofrequency ablation of hepatocellular carcinoma: pros and cons. Gut Liver. 2010;4(Suppl 1):S113–8.
35. Dawson LA. Overview: where does radiation therapy fit in the spectrum of liver cancer localregional therapies? Semin Radiat Oncol. 2011;21:241–6.
36. Scorsetti M, Arcangeli S, Tozzi A, et al. Is stereotactic body radiation therapy an attractive option for unresectable liver metastases? A preliminary report from a phase 2 trial. Int J Radiat Oncol Biol Phys. 2013;86:336–42.
37. Dawood O, Mahadevan A, Goodman KA. Stereotactic body radiation therapy for liver metastases. Eur J Cancer. 2009;45:2947–59.
38. Kirkpatrick JP, Kelsey CR, Palta M, et al. Stereotactic body radiotherapy: a critical review for nonradiation oncologists. Cancer. 2014;120:942–54.
39. Mohnike K, Wieners G, Schwartz F, et al. Computed tomography-guided high-dose-rate brachytherapy in hepatocellular carcinoma: safety, efficacy, and effect on survival. Int J Radiat Oncol Biol Phys. 2010;78:172–9.
40. Van Tilborg AA, Meijerink MR, Sietses C, et al. Long-term results of radiofrequency ablation for unresectable colorectal liver metastases: a potentially curative intervention. Br J Radiol. 2011;84:556–65.
41. Morris E, Treasure T. If a picture is worth a thousand words, take a good look at the picture: survival after liver metastasectomy for colorectal cancer. Cancer Epidemiol. 2017;49:152–5.
42. Berber E, Pelley R, Siperstein AE. Predictors of survival after radiofrequency thermal ablation of colorectal cancer metastases to the liver: a prospective study. J Clin Oncol. 2005;23:1358–64.
43. Nahum Goldberg S, Dupuy DE. Image-guided radiofrequency tumor ablation: challenges and opportunities—part I. J Vasc Interv Radiol. 2001;12:1021–32.

44. Nakazawa T, Kokubu S, Shibuya A, et al. Radiofrequency ablation of hepatocellular carcinoma: correlation between local tumor progression after ablation and ablative margin. AJR Am J Roentgenol. 2007;188:480–8.
45. Weichselbaum RR, Hellman S. Oligometastases revisited. Nat Rev Clin Oncol. 2011;8:378–82.
46. Badakhshi H, Grun A, Stromberger C, Budach V, Boehmer D. Oligometastases: the new paradigm and options for radiotherapy. A critical review. Strahlenther Onkol. 2013;189:357–62.
47. Palma DA, Salama JK, Lo SS, et al. The oligometastatic state—separating truth from wishful thinking. Nat Rev Clin Oncol. 2014;11:549–57.
48. Ost P, Reynders D, Decaestecker K, et al. Surveillance or metastasis-directed therapy for oligometastatic prostate cancer recurrence: a prospective, randomized, multicenter phase II trial. J Clin Oncol. 2018;36:446–53.
49. Aprile G, Fontanella C, Bonotto M, et al. Timing and extent of response in colorectal cancer: critical review of current data and implication for future trials. Oncotarget. 2015;6:28716–30.
50. Alunni-Fabbroni M, Ronsch K, Huber T, et al. Circulating DNA as prognostic biomarker in patients with advanced hepatocellular carcinoma: a translational exploratory study from the SORAMIC trial. J Transl Med. 2019;17:328.
51. Diehl F, Schmidt K, Choti MA, et al. Circulating mutant DNA to assess tumor dynamics. Nat Med. 2008;14:985–90.
52. Iizuka N, Sakaida I, Moribe T, et al. Elevated levels of circulating cell-free DNA in the blood of patients with hepatitis C virus-associated hepatocellular carcinoma. Anticancer Res. 2006;26:4713–9.
53. Tokuhisa Y, Iizuka N, Sakaida I, et al. Circulating cell-free DNA as a predictive marker for distant metastasis of hepatitis C virus-related hepatocellular carcinoma. Br J Cancer. 2007;97:1399–403.
54. Blackhall F, Frese KK, Simpson K, Kilgour E, Brady G, Dive C. Will liquid biopsies improve outcomes for patients with small-cell lung cancer? Lancet Oncol. 2018;19:e470–e81.

Summary

Stefanie Corradini, Jens Ricke, and Konrad Mohnike

Oligometastatic disease has a potential for curative outcomes following local thera-pies or surgery [1–4]. However, depending on the underlying tumour entity, only a small proportion of patients meet the criteria for oligometastatic disease, and tech-nical limitations of surgical techniques likewise reduce the number of amenable patients [5, 6]. Modern interventional radiological techniques have led to the devel-opment of minimally invasive therapies such as radio-frequency ablation (RFA), which currently is the most widely used of these and has the strongest evidence base [7–10]. However, RFA and other thermoablative local therapies are technically lim-ited in respect of location and size of the tumour. Local recurrence rates increase with tumour size, and the proximity to large blood vessels or thermosensitive struc-tures limit its applicability [11–13]. Radiation therapy techniques can overcome these limitations. Radiotherapy of the liver, lungs and other inner organs can be delivered by using dedicated non-invasive external-beam techniques, such as advanced stereotactic body radiotherapy (SBRT) strategies. The efficacy of these non-invasive approaches has been demonstrated in numerous tumour locations [14–19]. Another option for applying high single doses is interstitial brachytherapy (iBT). iBT allows the delivery of very high doses of radiation in a single fraction, and owing to the steep dose gradient organs at risk can be efficiently spared.

S. Corradini
Department of Radiation Oncology, Ludwig Maximilian University (LMU) Hospital Munich, Munich, Germany
e-mail: stefanie.corradini@med.uni-muenchen.de

J. Ricke
Department of Radiology, Ludwig Maximilian University (LMU) Hospital Munich, Munich, Germany
e-mail: Jens.Ricke@med.uni-muenchen.de

K. Mohnike
Department of Diagnostics, Department of Interventional Oncology & Radionuclide Therapy, Diagnostic Therapeutic Center Berlin, Berlin, Germany

Department of Radiology and Nuclear Medicine, University Hospital Magdeburg, Magdeburg, Germany
e-mail: konrad.mohnike@berlin-dtz.de

K. Mohnike et al. (eds.), *Manual on Image-Guided Brachytherapy of Inner Organs*, https://doi.org/10.1007/978-3-030-78079-1

Numerous pilot studies and randomised comparisons have shown that interstitial brachytherapy (iBT) is capable of achieving high to very high rates of tumour control for various tumour entities. These rates vary up to >90% after 12 months in liver malignancies, even for large or very large tumours [20, 21]. A dose dependence has been demonstrated, and hepatic metastases of most tumour entities, including primary liver tumours, could be excellently controlled with a prescription dose of 15–20 Gy [20–28]. A major limiting factor in the radiotherapy of liver malignancies is the relatively low tolerance of the liver parenchyma to radiation exposure. This can lead to subclinical focal or a generalised injury of the liver parenchyma following irradiation (radiation-induced liver disorder, RILD) [29]. Interstitial brachytherapy (iBT) is a procedure that is able to spare healthy liver tissue because of its inherently steep dose gradients. A classical RILD was not observed in our own studies and has not been reported in studies by other groups; only atypical cases of icteric elevations of liver enzymes and ascites have been reported in individual cases [24, 26]. The excellent ability of iBT to treat central liver tumours with a low rate of, e.g. biliary complications is a unique feature of iBT as compared with all other local procedures, including surgical resection [30]. Therefore, the available evidence suggests that this minimally invasive treatment is particularly advantageous in the treatment of large tumours (although substantial superiority of iBT compared with SBRT regarding the sparing of the surrounding tissue seems to decline with increasing lesion size) [31, 32]. Another major advantage of iBT is its repeatability [20–22, 24, 26].

Lung brachytherapy is associated with a low rate of severe adverse events, and in the treatment of early-stage lung cancer and lung metastases it has proven to be effective, safe and well tolerated, with promising results at a variety of centres [33]. For iBT of the kidneys, the adrenal glands, the pancreas and the retroperitoneum, evidence is still limited, but it suggests that iBT is a predominantly safe and effective option [34–36].

Regarding side effects, there is a strong correlation between severe bleeding complications and (1) secondary diagnosis of advanced liver cirrhosis and (2) peri-interventional administration of low-molecular-weight heparin [37, 38]. There are also indications that a history of biliodigestive anastomosis or papillotomy is a risk factor for the post-interventional development of cholangitis or liver abscesses [39]. The occurrence of gastroduodenal ulceration is associated with a dose exposure of the gastric or duodenal wall above 14–15 Gy (D1 cm^3). Therefore, in clinical practice, proton-pump inhibitors are administered for 6–8 weeks in cases of relevant gastroduodenal dose exposure [38, 40]. As an alternative, angiographic occlusion balloons can be placed between the stomach wall and the liver to avoid significant exposure of the stomach wall to radiation [41]. The risk of extrahepatic puncture-tract metastases is generally very low, and the local recurrence after iBT has no influence on overall survival [42, 43]. In appropriately designed studies, iBT was also used successfully for treating local recurrences [26, 42].

The key to a successful treatment is adequate patient selection with evaluation of all oncological factors. These include whether the disease is oligometastatic and whether a rapid polymetastatic progression can be expected without the potential to achieve local control. A second factor is the presence of a predisposition to severe complications. This aspect is critical in determining whether the treatment will be beneficial to the patient. The relative freedom of iBT from modality-related limitations makes adequate patient stratification particularly challenging. There is a need for clinical studies that incorporate different treatment modalities and local ablative techniques including surgery, RFA, SBRT and iBT (among others) as a part of multimodal treatment to address the issue of proper patient selection. Metastasis-directed multimodal therapy is successful with curative outcome in many patients. However, when the curative intent is not achieved, it can still lead to an increasingly long duration of palliation or intervals without systemic therapy. Therefore, there is a need to define new endpoints for patient stratification and for the assessment of initial response to therapy. These may serve as surrogate markers for the extent of tumour response and could include, for example, the quantification of biomarkers such as circulating tumour DNA obtained by liquid biopsy.

References

1. Fong Y, Cohen AM, Fortner JG, et al. Liver resection for colorectal metastases. J Clin Oncol. 1997;15:938–46.
2. Kopetz S, Chang GJ, Overman MJ, et al. Improved survival in metastatic colorectal cancer is associated with adoption of hepatic resection and improved chemotherapy. J Clin Oncol. 2009;27:3677–83.
3. Robertson DJ, Stukel TA, Gottlieb DJ, Sutherland JM, Fisher ES. Survival after hepatic resection of colorectal cancer metastases: a national experience. Cancer. 2009;115:752–9.
4. Simmonds PC, Primrose JN, Colquitt JL, Garden OJ, Poston GJ, Rees M. Surgical resection of hepatic metastases from colorectal cancer: a systematic review of published studies. Br J Cancer. 2006;94:982–99.
5. Khatri VP, Chee KG, Petrelli NJ. Modern multimodality approach to hepatic colorectal metastases: solutions and controversies. Surg Oncol. 2007;16:71–83.
6. Germer CT. [Hepatic metastases: an interdisciplinary therapy approach is desirable]. Chirurg. 2010;81:505–6.
7. Cucchetti A, Piscaglia F, Cescon M, et al. An explorative data-analysis to support the choice between hepatic resection and radiofrequency ablation in the treatment of hepatocellular carcinoma. Dig Liver Dis. 2014;46:257–63.
8. de Lope CR, Tremosini S, Forner A, Reig M, Bruix J. Management of HCC. J Hepatol. 2012;56(Suppl 1):S75–87.
9. Ruers T, Punt C, Van Coevorden F, et al. Radiofrequency ablation combined with systemic treatment versus systemic treatment alone in patients with non-resectable colorectal liver metastases: a randomized EORTC Intergroup phase II study (EORTC 40004). Ann Oncol. 2012;23:2619–26.
10. Ruers T, Van Coevorden F, Punt CJ, et al. Local treatment of unresectable colorectal liver metastases: results of a randomized phase II trial. J Natl Cancer Inst. 2017;109:djx015.
11. Tanis E, Nordlinger B, Mauer M, et al. Local recurrence rates after radiofrequency ablation or resection of colorectal liver metastases. Analysis of the European Organisation for Research and Treatment of Cancer #40004 and #40983. Eur J Cancer. 2014;50:912–9.
12. Kunzli BM, Abitabile P, Maurer CA. Radiofrequency ablation of liver tumors: actual limitations and potential solutions in the future. World J Hepatol. 2011;3:8–14.
13. Rhim H, Lim HK. Radiofrequency ablation of hepatocellular carcinoma: pros and cons. Gut Liver. 2010;4(Suppl 1):S113–8.
14. Andratschke N, Alheid H, Allgauer M, et al. The SBRT database initiative of the German Society for Radiation Oncology (DEGRO): patterns of care and outcome analysis of stereotactic body radiotherapy (SBRT) for liver oligometastases in 474 patients with 623 metastases. BMC Cancer. 2018;18:283.

15. Boda-Heggemann J, Jahnke A, Chan MKH, et al. In-vivo treatment accuracy analysis of active motion-compensated liver SBRT through registration of plan dose to post-therapeutic MRI-morphologic alterations. Radiother Oncol. 2019;134:158–65.
16. Gkika E, Strouthos I, Kirste S, et al. Repeated SBRT for in- and out-of-field recurrences in the liver. Strahlenther Onkol. 2019;195:246–53.
17. Han S, Yin FF, Cai J. Evaluation of dosimetric uncertainty caused by MR geometric distortion in MRI-based liver SBRT treatment planning. J Appl Clin Med Phys. 2019;20:43–50.
18. Ibragimov B, Toesca DAS, Yuan Y, Koong AC, Chang DT, Xing L. Neural networks for deep radiotherapy dose analysis and prediction of liver SBRT outcomes. IEEE J Biomed Health Inform. 2019;23:1821–33.
19. Scorsetti M, Comito T, Clerici E, et al. Phase II trial on SBRT for unresectable liver metastases: long-term outcome and prognostic factors of survival after 5 years of follow-up. Radiat Oncol. 2018;13:234.
20. Collettini F, Schnapauff D, Poellinger A, et al. Hepatocellular carcinoma: computed-tomography-guided high-dose-rate brachytherapy (CT-HDRBT) ablation of large (5-7 cm) and very large (>7 cm) tumours. Eur Radiol. 2012;22:1101–9.
21. Tselis N, Chatzikonstantinou G, Kolotas C, Milickovic N, Baltas D, Zamboglou N. Computed tomography-guided interstitial high dose rate brachytherapy for centrally located liver tumours: a single institution study. Eur Radiol. 2013;23:2264–70.
22. Collettini F, Singh A, Schnapauff D, et al. Computed-tomography-guided high-dose-rate brachytherapy (CT-HDRBT) ablation of metastases adjacent to the liver hilum. Eur J Radiol. 2013;82:e509–14.
23. Mohnike K, Wieners G, Pech M, et al. Image-guided interstitial high-dose-rate brachytherapy in hepatocellular carcinoma. Dig Dis. 2009;27:170–4.
24. Mohnike K, Wieners G, Schwartz F, et al. Computed tomography-guided high-dose-rate brachytherapy in hepatocellular carcinoma: safety, efficacy, and effect on survival. Int J Radiat Oncol Biol Phys. 2010;78:172–9.
25. Pech M, Wieners G, Kryza R, et al. CT-guided brachytherapy (CTGB) versus interstitial laser ablation (ILT) of colorectal liver metastases: an intraindividual matched-pair analysis. Strahlenther Onkol. 2008;184:302–6.
26. Ricke J, Mohnike K, Pech M, et al. Local response and impact on survival after local ablation of liver metastases from colorectal carcinoma by computed tomography-guided high-dose-rate brachytherapy. Int J Radiat Oncol Biol Phys. 2010;78:479–85.
27. Ricke J, Wust P, Wieners G, et al. Liver malignancies: CT-guided interstitial brachytherapy in patients with unfavorable lesions for thermal ablation. J Vasc Interv Radiol. 2004;15:1279–86.
28. Ricke J, Wust P, Wieners G, et al. CT-guided interstitial single-fraction brachytherapy of lung tumors: phase I results of a novel technique. Chest. 2005;127:2237–42.
29. Sanuki N, Takeda A, Oku Y, et al. Influence of liver toxicities on prognosis after stereotactic body radiation therapy for hepatocellular carcinoma. Hepatol Res. 2015;45:540–7.
30. Powerski M, Penzlin S, Hass P, et al. Biliary duct stenosis after image-guided high-dose-rate interstitial brachytherapy of central and hilar liver tumors: a systematic analysis of 102 cases. Strahlenther Onkol. 2019;195:265–73.
31. Hass P, Mohnike K, Kropf S, et al. Comparative analysis between interstitial brachytherapy and stereotactic body irradiation for local ablation in liver malignancies. Brachytherapy. 2019;18(6):823–8.
32. Wust P, Beck M, Dabrowski R, et al. Radiotherapeutic treatment options for oligotopic malignant liver lesions. Radiat Oncol. 2021;16:51.
33. Peters N, Wieners G, Pech M, et al. CT-guided interstitial brachytherapy of primary and secondary lung malignancies: results of a prospective phase II trial. Strahlenther Onkol. 2008;184:296–301.
34. Damm R, Streitparth T, Hass P, et al. Prospective evaluation of CT-guided HDR brachytherapy as a local ablative treatment for renal masses: a single-arm pilot trial. Strahlenther Onkol. 2019;195(11):982–90.

35. Mohnike K, Neumann K, Hass P, et al. Radioablation of adrenal gland malignomas with interstitial high-dose-rate brachytherapy: efficacy and outcome. Strahlenther Onkol. 2017;193:612–9.
36. Omari J, Heinze C, Wilck A, et al. Efficacy and safety of CT-guided high-dose-rate interstitial brachytherapy in primary and secondary malignancies of the pancreas. Eur J Radiol. 2019;112:22–7.
37. Mohnike K, Sauerland H, Seidensticker M, et al. Haemorrhagic complications and symptomatic venous thromboembolism in interventional tumour ablations: the impact of peri-interventional thrombosis prophylaxis. Cardiovasc Intervent Radiol. 2016;39:1716–21.
38. Mohnike K, Wolf S, Damm R, et al. Radioablation of liver malignancies with interstitial high-dose-rate brachytherapy : complications and risk factors. Strahlenther Onkol. 2016;192:288–96.
39. Wieners G, Schippers AC, Collettini F, et al. CT-guided high-dose-rate brachytherapy in the interdisciplinary treatment of patients with liver metastases of pancreatic cancer. Hepatobiliary Pancreat Dis Int. 2015;14:530–8.
40. Streitparth F, Pech M, Bohmig M, et al. In vivo assessment of the gastric mucosal tolerance dose after single fraction, small volume irradiation of liver malignancies by computed tomography-guided, high-dose-rate brachytherapy. Int J Radiat Oncol Biol Phys. 2006;65:1479–86.
41. Hass P, Steffen IG, Powerski M, et al. First report on extended distance between tumor lesion and adjacent organs at risk using interventionally applied balloon catheters: a simple procedure to optimize clinical target volume covering effective isodose in interstitial high-dose-rate brachytherapy of liver malignomas. J Contemp Brachytherapy. 2019;11:152–61.
42. Damm R, Zorkler I, Rogits B, et al. Needle track seeding in hepatocellular carcinoma after local ablation by high-dose-rate brachytherapy: a retrospective study of 588 catheter placements. J Contemp Brachytherapy. 2018;10:516–21.
43. Denecke T, Stelter L, Schnapauff D, et al. CT-guided interstitial brachytherapy of hepatocellular carcinoma before liver transplantation: an equivalent alternative to transarterial chemoembolization? Eur Radiol. 2015;25:2608–16.

Index